Gynaecological Oncology for the MRCOG

Edited by

Mahmood Shafi
Addenbrooke's Hospital, Cambridge

Helen Bolton
Addenbrooke's Hospital, Cambridge

Ketankumar Gajjar
Nottingham University Hospitals NHS Trust

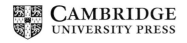

CAMBRIDGE
UNIVERSITY PRESS

University Printing House, Cambridge CB2 8BS, United Kingdom

One Liberty Plaza, 20th Floor, New York, NY 10006, USA

477 Williamstown Road, Port Melbourne, VIC 3207, Australia

314–321, 3rd Floor, Plot 3, Splendor Forum, Jasola District Centre, New Delhi – 110025, India

79 Anson Road, #06-04/06, Singapore 079906

Cambridge University Press is part of the University of Cambridge.

It furthers the University's mission by disseminating knowledge in the pursuit of education, learning, and research at the highest international levels of excellence.

www.cambridge.org
Information on this title: www.cambridge.org/9781316638712
DOI: 10.1017/9781316986844

© Cambridge University Press 2018

First published 2018

Printed in the United Kingdom by Clays, St Ives plc

A catalogue record for this publication is available from the British Library.

ISBN 978-1-316-63871-2 Paperback

Cambridge University Press has no responsibility for the persistence or accuracy of URLs for external or third-party internet websites referred to in this publication and does not guarantee that any content on such websites is, or will remain, accurate or appropriate.

Every effort has been made in preparing this book to provide accurate and up-to-date information that is in accord with accepted standards and practice at the time of publication. Although case histories are drawn from actual cases, every effort has been made to disguise the identities of the individuals involved. Nevertheless, the authors, editors and publishers can make no warranties that the information contained herein is totally free from error, not least because clinical standards are constantly changing through research and regulation. The authors, editors and publishers therefore disclaim all liability for direct or consequential damages resulting from the use of material contained in this book. Readers are strongly advised to pay careful attention to information provided by the manufacturer of any drugs or equipment that they plan to use.

We are grateful for the love and support that we enjoy from our respective partners who made writing this book possible, namely, Naseem Shafi, Mark Slack and Amita Mahendru. We are in gratitude to our loving children who bear the consequences of our commitment to writing.

—Imran, Omar & Mohsin Shafi;
Toby and Cosmo Slack;
Aryaman Gajjar

Gynaecological Oncology
for the MRCOG

Contents

List of Contributors   ix
Preface   xi
List of Abbreviations   xiii

1   **Epidemiology of Gynaecological Cancers**   1
Anjum Memon and Aisha El-Turki

2   **Pathology of Gynaecological Cancers**   11
Raji Ganesan and Jo Vella

3   **Imaging in Gynaecological Oncology**   23
Susan Freeman, Helen Addley and
Penelope Moyle

4   **Concepts of Treatment Approaches in Gynaecological Oncology**   34
Mohamed Khairy Mehasseb

5   **Radiation Therapy for Gynaecological Malignancies**   41
Christopher Stephen Kent and Paul Symonds

6   **Systemic Therapy in Gynaecological Cancers**   52
Benjamin Masters and Anjana Anand

7   **Preinvasive Disease, Screening and Hereditary Cancer**   62
Dhivya Chandrasekaran, Faiza Gaba
and Ranjit Manchanda

8   **Surgical Principles in Gynaecological Oncology**   77
Jane Borley and Maria Kyrgiou

9   **Role of Laparoscopic Surgery**   88
Hans Nagar

10   **Ovarian, Fallopian Tube and Primary Peritoneal Cancer (including Borderline)**   98
Hilary Turnbull and Timothy Duncan

11   **Endometrial Cancer**   112
Cathrine Holland

12   **Cervical and Vaginal Cancer**   126
Claire Louise Newton and Tim Mould

13   **Vulval Cancer**   138
Carmen Gan and Ketan Gajjar

14   **Uterine Sarcomas**   147
Helen Bolton and Mahmood Shafi

15   **Non-epithelial Ovarian Tumours and Gestational Trophoblastic Neoplasia**   153
Michael J. Seckl and Christina Fotopoulou

16   **Palliative Care**   165
Sara Booth and Mary McGregor

17   **Living with Cancer**   179
Andy Nordin and Manas Chakrabarti

18   **Communication in Gynaecological Oncology**   188
Nicholas Wood and Georgios Theophilou

Appendix   197
Index   207

Contributors

Dr Helen Addley
Addenbrookes Hospital, Cambridge

Dr Anjana Anand, MBBS, MSc, MRCP (UK), FRCR
Nottingham University Hospitals
NHS Trust, Nottingham, UK

Sara Booth
Addenbrookes Hospital, Cambridge

Jane Borley, MRCOG, PhD
Imperial College NHS Trust, Hammersmith
Hospital, London, UK

Manas Chakrabarti
East Kent Gynaecological Centre,
QEQM Hospital, Margate

Dhivya Chandrasekaran
Queen Mary University of London, UK

Timothy Duncan
Norfolk and Norwich University
Hospital, Norwich, UK

Aisha El-Turki, PhD
Universities of Brighton and Sussex, Brighton, UK

Christina Fotopoulou
Imperial College NHS Trust, Hammersmith
Hospital, London, UK

Dr Susan Freeman
Addenbrookes Hospital, Cambridge

Faiza Gaba
Queen Mary University of London, UK

Ketan Gajjar, MD, MRCOG
Nottingham University Hospitals
NHS Trust, Nottingham, UK

Carmen Gan, MRCOG
Nottingham University Hospitals
NHS Trust, Nottingham, UK

Raji Ganesan
Birmingham Women's and Children's
NHS Trust, Birmingham, UK

Cathrine Holland, BMBS, PhD, FRCOG
Central Manchester University Hospitals
NHS Foundation Trust, Manchester, UK

Dr Christopher Stephen Kent, MBChB, MRCP, MSc, FRCR
University Hospitals of Leicester
NHS Trust, Leicester, UK

Maria Kyrgiou, MRCOG, MSc, PhD
Imperial College NHS Trust, Hammersmith
Hospital, London, UK

Ranjit Manchanda
Queen Mary University of London, UK

Dr Benjamin Masters, BM, BSc, MRCP (UK)
Nottingham University Hospitals
NHS Trust, Nottingham, UK

Mary McGregor
Addenbrookes Hospital, Cambridge

Mohamed Khairy Mehasseb, MSc, MD, MRCOG, PhD
Glasgow Royal Infirmary, Glasgow, UK

Anjum Memon, MBBS, DPhil (Oxon), FFPH
Universities of Brighton and Sussex, Brighton, UK

Tim Mould, MBBS, MA, DM, FRCOG
University College Hospital, London, UK

Dr Penelope Moyle
Addenbrookes Hospital, Cambridge

Hans Nagar
Belfast Health

Claire Louise Newton, MBBS, BSc, MRCOG, MD
University College Hospital, London, UK

Andy Nordin
East Kent Gynaecological Centre,
QEQM Hospital, Margate

Professor Michael J. Seckl
Imperial College NHS Trust, Hammersmith
Hospital, London, UK

Professor Paul Symonds, MD, FRCR, FRCP
University of Leicester, Leicester, UK

Georgios Theophilou
St James's University Hospital, Leeds

Hilary Turnbull
Norfolk and Norwich University
Hospital, Norwich, UK

Jo Vella
Birmingham Women's and Children's
NHS Trust, Birmingham, UK

Nicholas Wood
Lancashire Teaching Hospitals NHS
Foundation Trust, Preston

Preface

Women with gynaecological cancers are managed by multidisciplinary teams, with many professionals from different backgrounds contributing to patients' health care. As outcomes for patients continue to improve, there has been a shift towards understanding survivorship issues and tailoring treatments to achieve the best possible outcomes while minimising the impact of treatment on quality of life. This book addresses all aspects of caring for women with gynaecological malignancy, covering general topics as well as specific issues faced by patients.

This book is aimed at trainees in gynaecology and oncology and at consultants with a special interest in gynaecological cancers. Although this book covers the syllabus for the MRCOG examination, it is also written to provide a comprehensive foundation for all healthcare professionals caring for women with gynaecological cancers, beyond the basics. Allied medical staff, palliative care professionals and nurse specialists will also find this book a useful resource for up-to-date information on the whole range of gynaecological cancers.

Chapters 1–9 and 16–18 cover the broad issues in gynaecological oncology whereas Chapters 10–15 cover site-specific tumours. The chapters are intended to be clinically focused and are based upon published facts. Wherever possible, the reader is directed to national guidelines and standards. Boxed information, key facts and tips are highlighted to assist the reader. Each chapter lists further reading recommendations to guide the interested reader to seek further information about the topics covered in the chapter.

We have had the pleasure of working with experts who have kindly contributed to this book. This is always one of the nicest aspects of writing a book in that there is collaboration with colleagues and friends whom we admire and respect for their expertise.

Abbreviations

ADC	Apparent diffusion coefficient	EORTC	European Organisation for Research in Treatment of Cancer
AFP	Alpha-fetoprotein		
AIN	Anal intraepithelial neoplasia	EPD	Extra-mammary Paget's disease
AS	Age standardised	ESGO	European Society of Gynaecological Oncology
ASCUS	Atypical squamous cells of undetermined significance		
		ETT	Epithelioid trophoblasic tumour
ASR	Age-standardised incidence (or mortality) rate	EUA	Examination under anaesthesia
		FDG	2-[^{18}F]-fluoro-2-deoxy-D-glucose
ASTEC	A Study in the Treatment of Endometrial Cancer	FIGO	International Federation of Gynaecology and Obstetrics
BCC	Basal cell carcinoma	FNA	Fine needle aspiration
BEP	Bleomycin, etoposide, cisplatin	FSH	Follicle stimulating hormone
BMI	Body mass index	GCT	Granulosa cell tumour
BOT	Borderline ovarian tumour	GOG	Gynaecologic Oncology Group
BRCA	Breast cancer-associated antigen	GTD	Gestational trophoblastic disease
BSO	Bilateral salpingo-oophorectomy	GTN	Gestational trophoblastic neoplasia
BT	Brachytherapy	GTT	Gestational trophoblastic tumour
CA125	Cancer-associated antigen 125	hCG	Human chorionic gonadotrophin
CA19.9	Cancer-associated antigen 19.9	β-hCG	Beta human chorionic gonadotrophin
CEA	Carcinoembryonic antigen	HDR	High dose rate
CGIN	Cervical glandular intraepithelial neoplasia	HES	Hospital Episode Statistics
		HGSOC	High-grade serous ovarian carcinoma
CHM	Complete hydatidiform mole	HIPEC	Hyperthermic intraperitoneal chemotherapy
CIN	Cervical intraepithelial neoplasia		
CNS	Clinical nurse specialist	HIV	Human immunodeficiency virus
CO	Cyclophosphamide and vincristine	HNA	Holistic needs assessment
CRS	Cytoreductive surgery	HNPCC	Hereditary non-polyposis colorectal cancer
CSCI	Continuous subcutaneous infusion		
CT	Computed tomography	HPV	Human papillomavirus
CTC	Common toxicity criteria	HRT	Hormone replacement therapy
DALY	Disability-adjusted life-years	ICCR	International Collaboration on Cancer Reporting
DCE	Dynamic contrast enhanced		
DES	Diethylstilboestrol	ICD	International Classification of Disease
DVT	Deep vein thrombosis	ICD-O	International Classification of Diseases for Oncology
DWI	Diffusion-weighted images		
EBRT	External beam radiotherapy	ICG	Indocyanine green
EEC	Endometrioid endometrial cancer	IHC	Immunohistochemistry
EMA	Etoposide, methotrexate and actinomycin D	IMRT	Intensity-modulated radiotherapy
		IOTA	International Ovarian Tumour Analysis
EOC	Epithelial ovarian cancer		

IUS	Intra-uterine system	PVP	Predictive value positive
LGSOC	Low-grade serous ovarian carcinoma	QALY	Quality-adjusted life-years
LH	Luteinising hormone	QOL	Quality of life
LINAC	Linear accelerator	RMI	Risk of malignancy index
LLETZ	Large loop excision of the transformation zone	RRESDO	Risk reducing early salpingectomy and delayed oophorectomy
LND	Lymph node dissection	RRS	Risk reducing surgery
LNG	Levonorgestrel	RRSO	Risk reducing salpingo-oophorectomy
LS	Lynch syndrome or lichen sclerosis	SABR	Stereotactic ablative radiotherapy
LVSI	Lymphovascular space invasion	SBRT	Stereotactic body radiotherapy
MAS	Minimal access surgery	SCC	Squamous cell cancer
MDT	Multidisciplinary team	SEE-FIM	Sectioning and extensively examining the fimbrial end
MDTM	Multidisciplinary team meeting	sEIC	Serous endometrial intraepithelial carcinoma
MMR	Mismatch repair		
MR(I)	Magnetic resonance (imaging)	SIGN	Scottish Intercollegiate Guidelines Network
MSI	Microsatellite instability		
NACT	Neoadjuvant chemotherapy	SIL	Squamous intraepithelial lesion
NCAT	National Cancer Action Team	SLN	Sentinel lymph node
NCDR	National Cancer Data Repository	SLND	Sentinel lymph node dissection
NCI	National Cancer Institute	SMILE	Stratified mucinous intraepithelial lesion
NCIN	National Cancer Intelligence Network		
NEOT	Non-epithelial ovarian tumour	SNP	Single nucleotide polymorphisms
NGO	Non-governmental organisations	STD	Sexually transmitted disease
NHSCSP	National Health Service Cervical Screening Programme	STIC	Serous tubal intraepithelial carcinoma
		STUMP	Smooth muscle tumour of uncertain malignant potential
NICE	National Institute for Health and Care Excellence		
		TAH	Total abdominal hysterectomy
NSAID	Non-steroidal anti-inflammatory drug	TAUS	Transabdominal ultrasound scan
OC	Ovarian cancer	TCGA	The Cancer Genome Atlas
OGCT	Ovarian germ cell tumours	TLH	Total laparoscopic hysterectomy
PA	Para-aortic	TNM	Tumour, node, metastases (staging system)
PARP	Poly-ADP ribose polymerase		
PBO	Partial bowel obstruction	TSH	Thyroid-stimulating hormone
PCB	Post-coital bleeding	TVUS	Transvaginal ultrasound scan
PCOS	Polycystic ovarian syndrome	T1WI	T1-weighted images
PET	Positron emission tomography	T2WI	T2-weighted images
PET/CT	Positron emission tomography/ computerised tomography	UKCTOCS	UK Collaborative Trial on Ovarian Cancer Screening
PHM	Partial hydatidiform mole	US	Ultrasound scan
PLCO	Prostate, lung, colorectal and ovarian cancer screening trial	VaIN	Vaginal intraepithelial neoplasia
		VIN	Vulval intraepithelial neoplasia
PMB	Postmenopausal bleeding	VTE	Venous thromboembolism
PND	Pelvic node dissection	WHO	World Health Organisation
PROMS	Patient reported outcome measures	WI	Weighted images
PSTT	Placental site trophoblastic tumour	WLE	Wide local excision
PVN	Predictive value negative		

Epidemiology of Gynaecological Cancers

Anjum Memon and Aisha El-Turki

Epidemiological Understanding

Epidemiology is the basic science underpinning public health and clinical medicine. It describes the occurrence of health-related states or events (incidence, prevalence), quantifies the risk of disease (relative risk, attributable risk, odds ratio) and its outcome (prognosis, survival, mortality), and postulates causal mechanisms for disease in populations (aetiology, prevention). The main function of epidemiology is to provide evidence to guide public health policy and clinical practice to protect, restore, and promote health of individuals and populations.

Public health is the collective and organised action by the society to improve the health of populations. This involves collaborative working between doctors, nurses, engineers, environmental scientists, health educators, social workers, nutritionists, administrators, and an effective partnership with non-governmental organisations (NGOs), corporations, and all levels of the government.

The applications of epidemiology in public health and clinical practice can be summarised as follows:

- **To describe the spectrum and extent of disease in the population** – e.g. what is the prevalence of human papilloma virus (HPV) infection among young girls?
- **To identify factors that increase or decrease the risk of disease** – e.g. what factors increase the risk of, or protect against, endometrial cancer?
- **To study the natural history and prognosis of disease** – e.g. does early diagnosis of cervical intraepithelial neoplasia (CIN) through cytological screening prevent future morbidity and improve survival?
- **To monitor and predict disease trends in the population** – e.g. what impact will the increasing prevalence of obesity in women have on future disease trends and healthcare needs?
- **To provide evidence for developing public health policy and making regulatory decisions** – e.g.

will a smoking ban in public places promote smoking cessation and reduce the incidence of smoking-related disease?

- **To evaluate the efficacy of preventive and therapeutic interventions** – e.g. does postmenopausal hormone replacement therapy (HRT) do more harm than good?
- **To evaluate public health programmes** – e.g. will vaccination of schoolgirls against oncogenic HPV prevent vulvar/vaginal/cervical cancers and save lives?
- **To evaluate the effectiveness of health services** – e.g. are known contacts of persons with sexually transmitted diseases (STDs) followed up and treated?

Classification of Gynaecological Cancers

The *International Statistical Classification of Diseases and Related Health Problems* (ICD-10) is the global standard diagnostic classification for epidemiological, clinical, and health service data. It is used by hospital records departments, cancer registries, and government agencies responsible for collection of health statistics (e.g. the Office for National Statistics in the United Kingdom) to classify diseases and other health problems recorded on many types of health and vital records. The ICD is essential for compilation of morbidity (e.g. cancer incidence) and mortality statistics (e.g. underlying cause of death) and allows comparison at an international level of health data collected in different countries at different times. In the tenth revision of the ICD (ICD-10, version 2016), malignant neoplasms of female genital organs are coded from C51 to C58. The category C57 (malignant neoplasm of other and unspecified female genital organs) includes neoplasms of the fallopian tube, broad and round ligaments, parametrium, uterine adnexa, and overlapping lesions (e.g. tubo-ovarian, utero-ovarian) (Table 1.1).

Table 1.1 ICD-10 codes and morphological classification of malignant neoplasms of female genital organs

ICD-10 code	Organ	Morphological subtypes
C51	Vulva	Squamous cell carcinoma
		Extramammary Paget's disease
		Malignant melanoma
C52	Vagina	Squamous cell carcinoma
		Adenocarcinoma
		Botryoid rhabdomyosarcoma
C53	Cervix uteri	Squamous cell carcinoma
		Neuroendocrine carcinoma
		Adenocarcinoma
C54	Corpus uteri	Endometrial adenocarcinoma
		Malignant mixed Müllerian tumours
		Leiomyosarcoma
C55		Uterus (part unspecified)
C56	Ovary	Surface epithelial tumours
		Serous adenocarcinoma
		Endometrioid adenocarcinoma
		Mucinous adenocarcinoma
		Clear cell carcinoma
		Germ cell tumours
		Dysgerminoma
		Yolk sac tumour
		Choriocarcinoma
		Mature and immature teratoma
		Sex cord-stromal tumours
		Granulosa cell tumour
		Sertoli–Leydig cell tumour
C57		Other and unspecified female genital organs
C58	Placenta	Hydatidiform mole
		Placental site trophoblastic tumour
		Choriocarcinoma

The *International Classification of Diseases for Oncology* (ICD-O-3) is used principally by cancer registries for coding the site (topography) and the histology (morphology) of the neoplasm, usually obtained from a pathology report.

The *Tumour Node Metastasis Classification of Malignant Tumours* (TNM-8) is an international standard cancer staging system used for describing the anatomical extent and progression of cancer. It is based on the assessment of three components:

T – describes the extent of the primary tumour

N – describes the absence/presence and extent of the regional lymph node involvement/metastasis

M – describes the absence/presence of distant metastasis.

The classification is used to: (i) aid the clinician in the planning and management of treatment; (ii) assist in evaluation of the results of treatment; (iii) provide some indication of individual prognosis;

(iv) facilitate the exchange of information between clinicians/treatment centres; (v) inform and evaluate treatment guidelines, national cancer planning and research; and (vi) evaluate population-based screening and early detection programmes. The TNM system is approved by the International Federation of Gynaecology and Obstetrics (FIGO), and its categories have been defined to correspond to the FIGO classification.

Measuring the Risk or Burden of Gynaecological Cancers

Incidence

Incidence (or *incident cases*) is a count of *new cases* of cancer in the population during a specified time period. The incidence rate is the number of *new cases* of cancer in a defined population within a specified time period (usually a calendar year), divided by total number of persons in that population. Cancer incidence rates in adults are typically expressed as per 100,000 population.

Incidence rate measures the rapidity (or 'speed') of the occurrence of new cases of cancer in the population within a time period. Increase in incidence of a cancer in the population can be due to a variety of factors, which may include: in-migration of susceptible people, a change in diagnostic criteria, improved case ascertainment, introduction of a new screening/diagnostic test, introduction of new, or changes in exposure to existing (e.g. enhanced transmission of HPV), infectious/aetiologic agent(s). Incidence rate is used to:

- predict the average risk (probability) of developing cancer
- research the causes and treatment of cancer
- describe trends of cancer over time
- evaluate the effectiveness of primary prevention and early detection and/or population-based screening (secondary prevention) programmes
- inform and guide health planning, resource allocation and commissioning of clinical and community-based services.

Age-Standardised Incidence (or Mortality) Rate

As the risk of cancer increases exponentially with age, the crude incidence rate (which is influenced by the population age structure) cannot be used to evaluate whether the risk/burden of cancer differs between populations. It is therefore necessary to use age-standardised incidence (or mortality) rates (ASRs) when comparing incidence rates between populations that have different age structures (e.g. the United Kingdom and India). The ASR is obtained by applying the (crude) age-specific rates in the observed population to the age-specific population counts (or weights) of a fixed reference (or standard) population. The most commonly used standard population is the *world* (and also *European*) *standard population* proposed by Sir Richard Doll – the eminent epidemiologist who discovered the main hazards of smoking. Age-standardisation controls for the confounding effect of age on cancer incidence and therefore allows a more direct comparison between different populations.

Cumulative Incidence (or Cumulative Risk)

Cumulative incidence is the probability or risk of developing cancer during a specified period (e.g. lifetime). It measures the number or proportion of people (out of 100 or 1,000) who would be expected to develop a particular cancer by the age of 64 (or 74) if they had the rates (i.e. risk) of cancer currently observed. Like the ASR, cumulative incidence permits comparisons between populations of different age structures. For example, the cumulative incidence of a woman in England developing ovarian cancer by age 74 is about 15/1,000, which can be interpreted as 1.5% (1 in 67) probability or (lifetime) risk of developing ovarian cancer by the time she completes 74 years.

Prevalence

Prevalence is the number of *existing cases* of cancer in a defined population at a notional point in time, divided by the total number of people in the population at that time. It is usually expressed as an absolute number of existing cases or as the proportion of a population with the disease. For example, the prevalence of cervical cancer can be defined as the number of women in a defined population who have been diagnosed with cancer, and who are still alive at a given point in time. Prevalence is a function of both the incidence of the disease and survival.

Mathematically prevalence can be defined as follows:

$$Prevalence = a/a + b$$

where a is the number of individuals in the population with the disease at a given time and b is the number of individuals in the population without the disease at a given time.

Therefore prevalence is a measure of the burden of cancer in the population, and it is most useful for describing diseases with a gradual onset and long duration. Increase in prevalence of a cancer in the population can be due to a variety of factors, which may include in-migration of cases, increase in incidence, and/or improved prognosis/survival (e.g. due to better treatment). Prevalence data are used for

- health planning, resource allocation and commissioning of clinical and community-based services
- estimation of cancer survivorship
- organisation of prevention programmes.

Partial (or limited duration) prevalence is the estimation of the number of cases of cancer diagnosed within 1, 3, and 5 years to indicate the number of patients undergoing initial treatment (cases within 1 year of diagnosis), clinical follow-up (within 3 years), or not considered cured (before 5 years). Patients alive 5 years after diagnosis are usually considered cured because, for most cancers, the death rates of such patients are similar to those in the general population.

Complete prevalence represents the proportion of patients alive on a certain day who previously had a diagnosis of cancer, regardless of how long ago the diagnosis was, still under treatment, or are considered cured.

Survival

Survival is the proportion (or percentage) of people still alive 1, 3, 5, and 10 years after they have been diagnosed with cancer. This *observed* survival probability is influenced by mortality both from the cancer itself and from other causes. For this reason, relative survival (%) is usually calculated (ratio of the observed survival in a particular group of patients to the survival expected in a group of people in the general population).

Quality-Adjusted Life-Years (Lost)/ Disability-Adjusted Life-Years (Lost)

Quality-adjusted life-years (QALYs) and disability-adjusted life-years (DALYs) quantify the spectrum of morbidity (between the diagnosis and cure/death) due to cancer in terms of its duration and severity. The calculation of these indices requires three elements:

1. the incidence of cancer
2. its mean duration (survival probability) and
3. a measure of life 'quality' between the diagnosis and cure/death.

These indices are used to estimate the impact of cancer on the individual and society and to establish priorities for healthcare programmes.

Mortality

Mortality is the number of deaths occurring, and the mortality rate is the number of deaths in a defined population within a specified time period (usually a calendar year), divided by total number of persons in that population. Cancer mortality rates are typically expressed as per 100,000 persons per year. Mortality is the product of the incidence and the fatality of a given cancer, and measures the average risk to the population dying from a specific cancer within a specified period. Fatality, the complement of per cent survival, is the probability (%) that a cancer patient will die from the disease.

Cancer Screening

Definition

Screening is the presumptive identification (detection) of an unrecognised or hidden disease or defect by the application of tests, examinations or other procedures that can be applied rapidly.

Cancer screening is the testing of apparently healthy volunteers from the general population for the purpose of separating them into high and low probabilities of having a specific cancer. The rationale behind cancer screening is that the disease has a natural history (i.e. phases of pathological progression/cellular transformation) that includes a clearly defined preclinical phase with biological characteristics, which allows for detection of the disease in an early (presumably) treatable stage that, in turn, will reduce the risk of future morbidity and improve survival. For example, cytological screening can detect preinvasive cervical disease, which if followed by treatment can be possibly cured, thereby reducing the risk of invasive cervical cancer. Randomised controlled trials and both case–control and cohort observational study designs are used to evaluate cancer screening programmes.

Screening Test Performance

The performance of a screening test is based on its sensitivity, specificity, and predictive value (Table 1.2).

Table 1.2 Calculation of sensitivity, specificity, and predictive value of a screening test

		Disease according to gold standard		
		Present	Absent	Total
Screening test result	Positive	A (True +)	B (False +)	A + B
	Negative	C (False −)	D (True −)	C + D
	Total	A + C	B + D	A + B + C + D

Sensitivity = A/(A + C) × 100 (%).
Specificity = D/(B + D) × 100 (%).
Positive predictive value = A/(A + B) × 100 (%).
Negative predictive value = D/(C + D) × 100 (%).
Prevalence of disease = A + C/(A + B + C + D) × 100 (%).

- **Sensitivity** – this is the ability of the test to identify correctly those who *have* the disease (true positives).
- **Specificity** – this is the ability of the test to identify correctly those who *do not have* the disease (true negatives).
- **Predictive value positive (PVP)** – this is the proportion of individuals who test *positive* and actually have the disease. PVP is a function of sensitivity, specificity and prevalence of the detectable preclinical phase. A high PVP is essential for a successful population-based screening programme (e.g. cervical cancer), whereas a low PVP implies that resources are being wasted on diagnostic follow-ups of false-positive individuals.
- **Predictive value negative (PVN)** – this is the proportion of individuals who test *negative* and actually do not have the disease.

Ovarian Cancer

Incidence and Mortality

Ovarian cancer is the seventh most common cancer among women worldwide, with an estimated 239,000 new cases (3.6% of cancer in women) and 152,000 deaths (4.3% of cancer deaths in women) in the year 2012, and a 5-year prevalence of 587,000 cases (3.4% of women with cancer). The incidence rates of ovarian cancer vary from a low of about 2/100,000 women in Tanzania to a high of 14/100,000 in Latvia. In general, incidence rates are relatively higher in developed countries – the highest rates (10–14/100,000 women) are observed in European populations, intermediate rates (7–10/100,000 women) are observed in North America, Australia/New Zealand, and some populations in Asia and the lowest rates (2–7/100,000 women) are observed in Africa, South America, the Caribbean, the Middle East, and parts of Asia. Data from the United Kingdom and the United States suggest that ovarian cancer is relatively more common in White than in Asian or Black women. In the United Kingdom, incidence rates for White women range from 17 to 18/100,000, rates for Asian women range from 9 to 16/100,000 and rates for Black women range from 7 to 12/100,000.

In the United Kingdom, ovarian cancer is the second most common gynaecological cancer (after uterine cancer). It is the sixth most common cancer among women, with about 7,400 new cases in the year 2014 accounting for around 4% of all cancers in women, with a cumulative risk of 1.5% (1 in 67) by age 74 (Figure 1.1). In most European populations, the incidence rates of ovarian cancer generally increase exponentially with age, with a sharp increase after about 40 years of age. It is predominantly a disease of older, postmenopausal women: about 82% of cases occur in women aged over 50 years (Figure 1.2). In 2014, 4,100 women in the United Kingdom died from ovarian cancer, accounting for around 5% of female deaths from cancer. Ovarian cancer has a relatively poor prognosis as the large majority of cases are diagnosed at an advanced stage; overall, about 35% of women diagnosed with ovarian cancer survive their disease for 10 or more years. When diagnosed at its earliest stage (Stage 1), 9 in 10 (90%) women will survive their disease for 5 or more years, compared to 5-year relative survival of 3% for those diagnosed at Stage IV. In the United Kingdom, ovarian cancer survival has been

5

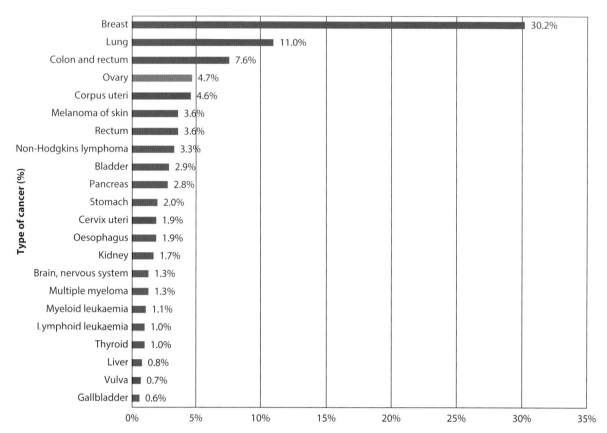

Figure 1.1 Frequency distribution (%) of the 22 most common cancers in women, England 2003–7
Source: Cancer Incidence in Five Continents Vol. X, IARC, 2013

steadily improving and has almost doubled in the last 40 years.

Trends in Incidence and Mortality

In most developed countries, there has been little change in the incidence of ovarian cancer over the past 40 or more years. In the United Kingdom, the incidence rates have remained stable since the early 1990s (22.9/100,000 in 1993; 23.3/100,000 in 2014), with a small (4%) decline in the last decade. In most populations, mortality rates have remained fairly stable or declined slightly over the past 40 years. In the United Kingdom, the ASRs (European standard) have decreased by about 20% in women between 2000 and 2014 (from 16 to 13/100,000 women).

Aetiology

Compared with other gynaecological cancers, little is known about the aetiology of ovarian cancer. In most

studies, family history of ovarian cancer, smoking, use of HRT, and body fatness have been associated with an increased risk, while states of anovulation (i.e. use of combined oestrogen–progestogen oral contraceptives, pregnancy), breastfeeding, tubal ligation, and hysterectomy have been associated with decreased risk.

Prevention

Apart from prophylactic oophorectomy, oral contraception, and (possibly) tubal ligation or salpingectomy, there are few readily modifiable risk factors for ovarian cancer. There is currently inconsistent evidence for a possible increase in risk with consumption of lactose/galactose-containing foods, saturated or animal fat intake, perineal talcum powder use and postmenopausal HRT and for a decrease in risk with vegetable intake. It is unclear whether obesity, body mass index (BMI) or physical activity influences ovarian cancer risk. It has been estimated that about 21% of ovarian cancer cases

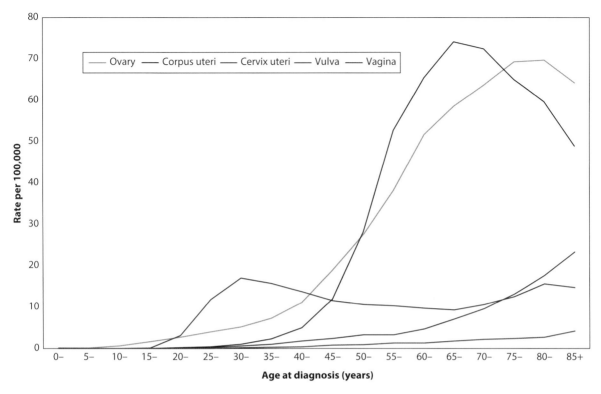

Figure 1.2 Age-specific incidence rates of gynaecological cancers, England 2003–7
Source: Cancer Incidence in Five Continents Vol. X, IARC, 2013

in the United Kingdom can be prevented by changes in lifestyle and risk factor modification.

Endometrial Cancer

Incidence and Mortality

Endometrial cancer is the fifth most common cancer among women worldwide, with an estimated 320,000 new cases (4.8% of cancer in women) and 76,000 deaths (2.1% of cancer deaths in women) in the year 2012, and a 5-year prevalence of 1,217,000 cases (7.1% of women with cancer). In contrast with cervical cancer, endometrial cancer is relatively more common in developed countries with incidence rates more than double those of the less developed countries (14.7/100,000 vs 5.5/100,000). In the United Kingdom, endometrial cancer is the most common gynaecological cancer. It is the fourth most common cancer among women, with about 9,300 new cases in the year 2014 accounting for around 5% of all cancers in women, with a cumulative risk of 1.7% (1 in 59) by age 74 (Figure 1.1). There is

no significant variation in the incidence of endometrial cancer by ethnicity in the United Kingdom. About 70% of the cases in the United Kingdom are diagnosed at Stage I. In most European and North American populations, the incidence rates of endometrial cancer begin to rise steadily 5–10 years before the menopause and reach a peak usually around the age of 70 years. It is essentially a cancer of postmenopausal women; over 90% of cases occur in women aged 50 or older, and very few cases are diagnosed under the age of 35 (Figure 1.2). The incidence rates of endometrial cancer vary from a low of 1.5/100,000 women in Algeria to a high of 26.7/100,000 women in Armenia. The highest rates are observed among women in North America, Europe, Australia/New Zealand, and Israel. Incidence rates are generally much lower in most countries in Latin America, Asia, and Africa. In developed countries, the mortality rates of endometrial cancer are substantially lower than the incidence rates (2.3/100,000 vs 14.7/100,000).

In 2014, about 2,200 women in the United Kingdom died from endometrial cancer, accounting for around

3% of female deaths from cancer. Endometrial cancer has a relatively better prognosis than ovarian and cervical cancers. Overall, about 78% (8 in 10) of women diagnosed with endometrial cancer survive their disease for 10 or more years. Five-year relative survival ranges from 95% at Stage I to 14% at Stage IV. In the United Kingdom, endometrial cancer survival has been steadily improving over the past 40 or more years.

Trends in Incidence and Mortality

In the United Kingdom, there has been a steady increase (by 63%) in the incidence of endometrial cancer since the early 1990s; the largest increase (89%) has been observed in women aged 70–9. The ASRs in the United Kingdom declined by 27% between 1971–3 (7.0/100,000) and 1997–9 (5.1/100,000) and then increased by 27% between 1997–9 and 2012–14 (6.5/100,000).

Aetiology

In contrast with cervical cancer, which is a model of viral carcinogenesis, endometrial cancer is a model of hormonal carcinogenesis. The 18-fold variation in ASRs across populations points to the role of modifiable factors in the aetiology of endometrial cancer. Among these, oestrogens and progestins are considered to play an important role in malignant transformation. Exposure to excessive oestrogen of endogenous as well as exogenous origin entailing continued/chronic stimulation of the endometrium is considered to be the main factor in this transformation and this is perhaps a common denominator for most of the established hormonal and reproductive risk factors (Table 1.3). The most compelling evidence has come from studies of HRT following the menopause; exposure to unopposed oestrogen for 10 or more years increases the risk about 10-fold. This excess risk can be counteracted substantially by combined use of oestrogens and progestins.

Prevention

Obesity (which increases peripheral production of oestrogens) and diabetes mellitus are associated with an increased risk of developing endometrial cancer, whereas past oral contraceptive use, childbearing and physical activity (potentially mediated by hormones) are associated with risk reduction. It is therefore possible to substantially reduce the incidence of endometrial cancer through modification of lifestyle, maintenance

Table 1.3 Factors associated with the risk of endometrial cancer

Factor	Effect	Strength (RR)
Early menarche	↑	(+) (2.4)
Late menopause	↑	+
Anovulation	↑	++
Nulliparity/low parity	↑	++ (2–3)
Infertility	↑	+ (2–3)
Obesity	↑	++ (2–11)
Metabolic syndrome/diabetes	↑	++ (1.3–2.7)
Alcohol	↑	(+)
Endogenous oestrogen	↑	+
Exogenous unopposed oestrogen-only therapy	↑	+++ (1.6–12)
Tamoxifen	↑	++ (1.7–7.0)
Oestrogen–progestin combined replacement	↑~↓	+
Combination oral contraceptives	↓	+++
High parity/breastfeeding	↓	+
Physical activity	↓	+

RR, Relative risk.
↑ Factor increasing the risk; ↓ factor decreasing the risk; ↑~↓ factor increasing or decreasing the risk.
(+) Inconsistent association; + week association; ++ moderate association; +++ strong association.

of normal weight and optimal use of oral contraceptive and postmenopausal HRT. It has been estimated that about 37% of endometrial cancer cases in the United Kingdom can be prevented by changes in lifestyle and risk factor modification.

Cervical Cancer

Incidence and Mortality

Cervical cancer is the fourth most common cancer among women worldwide, with an estimated 528,000 new cases (7.9% of cancer in women) and 266,000 deaths (7.5% of cancer deaths in women) in the year 2012, and a 5-year prevalence of 1.5 million cases (9% of women with cancer). About 85% of the cases occur in developing countries, where cervical cancer accounts for 12% of all cancers in women. The incidence rates of cervical cancer vary substantially between different regions, from a low of 3.6/100,000 women in Switzerland to a high of 75.9/100,000 in Malawi. The highest rates are observed among populations in sub-Saharan Africa, Melanesia, Latin America and the Caribbean, south-central and south-east Asia. Incidence rates are generally low in developed countries in Europe, North America, Australia/New Zealand, the Middle East, China, and Japan. In the United Kingdom, cervical cancer is the twelfth most common cancer among women, with about 3,200 new cases in the year 2014 accounting for around 1.8% of all cancers in women, with a cumulative risk of 0.62% (1 in 161) by age 74 (Figure 1.1). In most European populations, the incidence rates of cervical cancer begin to increase at 20–4 years and thereafter the risk increases rapidly to reach a peak usually around 35–9 years (Figure 1.2). In the United Kingdom, incidence rates of cervical cancer are similar for White and Black females but significantly lower in Asian females.

Almost nine out of ten (87%) cervical cancer deaths occur in the less developed regions. The mortality rates vary substantially between different regions of the world; from less than 2/100,000 in Western Europe to more than 20/100,000 in Africa. In 2014, 890 women in the United Kingdom died from cervical cancer (2.8/100,000), accounting for around 1% of female deaths from cancer. Cervical cancer generally has an excellent prognosis; overall, in the United Kingdom, about 63% of women diagnosed with cervical cancer survive their disease for 10 or more years. When diagnosed at its earliest stage (Stage I), almost all (96%) of the women will survive their disease for 5 or more years, compared to 5-year relative survival of 5% for those diagnosed at Stage IV. In the United Kingdom, the 5-year net survival has steadily improved from 51.5% in 1971–2 to 67.4% in 2010–11 (an increase of about 31% in the period).

Trends in Incidence and Mortality

Overall, the incidence and mortality from cervical cancer have declined considerably during the past 40 years in Western Europe, North America, Australia/New Zealand, China, and Japan. The decline has been attributed to a combination of factors including improved genital hygiene, increased use of condoms, improved treatment modalities, beneficial effects of organised population-based cytological screening programmes for early diagnosis and introduction of the vaccine against HPV infection. In the United Kingdom, the ASRs (European standard) of cervical cancer have declined by

around 28% since the early 1990s, whereas, in the same period, the mortality rates declined by around 62%.

Aetiology

A persistent infection with an oncogenic HPV type is now recognised as a causal factor for preceding precancerous changes and cervical cancer. However, infection with HPV is extremely common compared with the relatively rare development of cervical cancer. There is compelling evidence that HPV is necessary for cervical carcinogenesis, but infection alone is not sufficient for the cancer to develop. A number of cofactors have been identified as possible modifiers of HPV infection during the developmental stages of cervical cancer, including early sexual debut, increasing number of sexual partners, smoking, long-term oral contraceptive use, high parity, dietary factors, certain human leucocyte antigen (HLA) types, and co-infection with other sexually transmitted agents such as *Chlamydia trachomatis*, herpesvirus type 2, and human immunodeficiency virus (HIV).

Prevention

Cervical cancer is one of the most preventable forms of cancer on a global scale. Prevention efforts include increased public awareness about sexually transmitted infections, early detection of precursor lesions by regular cytological screening, HPV testing, and the recently developed vaccine against certain high-risk types of HPV. In the United Kingdom, all girls aged 12–13 are now offered HPV vaccination as part of the childhood immunisation programme. It has been estimated that almost all the cases of cervical cancer in the United Kingdom can be prevented by changes in lifestyle and risk factor modification.

Vulvar and Vaginal Cancers

Incidence and Mortality

Vulvar and vaginal cancers are rare throughout the world and constitute less than 5% of all gynaecological cancers. The ASRs of vulvar cancer vary from a low of 0.3/100,000 women in Republic of Korea to a high of 4.1/100,000 in Saarland, Germany. In general, incidence rates are relatively higher in developed countries; the highest rates are observed in European, North American, and Australia/New Zealand populations and the lowest rates (<1/100,000 women) are observed in parts of Asia, Africa, the Middle East, and South America. In the United Kingdom, there were about 1,300 new cases of vulvar cancer in the year 2014, accounting for 0.7% of all cancers in women, with a cumulative risk of 0.17 (1 in 588 women) by age 74 (Figure 1.1). Vulvar cancer is predominantly a disease of older women, with a steep rise in incidence after 60–4 years from 6.2/100,000 to 19.7/100,000 women by 85–9 years, and over half of the cases (55%) are diagnosed in women aged over 70 years (Figure 1.2). In 2014, there were about 450 deaths from vulvar cancer in the United Kingdom.

In most world regions, the overall incidence rates of vaginal cancer do not exceed 1/100,000 women. In the United Kingdom, there were about 250 new cases of vaginal cancer in the year 2014, accounting for around 0.1% of all cancers in women, with a cumulative risk of 0.05 (1 in 2,000 women) by age 74 (Figure 1.1). Like vulvar cancer, it is predominantly a disease of older women, with a steep rise in incidence after 60–4 years: from 1.4/100,000 to 3.4/100,000 women by 85–9 years, and about half of the cases (48%) are diagnosed in women aged over 70 years (Figure 1.2). In 2014, there were 110 deaths from vulvar cancer in the United Kingdom. Survival rates for vulvar and vaginal cancers vary significantly by stage of disease and age at diagnosis; overall, about 53% of women diagnosed with vulvar or vaginal cancer survive their disease for 10 or more years.

Trends in Incidence and Mortality

In most developed countries, there has been little change in the overall (i.e. all ages combined) incidence of vulvar and vaginal cancers over the past 40 or more years. In the United Kingdom, the incidence rate of vulvar cancer has remained steady at around 3–4/100,000 women and of vaginal cancer around 0.8–0.9/100,000. However, recently there has been some increase in the rates of vulvar cancer among young women (age <50 years) in some countries, which has been linked to increasing incidence of vulvar intraepithelial neoplasia (VIN) in young women caused by infection with HPV. In most populations, the mortality rates of vulvar and vaginal cancers have declined steadily over the past 40 or more years. In the United Kingdom, the ASRs (European standard) for vulvar and vaginal cancers declined by 44% and 50%, respectively.

Aetiology

A persistent infection with an oncogenic HPV type is now considered to play a central role in the initiation and promotion of the majority of vulvar and vaginal cancers. HPV is more strongly associated with cancers in younger women and about 70% of VIN3 and 20–50% of invasive vulvar cancers contain HPV DNA. About 80% of VaIN3 and 60% of invasive vaginal squamous cell carcinomas contain HPV DNA. A history of cervical intraepithelial neoplasia (CIN) or cervical cancer is considered a strong risk factor for vulvar and vaginal cancers. A number of HPV cofactors have been identified, including a history of genital warts (which are caused most commonly by non-oncogenic HPV types), smoking, and infection with other sexually transmitted agents such as herpes virus type 2 and HIV. Many cases of vulvar cancer are not associated with HPV infection. Chronic vulvar skin conditions, including lichen sclerosus, lichen planus, and Paget's disease, are associated with an increased risk of VIN3 and invasive vulvar cancer. Iatrogenic immune suppression in transplant patients has been associated with a 100-fold increased risk of vulvar cancer.

Prevention

Increased public awareness about sexually transmitted infections, surveillance for precancerous lesions, self-awareness, smoking cessation, HPV testing, and HPV vaccination make vulvar and vaginal cancers one of the most preventable forms of cancer. It has been estimated that about 40% of vulvar cancers and 63% of vaginal cancers in the United Kingdom can be prevented by changes in lifestyle and risk factor modification.

Further Reading

Cancer Research UK. www.cancerresearchuk.org/health-professional/cancer-statistics.

GLOBOCAN. (2012). Estimated cancer incidence, mortality and prevalence worldwide in 2012, International Agency for Research on Cancer (IARC), WHO. http://globocan.iarc.fr/Default.aspx.

Ferlay J, Soerjomataram I, Dikshit R et al. (2015). Cancer incidence and mortality worldwide: sources, methods and major patterns in GLOBOCAN 2012. *Int J Cancer.* 136(5): E359–86.

Forman D, Bray F, Brewster DH et al., eds. (2013). *Cancer Incidence in Five Continents*, Vol. X (electronic version). Lyon: International Agency for Research on Cancer. http://ci5.iarc.fr.

International Union Against Cancer. *Tumour Node Metastasis Classification of Malignant Tumours (TNM-8).* www.uicc.org/resources/tnm.

Chapter 2

Pathology of Gynaecological Cancers

Raji Ganesan and Jo Vella

Background

Pathology literally means the study (logos) of suffering (pathos). It is a science that deals with causes and mechanisms of disease that result in manifestation of illness. Also, it is the bridge between basic science and clinical practice. A cure for malignancy is a major challenge for medicine. Understanding of pathology of malignancy will assist in the clinical understanding of the disease.

A neoplasm is defined as a new growth that is composed of cells that grow abnormally and in an uncoordinated fashion, such that they exceed the growth of the surrounding normal tissues. Neoplasms may be benign or malignant. A malignant neoplasm is characterised by its ability to invade normal tissues and to spread to distant sites (metastasis). While strictly speaking the term cancer or carcinoma refers to a malignancy arising in epithelial tissues, it is often used as a generic term to describe all malignant neoplasms.

Cancer is a result of genetic mutations that are acquired, usually spontaneously. These genetic mutations alter the function of the cells such that the cells acquire self-sufficiency and become unresponsive to normal control mechanisms to evade cell death and gain limitless replicative potential. These cellular changes that result in malignancy can be linked to environmental insults, infections by viruses, inherited genetic mechanisms and a combination of these processes. The malignancies in the female genital tract exemplify many of these different pathways. In the developed world, the most frequent malignancy of the female genital tract is endometrial carcinoma; the most common sub-type is linked to unopposed oestrogen stimulation and a resultant alteration in the cellular micro-environment. Cervical cancer is caused by infection with high-risk human papilloma virus (HPV). The virus infects the cell by entering into the basal cells in the cervical transformation zone. The viral DNA integrates with the DNA of the epithelial cells, particularly when there is a persistent infection with high-risk strains (notably types 16 and 18). This results in inactivation of important regulatory mechanisms and confers immortality on the cell, thus allowing progression to neoplasia. Some ovarian, tubal and endometrial cancers are associated with genetic abnormalities. Mutations in the *BRCA-1* and *2* genes are the cause of about 10% of breast, tubal and ovarian cancers. Lynch syndrome, which is associated with defects in DNA repair, is associated with an increased risk of endometrial and ovarian cancers.

Summary

- Cancer results from genetic mutations that alter the cell and result in limitless growth.
- Cancers can be inherited or acquired.
- Cancers of the female genital tract exemplify some of these mechanisms.

Role of Pathologist in the Management of Malignancies of the Female Genital Tract

Pathologists receive samples of tumours during diagnostic biopsy and excision. Sampling methods include small biopsy, excision biopsy, fine needle aspiration, Pipelle sampling, drained fluids (e.g. ascites) and cytology samples (such as sampling from cervical screening). These samples are processed in the laboratory and glass slides containing a piece of the tissue or cell are produced. The pathologist examines these samples under the microscope and makes a diagnosis that includes several parameters that provide guidance for management of the tumour. These parameters include:

Tumour type: There are different types of tissues from which a neoplasm can develop. A neoplasm is allocated a tissue type and its name based on its appearance under the microscope. A pathologist uses her knowledge to differentiate the appearance of normal tissues from the tumour types known in any organ to assign a tumour type. In general, malignancies arising from epithelial cells are termed as carcinomas and those arising from connective tissue are termed as sarcomas. Further specific typing is done based on specific cell types. Tumour type determines management and therefore accurate tumour typing is essential for directing optimal management. For example, the diagnosis of high-grade serous carcinoma of the ovary in the context of a pelvic mass may result in neoadjuvant chemotherapy whereas the diagnosis of a sarcoma may result in preference for a primary surgical treatment.

Tumour grade: The grade of a tumour indicates how closely the tumour resembles the tissue it arises from and can be assigned only on microscopic examination. There are generally three grades: G1, G2 and G3. The closer the appearance of the malignant tissue to normal tissue, the lower the grade. Low-grade tumours generally tend to grow and spread at a slower rate than high-grade tumours. They tend to be less responsive to non-surgical treatment modalities. The malignant cells in high-grade tumours are highly abnormal and usually show brisk mitotic activity indicative of their proliferative potential. Grading a tumour on small biopsies can be difficult and sometimes a pathologist will assign GX as the tumour grade to indicate that the grade could not be assigned in a small sample. In some malignancies, such as in an immature teratoma, the distant implants appear well differentiated and are referred to as G0.

Tumour stage: The stage of a cancer can be assigned clinically (as in cervical carcinoma) or pathologically (as in endometrial carcinoma). The parameters used are similar and consist of the size of tumour and the extent of spread. When the extent of spread is assessed, only tissue invasion is taken into consideration. So, an endometrial cancer that invades the inner half of the uterine wall but has tumour emboli in parametrial vessels is still a stage 1 cancer. The two staging systems used in cancers of the female genital tract are the tumour, node and metastatic (TNM) system and the International Federation of Gynecology and Obstetrics (FIGO) system. In the TNM system, T describes the size of the tumour. N describes whether the cancer has

spread to the lymph nodes and which nodes are involved. For example, N0 means no lymph nodes are affected while N1 means there are cancer cells in the lymph nodes. M describes if the cancer has spread to another part of the body. For example, M0 means the cancer has not spread (metastasised) to other parts of the body. FIGO system is similar to the TNM system and, in the United Kingdom, it is used more widely in the context of female genital tract malignancies.

The purpose of staging by a uniform system is to provide consistent terminology for better communication among health professionals, to compare research outcomes and to provide comparable prognosis to the patients, no matter where they have been treated.

In the United Kingdom, the Royal College of Pathologists publishes datasets for various cancers in which guidance is provided for pathologists. All reports on cancers should contain the minimum data recommended in these datasets. On the international stage, datasets are provided by International Collaboration on Cancer Reporting (ICCR).

Vascular invasion/lymphovascular invasion: Access to the vascular space by a malignant cell indicates that the cell has acquired the capacity to travel beyond the site of origin and for distant spread. This is, therefore, an important indicator of prognosis. The presence and quantification of the extent of lymphovascular involvement is dependent on several factors including sampling of tissue and observer variation. In endometrial cancers, it has been shown that significant vascular invasion is associated with risk of recurrence.

Lymph node involvement: Removal of lymph nodes is often carried out as the part of radical surgical treatment for cancers. Sentinel node biopsy can be performed instead of lymph node dissection. The sentinel lymph node is defined as the first lymph node to which the lymphatics from a cancer drain into. The surgeon injects a coloured dye/radioactive tracer and then detects the sentinel node by tracing the path of spread. The pathologist examines this node by looking at thin slices of tissue. If the node does not contain metastatic cancer, the patient may not require full lymph node dissection thus avoiding increased surgical time and greater postoperative morbidity. Molecular tests can be carried out on sentinel nodes and these may yield results intraoperatively.

It is understood that the number of lymph nodes removed at surgery is related to survival in some cancers. When smaller number is removed, patients tend to have lower survival. Based on this, optimal numbers of lymph nodes have been defined. The number of lymph nodes retrieved at cancer surgery is a combination of surgical skill and pathologists' meticulousness.

Summary

- Pathological examination of tumour tissue guides management of malignancy.
- Tumour type, grade, stage, vascular invasion and lymph node involvement are assessed by the pathologist.
- Sentinel node sampling and evaluation is increasingly used in decision making.

Frozen Sections

Frozen sections are a method of rapidly solidifying small pieces of tissue to make tissue sections suitable for microscopic examination. An intraoperative consultation in gynaecological pathology is indicated:

- To determine the nature of a disease process: whether benign or malignant
- To type the tumour, if malignancy is confirmed
- To assess margins
- To ensure that the tissue sampled is adequate for diagnosis
- To obtain tissue for research and additional molecular studies.

The information from a frozen section is limited by sampling as only small amounts of tissue can be studied in the available period. Challenging situations in intraoperative consultation in gynaecological pathology are:

- Diagnosis of malignancy in mucinous tumours
- Distinction of an ovarian carcinoma from borderline tumours
- Determination of margins in Paget's disease
- Distinction between lymphomas and dysgerminoma
- Distinction between yolk sac tumour and juvenile granulosa tumour
- Lesions biopsied in pregnant women.

Pathology of Preinvasive and Invasive Neoplastic Disease of the Female Genital Tract

Vulva

Vulval Intraepithelial Neoplasia

The term vulval intraepithelial neoplasia (VIN) encompasses a spectrum of intraepidermal changes of the vulval skin or mucosa, ranging from mild atypia to severe abnormalities amounting to carcinoma in situ. Aetiologically and morphologically, two types of VIN are recognised. Classical/usual (warty or basaloid) VIN occurs in younger women and is caused by infection with HPV. It is diagnosed by noting full thickness abnormality of the squamous cells in the epithelium. Differentiated or simplex VIN is seen in older women. It is not associated with HPV but is associated with lichen sclerosus. The changes are seen only in basal cells and may be difficult to recognise. The pertinent histological features of VIN are outlined in Table 2.1. Classical VIN is graded as 1, 2 or 3. Differentiated VIN is always high grade.

Grading of classical VIN
VIN1   Abnormalities confined to lower one-third
VIN2   Abnormalities confined to lower two-thirds
VIN3   Abnormality involving full thickness of epithelium

Vulval Squamous Cell Carcinoma

Squamous cell carcinoma (SCC) is an invasive tumour showing differentiation towards squamous cells. It is the most common malignancy of the vulva and presents as an area of hyperkeratosis or as a small ulcer. Based on the extent on differentiation, SCC is graded as well, moderately or poorly differentiated (G1, G2 or G3). The strongest correlate of outcome is lymph node status and the most important factor predicting lymph node metastases is tumour depth.

Table 2.1 Histological features of VIN

Type of VIN		Histological features
Classical/ usual	Warty	- Prominent koilocytic change (indicative of HPV)
	Basaloid	- Small uniform cells resembling basal cells - Minimal koilocytic change
Differentiated		- Abnormal cells confined to the basal and parabasal layers - Keratin pearl formation - No koilocytic change

Vulval Verrucous Carcinoma

Verrucous carcinomas are rare tumours and are defined as a well-differentiated and biologically low-grade neoplasm of squamous cell origin. To fit this category, strict histological criteria must be fulfilled. These include pushing borders, no frank destructive invasion and large keratinocytes with pale eosinophilic cytoplasm and sparse mitotic activity.

Vulval Extramammary Paget's Disease

The vulva is one of the most commonly involved sites in extramammary Paget's disease. The origin of this neoplasm is unclear. Histological features are nests or single pale cells in the epidermis. Invasive elements may be seen rarely. Paget's disease can mimic eczema clinically and often the margins of the disease process cannot be identified. It must be differentiated from melanoma, which the disease mimics histologically.

Vulval Melanoma

Melanoma accounts for about 9% of all malignant vulval tumours. Parameters used in melanomas elsewhere such as Clark's levels and Breslow's thickness can be applied to vulval melanomas. Poorer outcome is indicated by:

- Breslow's thickness greater than 0.76 mm
- Clark's level greater than II
- Vascular involvement.

Other Vulval Tumours

Malignancies that occur in the vulva may arise in the glands present in the region. The most common of these neoplasms arise in Bartholins duct and gland. Neoplasms also arise from the connective tissue in the vulva and may be malignant.

Cervix

Cervical Intraepithelial Neoplasia

Cervical intraepithelial neoplasia (CIN) is the term used to describe proliferative intraepithelial squamous lesions that display abnormal maturation and cyto-nuclear atypia. Mitotic activity is often increased and abnormal mitotic forms may be seen. The most important feature is abnormal maturation and this is manifested by loss of polarity and cellular disorganisation. CIN has a three-tier grading system based on the level of involvement of the squamous epithelium by the abnormality. Immature metaplasia and atrophy are

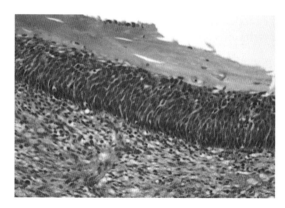

Figure 2.1 The squamous epithelium shows lack of maturation throughout its thickness, amounting to CIN3
(Haematoxylin eosin stain, 40× magnification)

benign lesions that are commonly difficult to differentiate from CIN. Immunohistochemistry (IHC) with p16 is used to facilitate grading of CIN. Strong, block staining with p16 is used as a surrogate indicator of the presence of high-risk HPV (Figure 2.1).

Grading of CIN

CIN1	Abnormality confined to basal third of epithelium
CIN2	Abnormality up to lower two-thirds of epithelium
CIN3	Abnormality involving superficial third of epithelium

Cervical Glandular Intraepithelial Neoplasia

Cervical glandular intraepithelial neoplasia (CGIN) refers to abnormalities of the glandular cells of the cervix and is divided into two tiers: high-grade CGIN, a relatively robust histopathological diagnosis with good inter-observer correlation and correlation with biological potential for malignancy, and low-grade CGIN, which is less understood and may be under-reported (Figure 2.2 and Table 2.2).

Distinguishing high-grade CGIN from invasive adenocarcinoma in its earliest stages is difficult and features that raise the possibility of invasion are back-to-back arrangement of glands with little intervening stroma, a cribriform gland pattern, a desmoplastic stromal response and increased cytoplasmic eosinophilia. There are a number of benign conditions that may mimic CGIN.

Stratified Mucinous Intraepithelial Lesion

Stratified mucinous intraepithelial lesion (SMILE) is a recently recognised variant of intraepithelial neoplasia

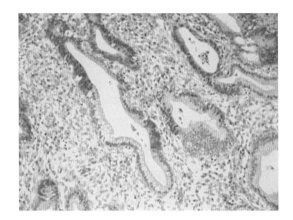

Figure 2.2 Endocervical epithelium shows crowding of nuclei with mitosis and apoptotic bodies – features of high-grade CGIN (Haematoxylin eosin stain, 40× magnification)

Table 2.2 Features of high-grade CGIN

Architectural	Cytological
• Gland crowding	• Cellular stratification
• Branching and budding	• Loss of cytoplasmic mucin
• Presence of intraluminal papillary projections	• Nuclear enlargement
	• Loss of polarity
	• Increased mitotic activity

Histological mimics of CGIN and endocervical adenocarcinoma

• Endometriosis
• Tuboendometrioid metaplasia
• Microglandular hyperplasia
• Hyperplasia of mesonephric remnants
• Arias-Stella reaction involving endocervical glands

identified by the presence of conspicuous cytoplasmic vacuoles in lesions otherwise resembling CIN.

Screening for the precursors – CIN and CGIN – reduces the occurrence of invasive cervical cancers. In England, screening for cervical cancers is offered to women between the ages of 25 and 64. Since its introduction, the screening program has helped halve the number of cervical cancer cases, and is estimated to save approximately 4,500 lives per year in England. The aim of the cervical cancer screening programme is to reduce the incidence of and mortality from cervical cancer. Presently cervical screening is performed by cytological examination of cervical cytology samples under the microscope which enables abnormalities in cervical epithelial cells to be picked up at the pre-invasive stage when treatment can be given to prevent

cancer. In recognition of the fact that the vast majority of screen-detected cervical cancers are caused by HPV, the screening programme will be adopting high-risk HPV screening protocols.

Cervical Squamous Cell Carcinoma

A simple two-tiered classification is recommended and this is based on whether the cells show keratin production and thus are keratinising, or lack keratin production and therefore are non-keratinising. Tumour type, presence of vascular invasion and depth of invasion (stage of disease) are the main pathological prognosticators. Histological grade does not appear to have a major influence on outcome.

FIGO Stage IA carcinoma
• Maximum size: 5 mm deep and 7 mm in horizontal dimension
• Stage IA1: maximum depth of invasion 3 mm
• Stage IA2: maximum depth of invasion 5 mm
• Vascular space involvement does not affect staging

The recommended treatment of FIGO Stage IA1 carcinomas is by local excision with resection margins that are clear of both CIN and invasive disease. Radical hysterectomy is usually undertaken for FIGO stage IA2 and IB1 carcinomas, although in some institutions IA2 carcinomas are treated by local excision. If fertility preservation is desired, trachelectomy may be considered for FIGO stage IA2 tumours and small stage IB1 carcinomas.

TIPS
• The risk of lymph node metastases is negligible in stage IA1 tumours.
• The most important prognostic factors are stage, size, depth of invasion, lymph node metastases and the presence of lymphovascular space invasion. Histological grade does not appear to influence prognosis.

Cervical Adenocarcinoma

Unlike its squamous counterpart, there are no clearly defined or easily reproducible criteria for diagnosis or early invasion in adenocarcinomas. The outcome in these cancers depends on size, stage and grade. There are several different histological subtypes. There may be difficulties in differentiating between endometrial and endocervical carcinoma in some instances and IHC may be helpful.

It is increasingly becoming recognised that there are cervical carcinomas that are not aetiologically associated with HPV. Minimum deviation adenocarcinoma (adenoma malignum) is a well-differentiated variant of endocervical adenocarcinoma that is not associated with HPV as a causative factor. It has the following features:

- Little or no cytological atypia
- Little mitotic activity
- Presence of glands deep within the cervical stroma beyond the normal crypt field
- Sometimes vascular and perineural invasion
- A known association with ovarian sex cord stromal tumour with annular tubules (in Peutz–Jeghers syndrome) and mucinous neoplasms.

Other non-HPV-associated cervical carcinomas include clear cell carcinomas and mesonephric carcinomas.

Cervical Adenosquamous Carcinoma

The adenosquamous carcinoma variant appears more frequently in younger women. The tumours contain malignant squamous and glandular cells and it may also be possible to identify adjacent CIN and CGIN.

Cervical Neuroendocrine Carcinoma

Neuroendocrine carcinoma (NEC) of the cervix accounts for less than 5% of all cervical carcinomas and are typically associated with a poorer prognosis than the more common histological subtypes due to a high incidence of early metastatic spread. The diagnosis is made by the pathologist who recognises certain morphological features including brisk mitotic activity, conspicuous apoptosis and necrosis. They are commonly positive for immunohistochemical markers of neuroendocrine differentiation.

Summary

- Common cervical cancers are aetiologically related to HPV.
- They have precursor lesions termed intraepithelial neoplasia.
- Precursor lesions can be detected by cervical screening.
- NEC of the cervix has an aggressive behaviour.

Endometrium

Endometrial Hyperplasia

Hyperplasia of the endometrium is characterised by an increase in glandular tissue relative to stroma, with

Table 2.3 Types of endometrial hyperplasia and their microscopic features

Type	Microscopic features	Notes
Endometrial hyperplasia without atypia	• Proliferation of glands of varying size and shape • Increased gland-to-stroma ratio • No cytological atypia	• Old terminology: Simple hyperplasia without atypia; complex hyperplasia without atypia
Atypical endometrial hyperplasia	• Similar features to those described above with superadded cytological atypia	• Old terminology: Simple atypical hyperplasia, complex atypical hyperplasia • Associated with a risk of synchronous or subsequent carcinoma

concomitant architectural and sometimes cytological abnormalities. The latest edition (2014) of the World Health Organisation (WHO) classification of neoplasms of the female genital tract simply subdivides endometrial hyperplasia as occurring with or without atypia. The features of the two categories of endometrial hyperplasia are outlined in Table 2.3.

It may be difficult to distinguish atypical hyperplasia from well-differentiated endometrioid carcinoma. Histological features which are suggestive of carcinoma include a complex cribriform pattern, intraglandular bridging, intraglandular neutrophils, abnormal mitotic activity and a fibroblastic stromal response.

Endometrial Carcinoma

Carcinoma of the endometrium has increased in frequency. In developed countries, it is now the most common gynaecological cancer. Morphologically, aetiologically and conceptually, there are two types of endometrial carcinomas: types 1 and 2. The characteristics of each of these types of endometrial cancer are outlined in Table 2.4. This classification is likely to be superceded by the TCGA classification in the near future, in which molecular subtyping of endometrial cancers provides guidance to management and prognosis.

Serous Endometrial Intraepithelial Carcinoma

Serous endometrial intraepithelial carcinoma (sEIC) is the term used when serous carcinoma is confined to the endometrial epithelium. It is characterised by

Table 2.4 Characteristics of types 1 and 2 endometrial carcinomas

	Type 1 Prototype: endometrioid carcinoma	Type 2 Prototype: serous carcinoma
Incidence	More common	Less common
Age predilection	Younger (including pre- and perimenopausal)	Older (postmenopausal)
Aetiologically associated with unopposed oestrogen stimulation	Yes	No
Other associations	Diabetes, hypertension, obesity, long-standing tamoxifen use, PCOS	None
Precursor lesion	Atypical endometrial hyperplasia	Serous endometrial intraepithelial carcinoma
Molecular abnormalities	PTEN and k-RAS mutations	p53 mutations
Prognosis	Relatively good	Relatively poor (more likely to present at an advanced stage)

mitotically active, markedly cytological atypical cells occupying the endometrial surface or glands. It is considered to be the precursor of uterine serous carcinoma. However, it is important to also recognise that sEIC itself has an aggressive behaviour similar to uterine serous carcinoma and can metastasize readily to extrauterine sites.

Mixed Tumours of the Uterus

Mixed tumours of the uterus contain a mixture of glands and mesenchymal tissue. Atypical polypoid adenomyomas are typically solitary, well-circumscribed, polypoid lesions occurring in reproductive-age women which contain endometrioid glands with varying degrees of architectural and cytological atypia, separated by myofibromatous stroma. In about 10% of cases, they are associated with endometrial carcinomas. On removal, atypical polypoid adenomyomas may recur in up to 45% of cases.

Adenosarcomas are tumours that contain benign glands and neoplastic stroma. Typically they are low-grade malignancies. They tend to recur and eventually may show distant metastasis. Uterine carcinosarcomas (previously referred to as malignant mixed Müllerian tumours) are highly aggressive and have traditionally been regarded as a subtype of uterine sarcoma. However, in recent years, convincing evidence has suggested that most, if not all, are monoclonal in origin rather than true collision tumours. Data confirm that the carcinomatous element is the 'driving force' and that the sarcomatous component is derived from the carcinoma or from a stem cell that undergoes divergent differentiation. Thus, uterine carcinosarcomas are best regarded as metaplastic carcinomas.

Summary

- Endometrial hyperplasia is classified as with or without atypia.
- Endometrial carcinomas are classified into two types: type 1 (prototype endometrioid carcinoma) and type 2. Type 1 generally presents at an early stage and has a good outcome.
- Tumours with epithelial and mesenchymal elements are referred to as mixed tumours.

Tumours of the Uterine Wall

Smooth Muscle Tumours of the Uterus

The most common tumour of the smooth muscle in the uterus is the benign leiomyoma (fibroid). Several variants have been described. Smooth muscle tumours of the uterus also include smooth muscle tumours of unknown malignant potential (STUMP) and leiomyosarcoma. The distinction between these types requires microscopic examination (Table 2.5).

Endometrial Stromal Tumours

Endometrial stromal tumours of the uterus are the second most common mesenchymal tumours of the uterus. According to the WHO classification, they are divided into endometrial stromal nodules, low-grade endometrial stromal sarcomas, high-grade endometrial stromal sarcomas and undifferentiated uterine sarcomas. Low-grade endometrial stromal sarcomas are the most common and typified by permeation through the wall of the uterus. They frequently contain chromosomal rearrangement that results in JAZF1–SUZ12 or equivalent genetic fusion.

Table 2.5 Smooth muscle tumours of the uterus

Name	Features	Comment
Cellular and highly cellular leiomyoma	• Cytologically bland • <5 mitoses per 10 high power fields (hpf)	Benign
Leiomyoma with bizarre nuclei	• Variable numbers of cytologically bizarre nuclei • <10 mitoses per 10 hpf • No coagulative tumour cell necrosis	Benign
Mitotically active leiomyoma	• 5–15 mitoses per 10 hpf • Often submucosal • Sometimes associated with hormone therapy	Benign
Smooth muscle tumour of uncertain malignant potential (STUMP)	• Other combination of features causing concern but falling short of leiomyosarcoma	Behaviour uncertain
Leiomyosarcoma	• Diffuse, moderate to marked cytological atypia • Usually high mitotic rate • Coagulative tumour cell necrosis	Malignant

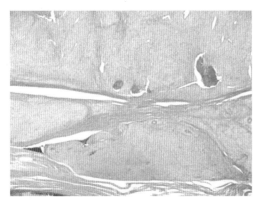

Figure 2.3 This is an endometrial stromal sarcoma showing typical myometrial vascular permeation
(Haematoxylin eosin stain, 40× magnification)

High-grade endometrial stromal sarcoma is pathologically and clinically a high-grade malignancy with poor outcome. It is characterised by the presence of YWHAE–NUTM2A/B genetic fusion (Figure 2.3).

Ovary and Fallopian Tube

Three groups of tumours comprise the majority of primary ovarian tumours, namely surface epithelial tumours, sex cord stromal tumours and germ cell tumours. The surface epithelial ovarian tumours comprise serous, mucinous, endometrioid and clear cell types. They are further classified as benign, borderline and malignant. Malignant serous tumours may be low grade or high grade and they are considered to represent two separate disease processes.

Carcinomas: Epithelial ovarian carcinomas have been divided into two broad categories, designated as type I and type II tumours that correspond to two main pathways of tumourigenesis. Type I tumours are usually low grade and include low-grade serous carcinoma, low-grade endometrioid carcinoma, mucinous carcinoma and clear cell carcinomas. They present at an early stage, behave in an indolent fashion and are characterised by mutations in a number of different genes, including *KRAS, BRAF, PTEN*, and beta-catenin. Type II tumours are high grade and include high-grade serous carcinoma, high-grade endometrioid carcinoma, carcinosarcoma and undifferentiated carcinoma. These tumours are highly aggressive neoplasms and usually present at an advanced stage. They are characterised by mutations of p53. High-grade serous carcinomas account for approximately 70% of ovarian cancers and have the highest mortality of the gynaecological malignancies due to the advanced stage at presentation. There is compelling evidence that a high percentage of so-called 'ovarian' high-grade serous carcinomas arise in the fimbrial end of the fallopian tube. Serous tubal intraepithelial carcinoma (STIC) is considered a precursor lesion. In order to reflect this in our clinical practice and in order to promote a uniform approach, criteria for primary site assignment of non-uterine high-grade serous carcinomas as tubal, ovarian, peritoneal or tubo-ovarian have recently been recommended. While the primary site does not currently alter therapy, consistency in primary site assignment allows accurate data collection for comparing disease outcomes in routine practice and clinical trials.

Ovarian mucinous carcinomas are usually well differentiated. They are of two types: intestinal and Mullerian mucinous (seromucinous) and they are histogenetically and clinically distinct. Mucinous carcinomas are uncommon and should only be diagnosed after the possibility of metastatic carcinoma is excluded clinically, on imaging and pathological examination. Endometrioid and clear cell carcinomas may be associated with endometriosis.

Summary

- Ovarian carcinomas are of two types based on morphological, clinical and molecular findings.
- The most common ovarian carcinoma is high-grade serous carcinoma and usually presents in advanced stage.
- Serous cancers are now believed to arise predominantly from the fallopian tube.
- Mucinous carcinoma of the ovary should be diagnosed only after exclusion of the possibility of metastasis from another organ.

Borderline Ovarian Tumours

These neoplasms, unique to the ovary, are relatively uncommon. The preferred WHO term is borderline, with atypically proliferative tumours as a synonym. These are tumours that display a greater degree of proliferation and atypia than benign tumours but lesser than that of a carcinoma. They are noninvasive. They occur over a wide age range and are often seen in young females where they pose management challenges if fertility is desired. They are mostly serous or mucinous in type. Extraovarian disease occurring with an ovarian serous borderline tumour is referred to as implants, a different terminology from other neoplasms where spread beyond the organ of origin is termed metastasis. Implants are present in approximately 20% of serous borderline tumours and most commonly occur in the omentum, peritoneal surfaces (including the serosa of the uterus) and the surface of the fallopian tube. A specific type of implant, defined as invasive implant, is associated with a malignant clinical behaviour and therefore in such instances a diagnosis of low-grade serous carcinoma is made. In mucinous borderline tumours, there may be subtle morphological changes that alter the diagnosis to a carcinoma. It is important that the pathologist carefully excludes metastatic mucinous carcinomas in the differential.

Staging of an ovarian borderline tumour is identical to that of invasive ovarian carcinomas. The prognosis in fully staged serous borderline tumours confined to the ovary is excellent with overall survival approaching 100%. With advanced stage neoplasms with noninvasive implants, the overall survival is in excess of 90%, although some patients will develop late recurrences. When invasive tumour is present in the omentum or peritoneum in association with a borderline tumour of the ovary, they are referred to as low-grade carcinoma. The extent of the omental or/and peritoneal disease determines prognosis in these cases.

Summary

- Borderline ovarian tumours are those that show proliferative activity higher than a benign tumour but lack evidence of invasion.
- Serous borderline tumours may be associated with extra ovarian disease or implants.
- When extra ovarian disease is invasive, then the tumour is termed low-grade serous carcinoma, irrespective of the nature of the ovarian tumour.

Germ Cell Tumours

The most common ovarian germ cell tumour is a mature cystic teratoma, which is also known as an ovarian dermoid cyst. They occur over a wide age range, most commonly in the reproductive-age group. Most usually present with symptoms related to the presence of a mass or torsion, although many are identified as incidental findings during imaging of the pelvis. Uncommonly paraneoplastic symptoms such as haemolytic anaemia, vasculitis and encephalitis may also be seen. On microscopy, a wide variety of mature tissues, commonly skin and adnexal structures, are seen. When neuroectodermal tubules and cellular mitotically active glia are seen, the diagnosis of an immature teratoma is made. Immature teratomas are malignant tumours. In patients with immature teratomas, mature glial tissue may be seen in extraovarian sites especially in the peritoneal cavity and is referred to as peritoneal gliomatosis. Sometimes ovarian teratomas may exhibit unidirectional differentiation and are then referred to as monodermal teratomas. The most common is struma ovarii in which thyroid tissue is seen. Struma ovarii can undergo all the malignant changes that are seen in eutopic thyroid. Struma may be pure, but is most commonly associated with a dermoid cyst. Less commonly, a carcinoid tumour (strumal carcinoid), a Brenner tumour or a mucinous tumour is seen. Carcinoids are the second most common monodermal teratoma.

The most common malignant germ cell tumour is dysgerminoma. These usually arise in the second and third decades of life. They are rarely bilateral and may be associated with raised serum HCG. This is because syncytiotrophoblast type cells (which secrete HCG) may be present admixed with the malignant cells. Yolk sac tumour is the second most common within the category of primitive germ cell tumours in women, and also peaks in the late teens and early twenties. It typically presents as a large bulky mass with a more variegated sectioned surface than dysgerminoma with prominent areas of haemorrhage and/or necrosis. Given its very primitive nature, it is enigmatic that sometimes it is associated with a dermoid cyst. Occasionally, it may be part of a mixed germ cell tumour.

Summary

- Dermoid cyst (correctly termed benign, mature, cystic teratoma) is the most common ovarian germ cell tumour.
- Teratomas may predominantly show the presence of thyroid tissue when they are termed struma ovarii.
- Immature teratomas are malignant tumours.
- Other malignant germ cell tumours include dysgerminoma and yolk sac tumour.

Sex Cord Tumours

These are a diverse group of neoplasms with a wide morphological spectrum. They are composed of ovarian and testicular stromal-type cells. They represent less than 10% of all primary ovarian neoplasms. The WHO classification divides them into four main categories:

- Granulosa stromal cell tumours, composed of ovarian-type cells
- Sertoli stromal cell tumours, composed of testicular-type cells
- Sex cord stromal tumours of mixed or unclassified cell types
- Steroid cell tumours.

The most common benign tumour in this category is the fibroma. These may occur at any age, but are seen most commonly in middle-aged women, with an average age at presentation in the fifth decade. They are often bilateral and are rarely present with ascites and pleural effusion (Meig's syndrome). The most common malignant tumour in this category is the adult granulosa cell tumour. They are most common in perimenopausal women. They are the most common tumour associated with oestrogenic manifestation and patients frequently present with abnormal vaginal bleeding. They can have concurrent endometrial hyperplasia or adenocarcinoma and patients must undergo endometrial evaluation. Adult granulosa cell tumours confined to the ovary have a good prognosis with a 10-year survival of 85%. These tumours have a propensity for late recurrences.

Summary

- The most common benign ovarian stromal tumour is fibroma.
- The most common ovarian sex cord stromal tumour is adult granulosa cell tumour.

Miscellaneous Tumours

The most important neoplasm in this category is the small cell carcinoma of the ovary, hypercalcaemic type. This is an aggressive ovarian tumour representing less than 1% of ovarian tumours and is mostly seen in the third decade of life. Nearly 50% of the women present at an advanced stage. About two thirds of the patients have raised serum calcium levels. Histological examination generally reveals a relatively monotonous appearance with tumour cells arranged in various architectural patterns. Follicle-like structures are present in 80% of cases and are a characteristic, but not pathognomonic, histological feature. Until recently, the pathogenesis of this tumour was unknown. Recently, mutations of the *SMARC A4* gene have been noted in this tumour.

Metastatic Tumours

Metastatic tumours to the ovary comprise about fifth of malignant ovarian tumours. The ovary is a common site for metastasis from other primary sites. Adenocarcinomas arising in the gastrointestinal tract are the most common site of origin. Ovaries may be involved in disseminated malignancy and from carcinomas of the breast, endometrium and the cervix. In many cases, the ovarian mass may be the first site to present clinically and the primary site is discovered later. Typically metastatic ovarian cancers are solid, bilateral and small in size. They usually show tumour on the capsule and have a nodular cut surface. On microscopy, there is often necrosis and lymphovascular space invasion. Prominent stromal luteinisation may be seen in some metastatic mucinous carcinomas and the patient may present with virilising symptoms. IHC is helpful in allocating or excluding a primary site. Non-epithelial malignancies such as lymphomas and melanomas may also present with ovarian masses.

Summary

- Ovary is a common site for metastases.
- The most common primary sites of origin are the gastrointestinal tract, breast and cervix.
- Typically metastatic tumours are bilateral, solid and small in size.
- Morphology and IHC are useful in allocating a primary site.

Peritoneum

Primary tumours of the peritoneum include mesothelial tumours (such as well-differentiated papillary mesothelioma and malignant mesothelioma) and epithelial tumours (low-grade serous carcinoma, high-grade serous carcinoma). Secondary tumours include metastatic carcinoma and low-grade mucinous neoplasm associated with pseudomyxoma peritonei. Tumour-like lesions of the peritoneum include mesothelial hyperplasia, endometriosis and endosalpingiosis.

Pseudomyxoma peritonei is the clinical term for the accumulation of mucinous material in the pelvic or abdominal cavity. Disseminated peritoneal adenomucinosis (DPAM) is the pathological term which refers to low-grade mucinous lesions. In contrast, peritoneal mucinous carcinomatosis (PMCA) refers to high-grade mucinous lesions. The low-grade lesions are typically associated with an appendiceal tumour and in many cases there is involvement of ovaries that may outsize an unremarkable appearing appendix. In these cases, the cellularity is low and the neoplastic cells are bland. These tumours typically have a better prognosis. The high-grade lesions show a pattern of spread typical of carcinoma including involvement of lymph nodes and metastases outside the abdominal cavity. On microscopy, the lesions are more cellular and the cells show obvious features of malignancy. The primary tumour is generally from the gastrointestinal tract.

The Relationship between Endometriosis and Carcinomas of the Female Genital Tract

Malignant transformation of endometriosis occurs at an estimated frequency of 1.1–3%. Endometrioid and clear cell carcinomas are the most common histological types of cancers that arise within endometriosis. The ovary is the most common site where malignancy may arise in association with endometriosis and accounts for 75% of cases.

The Specimen Pathway including Request Form, Report Contents and Cancer Datasets

Fixation

Most specimens are sent to the laboratory in fixative, most commonly 10% formalin (4% formaldehyde) solution. An adequate amount of fixative is considered to be 10–15 times the volume of the tissue. Usually 6 to 8 hours is required for adequate fixation in formalin. Fixation serves to:

- Preserve tissue by preventing autolysis
- Harden tissue to allow thin sectioning
- Inactivate infectious agents
- Enhance avidity for dyes.

When the tissue specimen is to be preserved for future use for research and cytogenetic analysis (for example, NHS Genomics study or Biobanking), the specimens may need to be sent fresh to specialist laboratories.

The Request Form

The request form accompanying the specimen contains vital information, such as patient details, to prevent misidentification and to prevent serious errors, as well as clinical details, with contact information. Accurate clinical details are essential, especially for the pathologist to respond to particular queries. The details should include:

- Date and type of procedure
- Clinical history including

    - The purpose of surgery
    - History of prior known disease
    - History of current disease and treatment
    - An indication of urgency of diagnosis
    - Menstrual history
    - Cytological screening history
    - Other relevant details.

21

Basic Information Required on the Pathologist's Report for Gynaecological Cancers

The report issued by the pathologist should include the following information where relevant:

- Clinical details
  - These are transcribed from the request form
- Macroscopy
  - Dimensions and description of the specimen
  - Description of any abnormalities
  - Block key
- Microscopy
  - Morphological description
  - Information for prognosis and staging as per the relevant Royal College of Pathologists Cancer Dataset
  - Results of any special stains or IHC
  - May include a discussion of the differential diagnosis, reasons for diagnostic interpretation, prognostic considerations
  - Diagnosis
  - Cancer dataset.

Cancer Datasets

The Royal College of Pathologists has published five datasets for malignancies of the female genital tract. These cancer datasets recommend core data items to include in the histology report for malignant resections. Core data items are items that are supported by robust published evidence and are required for cancer staging, optimal patient management and prognosis.

Markers Used in Diagnosis, Management and Prognostication

Diagnostic Immunohistochemistry

Diagnostic IHC is the process by which antigens (proteins) that are present in a cell are detected by the use of antibodies that bind to the antigens. This technique is widely used in diagnosis of the site of origin and type of cancer. For example, the profile of primary ovarian cancers differs from cancers that are metastatic to the ovary from the colon. In cases of undifferentiated cancers, IHC assists in primary site assignment.

Markers to Aid Management

IHC can aid patient management. For example, IHC testing for the presence of hormone receptors in cancers may direct towards hormone manipulation as a primary treatment tool in patients who are unfit for surgery. Testing for Her2 receptors on breast carcinoma cells is done by IHC and the results are used by oncologists to determine treatment with Her2 receptor blockers such as trastuzumab.

Molecular Pathology

Molecular techniques are increasingly used to diagnose, direct treatment and prognosticate on tumours. Examples in the female genital tract include the detection of genetic mutations in diagnosis of small cell carcinoma of the ovary, hypercalcaemic type and in typing of endometrial stromal neoplasms. In some circumstances, oncologists request HER2 testing which includes fluorescent in situ hybridisation (FISH) technique. Recognition that virtually all advanced tumours have circulating tumour cells and tumour DNA has led to an interest in mapping tumour burden by molecular tests. Detection of hereditary predisposition to cancer in some ovarian and endometrial cancers requires testing for germline mutations by molecular methods. Molecular tumour profiling methods include expression profiling and next-generation sequencing technology. The Cancer Genome Atlas (TCGA) is a comprehensive, multidimensional map of key genomic changes in various cancers.

Further Reading

Kurman RJ, Carcangiu ML, Herrington CS, Young RH. *WHO Classification of Tumours of the Female Reproductive Organs*, 4th ed. Lyon: IARC, 2014.

Lee CH, Nucci MR. Endometrial stromal sarcoma – the new genetic paradigm. *Histopathology* 2015 July; 67(1): 1–19.

Singh N, Gilks CB, Hirschowitz L, Wilkinson N, McCluggage WG. Adopting a uniform approach to site assignment in tubo-ovarian high grade serous carcinoma: the time has come. *Int J Gynecol Pathol* 2016; 35: 230–7.

Toledo G, Oliva E. Smooth muscle tumours of the uterus: a practical approach. *Arch Pathol Lab Med* 2008; 132: 595–605.

Vinay Kumar, Abbas AK and Aster JC. *Robbins and Cotran Pathologic Basis of Disease*, 9th ed. Philadelphia: Elsevier Saunders, 2014.

Chapter 3

Imaging in Gynaecological Oncology

Susan Freeman, Helen Addley and Penelope Moyle

Introduction

Diagnostic imaging has an important role in diagnosis, treatment planning and follow-up of gynaecological malignancies. Gynaecological imaging modalities include ultrasound (US), magnetic resonance imaging (MRI), computerised tomography (CT) and positron emission tomography (PET). These modalities have their own inherent strengths and weaknesses. By understanding these factors, the most appropriate investigation can be performed to provide the most useful information in different clinical scenarios.

Ultrasound

US has a pivotal role in gynaecological imaging as it is widely available and a relatively cheap imaging investigation. US images are created with high-frequency sound waves and therefore can be safely utilised in all patients. US is the imaging modality of choice in the initial investigation of patients presenting with abnormal vaginal bleeding, pelvic pain or suspected pelvic mass. Ideally US should be performed using both transabdominal and transvaginal methods, to ensure that all pathologies are detected and accurately characterised. Transabdominal US (TAUS) is performed with a 3.5–5.0 MHz transducer in patients with a full bladder, which serves to displace bowel loops (and therefore gas) from the pelvis and provides a sonographic window for clearer images. TAUS is particularly useful in patients with a bulky fibroid uterus or large volume adnexal masses that may extend from the pelvis into the abdominal cavity. TAUS also enables assessment of the upper abdomen for the presence of associated pathology such as ascites or hydronephrosis.

Transvaginal US (TVUS) is performed once the patient has emptied her bladder, which allows the pelvic organs to be closely apposed to the US probe. The smaller depth of field means that a higher frequency probe can be used (typically 5–7.5 MHz), which provides higher-resolution images. The high-resolution imaging of TVUS allows the assessment of endometrial thickness in patients with postmenopausal bleeding and characterisation of adnexal masses, with approximately 20% remaining indeterminate. TVUS is able to detect small papillary lesions and mural nodules within complex ovarian cysts. Colour and power Doppler are used to identify soft tissue vascularity.

US imaging has limitations in patients with a large body mass index (BMI), as it can be difficult to produce diagnostic images due to the increased distance between the probe and pelvic organs. Images can be obscured by bowel gas or by a poorly filled bladder in TAUS. These differences can lead to inter-observer variability.

US-guided biopsies and drainages can be performed both transabdominally and transvaginally. Real-time imaging with US is particularly useful in patients with small, mobile peritoneal disease.

Magnetic Resonance Imaging

MRI has an increasingly important role in gynaecological oncology imaging. MRI has excellent soft tissue and spatial resolution, which enables the detection of lesions within the pelvis. MRI does not require ionising radiation, which is particularly important in young patients. Multiplanar imaging, in conjunction with excellent soft tissue resolution, improves diagnostic capability.

Conventional Imaging Sequences

MRI uses specific sequences to characterise indeterminate adnexal masses seen on US. The most commonly used sequences are T1-weighted (T1WI) and T2-weighted images (T2WI). The contrast and brightness of the resulting images are predominantly determined by the sequence. T1WI with fat saturation are especially useful in differentiating between fat and haemorrhage. Lesions containing high signal intensity material on T1WI may represent fat or haemorrhage; therefore, the use of T1WI with fat saturation enables the presence of fat to be detected as a reduction in signal intensity and thereby differentiating between these two substances.

The sequences obtained are carefully tailored to answer a specific clinical question. For example in endometrial carcinoma, high-resolution T2WI will be perpendicular to the endometrial cavity to allow accurate assessment of depth of myometrial invasion.

Functional MRI

In addition to conventional MRI sequences, functional imaging with diffusion-weighted imaging (DWI) and dynamic contrast enhanced (DCE) imaging provides more information regarding staging and lesion characterisation. DCE imaging is often utilised in patients with endometrial cancer as it improves staging accuracy. Studies have shown that complex ovarian lesions can be investigated using DCE to distinguish between benign and malignant tumours.

DWI evaluates the variability of water movement with the soft tissues, which is due to changes in tissue cellularity, cell membrane permeability and fluid viscosity. Within tumour, the movement of water is restricted due to increased cellularity and increased permeability of cell walls, which is demonstrated as high signal intensity on DWI. It has been incorporated into many gynaecological MRI protocols as it has been shown to improve accuracy. It is particularly useful when intravenous gadolinium is contraindicated. DWI improves lesion detection, which is particularly useful in drop metastases and peritoneal disease.

Limitations of MRI

MRI is an expensive investigation as the machines are less numerous and the studies are more time-consuming. MRI should be considered a problem-solving modality directed to answer a question that could not be achieved with US or CT. MRI is subject to motion artefact and may require prolonged imaging times. Contraindications to MRI include:

- Medically unstable patients (necessary equipment may be unsuitable in the scanning room)
- First trimester of pregnancy (insufficient evidence on safety, therefore avoid if possible)
- Implanted metallic devices (ferromagnetic) – pacemakers, neural stimulators, cochlear implants
- Renal failure (if intravenous gadolinium is required for sequences)

- Claustrophobia or agitation
- Extreme obesity – which may require specialist scanners.

TIP
MRI should be considered as a problem-solving imaging modality, when CT or US cannot answer the specific clinical question.

Computerised Tomography

CT is an imaging modality that utilises X-rays to create cross-sectional images of the body. Contrast agents (intravenous or oral) are often used to aid detection of pathology by enhancing the contrast between a lesion and the normal surrounding structures. Oral contrast can be used to improve delineation of bowel loops, which enhances the detection of serosal disease on the surface of bowel. Intravenous contrast agents can be injected to enhance tissues according to their vascularity. It is important to know in which time 'phase' the CT image has been performed, so that the images can be interpreted appropriately:

- **Non-enhanced CT** – no intravenous contrast
- **Early arterial phase** (around 15–20 seconds after injection) – when the contrast is still in the arteries and has not yet enhanced the organs or other soft tissue
- **Later arterial phase** (around 35–40 seconds after injection) – when all of the structures that receive their blood supply from the arteries will show optimal enhancement
- **Portal venous phase** (around 70–80 seconds after injection) – when the liver parenchyma is enhanced
- **Delayed phase** – (around 6–10 minutes after injection) – when there is washout of the contrast from abdominal structures, except for fibrotic tissue.

CT is widely available in most of the radiology departments. It can provide fast, high-resolution imaging of the entire body. It is therefore useful in the assessment of metastatic spread of disease and detection of recurrent disease. Imaging of the abdomen and pelvis is performed following intravenous iodinated contrast medium in the portal venous phase. The contrast medium causes blood vessels and solid abdominal organs to enhance, which permits the detection of parenchymal metastases. Intravenous contrast medium should be avoided in patients with renal dysfunction and allergy to contrast medium.

CT has intrinsically poor soft tissue resolution, meaning that the evaluation of the female pelvis is limited, and it is usually not possible to differentiate benign from malignant lesions using this modality. CT requires the usage of ionising radiation and therefore the benefit of imaging must be weighed against the potential risks. In patients with incurable malignancy, this is less important but should be remembered in younger patients who are treated with curative intent. Image degradation occurs with increasing BMI (photon starvation) and metallic hip replacements (beam hardening artefact).

CT has a limited role in early-stage gynaecological malignancy but is frequently used in staging advanced tumours and in surveillance for recurrence.

CT-guided biopsies of omental disease and retroperitoneal lymph nodes are useful in both primary diagnosis and confirmation of recurrent disease.

Positron Emission Tomography/ Computerised Tomography

PET/CT detects metabolic activity using a radioactive isotope 2-[^{18}F]-fluoro-2-deoxy-D-glucose (FDG). This isotope is actively taken up by tissues undergoing glycolysis, a process that is commonly accelerated in malignant tumours. PET/CT has a role in staging cervical cancer and in the detection of recurrent disease to aid management decisions. PET/CT is particularly useful in detecting lymph nodes infiltrated with tumour that have not yet changed in size or morphology when assessed using other imaging modalities. Small tumours (less than 5 mm) will not be detected, and low-grade or cystic tumours will not necessarily demonstrate avid FDG uptake. False positives seen with PET/CT include inflammation, infection and postoperative changes. These possibilities must always be considered when interpreting PET/CT images.

Imaging in Endometrial Cancer

Endometrial carcinoma is the commonest gynaecological malignancy in the United Kingdom. The majority of patients typically present with symptoms of postmenopausal bleeding.

Diagnosis

US is the primary imaging modality of choice in the initial investigation of patients with postmenopausal bleeding. High-resolution imaging with TVUS allows accurate measurement of the endometrial thickness, identification of endometrial polyps and assessment of vascularity using Doppler.

The most common appearance of endometrial cancer on US is nonspecific endometrial thickening. In postmenopausal women, a threshold of >4 mm is used to triage patients into those who require endometrial sampling. The endometrial thickening seen in endometrial carcinoma cannot be distinguished from benign endometrial hyperplasia. However, the US features suspicious for the presence of malignancy include disruption of the endometrial/myometrial junction, irregularity of the endometrial surface and focal disruption of the inner myometrium. Colour Doppler may aid in identification of endometrial polyps by identifying the vascularity within its pedicle.

Beyond the identification of endometrial thickening and polyps, US has a limited role in endometrial cancer. The accuracy of TVUS in the assessment of depth of myometrial invasion has been reported as varying between 60 and 76%.

Once endometrial cancer is confirmed on histology, imaging with MRI provides tumour staging, which guides management decisions and provides prognostic information.

MRI can also have a diagnostic role in patients where endometrial biopsy is not possible or histology is inconclusive. Endometrial biopsies demonstrating complex atypical hyperplasia could represent a sampling error, missing an underlying malignancy. In these scenarios, the presence or absence of myometrial invasive tumour or other malignant features on MRI provides essential information to guide treatment. For example, in the medically unfit patient with no clear endometrial invasion with complex atypical hyperplasia on biopsy, conservative management with curettage and Mirena intrauterine system could be considered which would avoid the morbidity and mortality associated with surgery.

Staging

The FIGO staging system for endometrial cancers is surgical and does not include imaging. However, preoperative MRI plays an important role in risk stratification and treatment planning and is therefore recommended as an aid in assessing and staging endometrial cancers by the European Society for Urogenital Radiology. The prognosis of endometrial carcinoma has been shown to correlate with the depth of myometrial invasion, nodal involvement and tumour grade.

Standard endometrial cancer staging protocols for MRI include sagittal and axial oblique T2WI of the uterus to assess depth of myometrial invasion, axial whole pelvis T2WI and T1WI to identify pelvic lymph nodes and adnexal pathology and axial images of the upper abdomen to reveal abdominal lymphadenopathy. On DWI, endometrial cancers demonstrate restricted diffusion, seen as high signal intensity within the uterine cavity. The high signal intensity tumour means that tumour margins can be accurately discerned, including depth of myometrial invasion and cervical stromal invasion. DWI should be cross-correlated with T2WI and apparent diffusion coefficient (ADC) map to give anatomical location and accurate staging and to avoid the artefact 'T2 shine-through'. Studies have shown that MRI has an overall staging accuracy between 85 and 93%.

Stage I endometrial cancers are confined to the uterine body. Endometrial cancers are then subdivided into those invading less than 50% of the myometrium (stage IA) and those invading 50% or more of the myometrium (IB).

On T2WI, endometrial cancer typically demonstrates intermediate signal intensity, which replaces the high signal intensity of the normal endometrium (Figure 3.1). If intravenous gadolinium is administered, the endometrial cancer shows early enhancement compared with myometrium. However in later phases, the tumour is hypointense to the avidly enhancing myometrium.

Stage II represents cervical stromal invasion. The cervix usually has a low signal intensity stromal ring seen on axial oblique T2WI (obtained perpendicular to the endocervical canal). Cervical stromal invasion can be diagnosed once the black stromal ring has been disrupted by intermediate signal intensity tumour.

Stage III endometrial cancer denotes local or regional spread of tumour. This includes:

- Stage IIIa: deep myometrial invasion with extension through the serosa or adnexal involvement. This is detected when the smooth

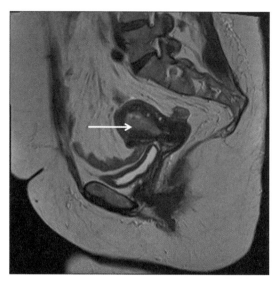

Figure 3.1 MRI imaging in endometrial cancer. Sagittal T2-weighted image through the centre of the anteverted uterus demonstrates increased endometrial thickness due to a polypoidal mass of intermediate signal intensity (white arrow). The tumour is seen invading the inner half of the myometrium consistent with stage IA endometrial carcinoma.

contour of the uterine serosa is disrupted with intermediate signal intensity tumour. In patients with fibroids or adenomyosis, DWI and/or post contrast imaging can improve assessment of depth of tumour invasion. Adnexal invasion is identified as unilateral or bilateral ovarian masses or soft tissue deposits outlining the pouch of Douglas and sigmoid serosa.

- Stage IIIb: vaginal or parametrial invasion. Vaginal invasion can be identified when the low signal intensity vaginal wall is disrupted either in direct contiguous spread from the primary tumour or as a focal lesion (drop metastasis). Conspicuity of these lesions is increased with DWI.

- Stage IIIc: pelvic (IIIC1) or para-aortic (IIIC2) lymphadenopathy. Metastatic lymph nodes are typically enlarged and rounded and the fatty hilum is replaced.

Stage IV disease represents direct invasion of the rectum and/or bladder (stage IVa) or distant metastasis (stage IVb). To diagnose stage IVa disease, the tumour must be seen to invade through to the mucosa. Involvement of the serosa does not equate to stage IVa disease and the presence of bullous oedema within the bladder should not be confused with tumour. Axial

T2WI images through the upper abdomen may reveal peritoneal disease within the upper abdomen, more commonly found in high-grade, clear-cell or serous papillary tumours. It should not be forgotten that inguinal lymph nodes represent stage IVB disease and can be readily identified on pelvic imaging.

CT has a role in evaluating advanced or high-grade disease. The strength of CT is in its speed of acquisition combined with large volume of coverage. CT is therefore capable of providing accurate nodal assessment of the chest, abdomen and pelvis. Supraclavicular and intra-thoracic lymphadenopathy is readily identified on CT imaging of the chest. Lung metastases are not common at presentation but should be considered during staging examinations before planning surgical treatment. Following intravenous contrast medium, liver metastases may be seen as ill-defined low attenuation lesions. Peritoneal disease is better identified after the administration of oral contrast medium, allowing tumour and bowel loops to be distinguished. The primary tumour can usually be seen as an irregular low attenuation mass within the endometrial cavity, in comparison to the enhancing myometrium. However, the poor soft tissue resolution of CT means that further local staging information is limited. There is no current role for PET/CT in endometrial staging.

Recurrence

CT imaging may be considered for patients at high risk of recurrence. In these situations, CT is useful in detecting lymph node, peritoneal and pulmonary metastases. However, tumour nodules at the vaginal vault can be difficult to detect and characterise, and in these situations MRI will be more helpful.

PET/CT has a role in assessing patients with pelvic recurrence who are potentially suitable for surgical resection. PET/CT is utilised to identify unsuspected distant disease beyond the pelvis, which would substantially alter the treatment strategy.

In summary:

- TVUS aids diagnosis by evaluating endometrial thickness.
- MRI assists in initial preoperative staging and aids treatment planning.
- CT can assess distant spread, and recurrence at distal sites.
- Pelvic tumour recurrence may require MRI imaging.

Imaging in Cervical Cancer
Diagnosis

Cervical cancer is usually diagnosed following clinical examination and biopsy, rather than imaging. However, occasionally cervical cancers are found incidentally on imaging. During pelvic US or CT, the primary tumour may be seen as an irregular soft tissue, mass centred on the cervix. Cervical cancer may also be suspected on imaging when patients present with secondary complications of the tumour such as ureteric obstruction causing hydronephroureter and the presence of lymphadenopathy.

Staging

Once the histological diagnosis of cervical cancer diagnosis is confirmed, radiological investigation is directed at staging the tumour for the purposes of risk stratification prior to treatment planning. It is helpful for the radiologist to know the histology of the tumour prior to reporting, as the pattern of disease can vary depending on tumour type. Squamous cell carcinomas are typically exophytic at the external os. Adenocarcinomas are seen in a higher position within the endocervical canal.

Cervical cancer staging is clinically based on the 2009 FIGO classification. Typically patients undergo examination under anaesthesia to evaluate the tumour size, the presence of parametrial and pelvic sidewall invasion and vaginal involvement. Assessment of the bladder and rectum with cystoscopy and sigmoidoscopy is also recommended to complete staging.

In addition to clinical staging, it is now well established that MRI has a central role in staging cervical cancers. MRI accurately predicts tumour size and also depth of invasion into the parametrium or pelvic sidewall. MRI is also able to detect lymph node metastases, which have an important prognostic value, although not included in the FIGO classification. The information provided by staging MRI is used to triage patients to the most appropriate treatment. Patients with early-stage disease may undergo surgery, while advanced tumours require treatment with chemoradiotherapy. Therefore, the detection of early parametrial invasion is critical in determining the management of this tumour.

Cervical tumours are identified by the disruption of normal cervical anatomy on T2WI due to its excellent soft tissue and spatial resolution. On T2WI, cervical stroma is low signal intensity with the mucosal glands in the endocervical canal seen as high signal intensity. T2WI is performed in three planes including sagittal, axial and axial oblique imaging (acquired perpendicular to the endocervical canal), which is important for the assessment of tumour extending into the parametria. Cervical tumours are identified as intermediate signal intensity on T2WI, which may be seen as interrupting the low signal intensity stromal ring or replacing the high signal intensity within the endocervical canal. T1WI is performed to assess for the presence of haemorrhage, lymph node metastases and bone lesions. The cervical tumour causes restriction of water molecule movement and is therefore clearly seen on DWI as high signal intensity. DWI can be particularly helpful in infiltrative cervical tumours with poorly demarcated boundaries on conventional T2WI and in the assessment of local invasion.

Stage I tumours are confined to the cervix. Stage IA tumours are small tumours diagnosed on microscopy and, by definition, are not visible on MRI. Therefore, the earliest stage tumour seen on MRI is stage IB subdivided into tumours measuring ≤4 cm (IB1) and >4 cm (IB2). The cervical tumour is seen as an intermediate to high signal intensity mass centred on the cervix, disrupting normal anatomical planes, as described above.

Stage II represents tumour growth beyond the cervix, but not extending to pelvic sidewall or lower third of vagina. On sagittal and axial T2WI, intermediate signal intensity tumour is seen replacing the high signal intensity of the vaginal mucosa (upper two thirds only); this is stage IIa which is also subdivided according to tumour size (≤4 cm and >4 cm). The suspicion of vaginal invasion on T2WI can be confirmed with matched and restricted diffusion on DWI.

Once the cervical tumour invades the parametria, this corresponds to stage IIb. On T2WI, there is disruption of the low signal intensity stroma (Figure 3.2). Often lobulated or spiculated intermediate signal intensity soft tissue can also be seen extending into the parametrial fat.

Stage IIIa disease describes tumour extension to the lower third of the vagina. On sagittal T2WI, the junction between the upper two thirds and the lower third is often taken as the level of the bladder base. Stage IIIb disease occurs when the tumour extends to pelvic sidewall and/or causes hydronephrosis (Figure 3.3).

Local invasion of bladder or bowel represents stage IVA disease, but intermediate signal intensity tumour

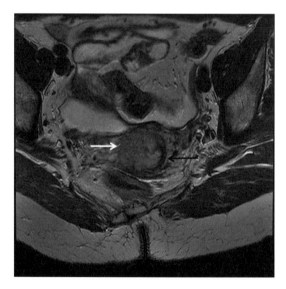

Figure 3.2 MRI imaging in cervical cancer. Axial oblique T2-weighted MR image of the cervix demonstrates disruption (white arrow) of the black line of the low signal intensity stromal ring (black arrow) due to intermediate signal intensity cervical tumour. This represents stage IIB cervical cancer.

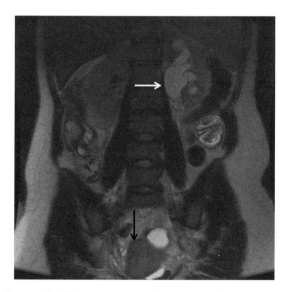

Figure 3.3 MRI imaging in cervical cancer. Coronal T2-weighted MR image of the abdomen demonstrates hydronephrosis of the left kidney (white arrow) due to a cervical tumour (black arrow) obstructing the distal left ureter in the pelvis caused by a stage IIIB tumour.

must be seen extending through to the mucosa. Serosal invasion of the bladder can often lead to bullous oedema of the urothelium, but this should not be over-interpreted as stage IV disease. Clear fat planes between the tumour and the adjacent organs can preclude the need for cystoscopy or sigmoidoscopy, which can be reserved for cases when there is suspected invasion. Distant metastases to organs such as lung, liver and bone represent stage IVB disease. It should be remembered that involved inguinal lymph nodes denote distant metastatic disease.

If the patient has been assessed to have stage IIB or beyond, then further imaging is recommended to assess distant disease. Thoracic CT imaging is recommended as a minimum to assess thoracic nodal involvement and pulmonary metastases. In squamous cell cervical cancers, pulmonary metastases may cavitate giving a typical imaging appearance. PET/CT may be helpful in the staging in patients with locally advanced cervical cancer who are being considered for radical treatment.

In patients with locally advanced disease treated with chemoradiation, repeated imaging is essential for assessing response during treatment. MRI is also used to assess optimal brachytherapy position, identify complications and aid in radiotherapy planning.

Recurrence

Following curative surgery or chemoradiation, MRI is performed only if there is suspicion of locally recurrent disease. MRI in post-treatment patients can be challenging as recurrent disease may be of small volume and difficult to identify on the background of tissue changes following surgery or radiotherapy. In particular, fibrotic radiation changes can be misinterpreted as recurrent disease in the early post-treatment period. For example, fibrosis around the distal ureters can cause hydronephrosis, which must be distinguished from tumour recurrence. DWI is very helpful in this situation, as recurrent disease will demonstrate restricted diffusion, seen as high signal intensity, whereas fibrosis will remain low signal intensity. Enlarged pelvic lymph nodes (>8 mm) of intermediate or high signal intensity (secondary to necrosis) are suspicious for disease recurrence.

CT imaging is typically used for the assessment of distant disease within the chest and abdomen enabling evaluation of para-aortic lymph nodes, lungs, liver and bones, which are the most common sites of extrapelvic tumour recurrence. PET/CT also has a role when deciding on local or regional treatment options due to its increased sensitivity of detecting distant disease.

In summary:

- Cervical cancer is a clinical diagnosis; however, staging with MRI is helpful in planning treatment.
- CT or PET/CT imaging is performed prior to radical treatment to ensure that disease has not spread beyond the pelvis.
- When recurrent disease is suspected, a combination of imaging modalities may be utilised. CT or PET/CT is crucial to identify distant metastases, as this will significantly alter the treatment strategy.

Imaging in Ovarian Cancer

Imaging plays a significant role in both the diagnosis and staging of ovarian carcinoma, and consequently in planning appropriate treatment.

Diagnosis

Adnexal masses are relatively common, with up to 10% of women having pelvic surgery for an ovarian lesion during their lifetime. The vast majority of ovarian masses in premenopausal women are benign, but the incidence of malignancy increases significantly after the menopause. The symptoms and signs of early ovarian cancer are nonspecific and consequently clinical suspicion must remain high so that patients can be adequately investigated. Since 2011, there has been a focus in the United Kingdom to improve early detection of ovarian cancer in patients with symptoms suggestive of ovarian cancer, combining blood CA125 levels and pelvic US. In combination with the patient's menopausal status and CA125 level, the US findings can be used to calculate the risk of malignancy index (RMI) summarised in Box 3.1.

Pelvic US should include both transabdominal and transvaginal examinations. TAUS is essential in large

---

Box 3.1 Calculation of the RMI

RMI I combines three presurgical features: serum CA125 (CA125); menopausal status (M) and ultrasound score (U).

The RMI is a product of the ultrasound scan score, the menopausal status and the serum CA125 level (IU/ml) as follows:

$$RMI = U \times M \times CA125.$$

Ultrasound score: The ultrasound result is scored 1 point for each of the following characteristics: multilocular cysts, solid areas, metastases, ascites and bilateral lesions. U = 0 (for an ultrasound score of 0), U = 1 (for an ultrasound score of 1), U = 3 (for an ultrasound score of 2–5).

The menopausal status is scored as 1 = premenopausal and 3 = postmenopausal.

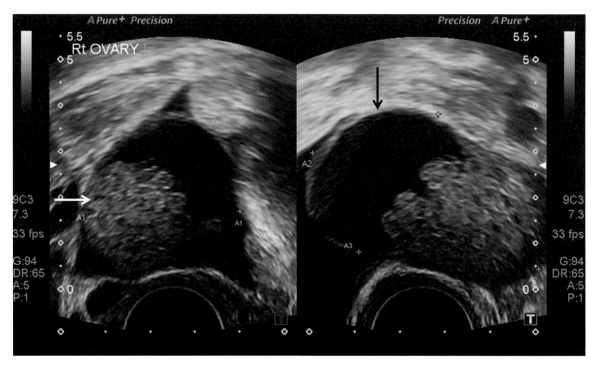

Figure 3.4 US imaging in ovarian cancer. US image of the right ovary in transverse and longitudinal sections demonstrates enlargement of the right ovary by a complex mass with cystic (black arrow) and solid mural components (white arrow). US appearances are suspicious for malignancy.

pelvic cysts as these often extend beyond the pelvis, and can also demonstrate the presence of ascites and peritoneal disease which are strongly suggestive signs of a malignant process. The kidneys should be imaged to identify any accompanying hydronephrosis. TVUS provides high-resolution imaging of the adnexa, and can accurately characterise approximately 80% of ovarian masses into benign or malignant lesions. The key sonographic features which enable the lesion to be characterised include septations (single, multiple, smooth, nodular), mural nodules, papillary projections (Figure 3.4). The use of power Doppler/colour Doppler distinguishes between vascular mural nodules and haematoma within cysts.

A simple ovarian cyst is defined as a round, oval shape, with thin wall, anechoic fluid, posterior acoustic enhancement and no internal septations or mural nodules. Simple cysts in premenopausal women measuring less than 5 cm are considered functional; cysts measuring 5–7 cm require follow-up for 1 year if being managed conservatively and cysts measuring greater than 7 cm should undergo further imaging with MRI or surgical intervention. Simple cysts in postmenopausal women are usually benign; however, those larger than

1 cm should undergo surveillance with repeated evaluation in 4–6 months. If the CA125 remains normal, and the cyst remains less than 5 cm, unchanged or reduced in size, then it is reasonable to consider discharge from follow-up after 1 year.

In comparison, a complex ovarian cyst is defined by the presence of one or more of the following features: internal septations, mural nodules or papillary projections, which are associated with an increased risk of malignancy.

Incidental ovarian masses are often detected on CT imaging, given the increasing usage of this modality across all clinical departments, particularly within the Emergency Department. However, characterisation of ovarian lesions is limited with CT due to its poor soft tissue resolution. In the majority of cases, further imaging with US is required to characterise further. Mature teratomas are an exception to this rule, as macroscopic fat and calcification can be seen on CT.

Patients with suspected ovarian cancer on US require CT examination to assess the potential extent of the disease. This information helps to guide management decisions into suitability for primary surgery or neoadjuvant chemotherapy prior to interval debulking surgery. When neoadjuvant chemotherapy is considered, it is essential to obtain a tissue biopsy to confirm underlying tissue histology prior to commencing treatment. In these cases, US or CT-guided ovarian or peritoneal biopsies can be carried out successfully in most cases. Image-guided biopsies are effective, with minimal associated complications.

MRI is a problem-solving tool, which is used to characterise adnexal masses that remain indeterminate following US examination. The MRI features predictive of malignancy replicate those in US and include the presence of septations, enhancing solid components, ascites and peritoneal disease. Intravenous gadolinium can be employed to demonstrate enhancement within increased neovascularity in malignant tissue. Using dynamic contrast techniques, a rapid uptake rate of contrast with high level of enhancement is suggestive of malignancy. DWI has a valuable role in MR imaging of the adnexal mass, as malignant soft tissue demonstrates restricted diffusion. By combining DWI with conventional MRI, the diagnostic confidence of adnexal mass characterisation is increased to approximately 95%.

PET/CT imaging is not currently recommended in the diagnosis of ovarian malignancy. Although increased FDG uptake can indicate the presence of malignancy, care should be taken due to its limitations including the physiological uptake seen in normal ovaries, uptake in common benign lesions such as teratomas and lack of uptake in cystic or necrotic tumours.

Staging

The FIGO staging system is most commonly utilised and has recently been updated in 2013, now also incorporating fallopian tube and primary peritoneal cancer. Staging is surgical.

CT is the modality of choice for radiological staging of ovarian carcinoma as it is quick, readily available and provides whole body imaging with a reported accuracy for all stages of ovarian cancer of 70–90%.

Stage I disease represents disease confined to the ovaries or fallopian tubes and is best demonstrated by TVUS or MRI. The primary ovarian tumour can have a variable appearance but often comprises a complex cystic/solid adnexal mass with thick, irregular septations and/or papillary projections. However, on CT, this is often demonstrated simply as a bulky ovary.

In stage II disease, the tumour spreads locally with direct extension to the surrounding pelvic tissues but not into the upper abdomen. It can be difficult to identify peritoneal disease localised within the pelvis on CT, leading to under-staging. If required, peritoneal disease can be identified as an intermediate signal intensity lesion on T2WI outlining the pouch of Douglas and pelvic sidewalls, with corresponding restricted diffusion on DWI.

Stage III disease reflects peritoneal disease beyond the pelvis and/or retroperitoneal lymph node metastases. The majority of patients diagnosed with ovarian cancer present with peritoneal metastases. Stage III disease is subdivided into IIIA, B and C. Stage IIIA disease represents histologically involved retroperitoneal lymph nodes. CT is not reliably able to diagnose small-volume stage IIIA disease, as it relies on size criteria to identify nodal disease. DWI in MRI is also unable to differentiate between benign and malignant nodes as all nodes demonstrate restricted diffusion, but can be used to improve detection of lymphadenopathy. Small volume retroperitoneal lymph node metastases can be detected with PET CT due to avid FDG uptake, but this modality is rarely used in staging.

Peritoneal metastasis outside the pelvis represents stage IIIB disease if the largest peritoneal lesion is less than 2 cm and stage IIIC if the largest lesion measures more than 2 cm. Peritoneal deposits are predominantly nodular or plaque-like. The omentum is the commonest site for peritoneal metastases and may be seen on CT as subtle fat stranding through to extensive soft thickening replacing the omental fat, or 'omental cake' (Figure 3.5). Plaque-like serosal disease of the bowel on CT imaging can be a challenge to radiologists, as it can manifest as subtle bowel wall thickening or irregularity. Therefore oral contrast medium is administered to help identify serosal disease, which appear as intermediate attenuation lesions against the high attenuation of the oral contrast medium. Small bowel obstruction is commonly seen as a complication of diffusely infiltrating serosal metastases. Infiltration of small bowel or sigmoid mesentery may produce a pleated or stellate pattern on CT, as intermediate attenuation tumour is seen to replace normal mesenteric low attenuation fat. Peritoneal deposits may contain calcification in up to 33% of cases; these are more apparent on CT as the high attenuation calcification is more readily visualised against the low attenuation of the peritoneal fat. Calcification is not easily seen on MRI as it causes signal voids.

Subcapsular peritoneal deposits of the liver and spleen typically cause scalloping of the parenchyma with

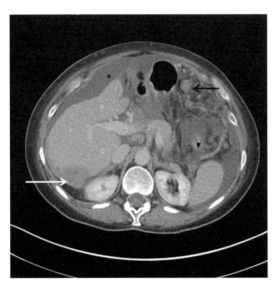

Figure 3.5 CT imaging in ovarian cancer. Axial CT image following the administration of intravenous contrast medium demonstrates ascites (*) with low attenuation subcapsular liver lesion adjacent to the right lobe of the liver (white arrow) and abnormal soft tissue within the omentum (black arrow) – stage IIIC ovarian cancer.

a smooth and well-defined margin. These lesions may be difficult to differentiate from an intra-parenchymal metastasis, particularly if the deposit is large, and therefore reformatting CT images to attain sagittal and coronal views is recommended. It is essential to differentiate between the two lesions because subcapsular deposits represent stage III disease whereas intra-parenchymal liver and splenic metastases represent stage IVB, and this can profoundly influence management. The presence of ascites, which is clearly identifiable on CT imaging, is an important predictor for stage IIIB/C disease. Even in the absence of peritoneal disease on CT, ascites is usually an indication of small size (miliary) peritoneal metastasis.

Stage IV disease represents distant metastases, excluding peritoneal metastases. Positive cytology must be obtained from a pleural effusion to assign stage IVA disease. Stage IVB disease occurs via haematogenous spread to the solid abdominal organs such as the liver, spleen, kidneys and adrenals, and very rarely brain and bone metastases may occur. These metastases are uncommon at presentation, but can be the sites of recurrence and up to 50% of patients are found to have haematogenous metastases at the time of postmortem examination. Intra-parenchymal disease can be identified as ill-defined low attenuation

lesions on CT, most commonly within liver and spleen, completely surrounded by normally enhancing parenchyma. Lymphatic spread to the cardiophrenic nodes and inguinal nodes also constitutes stage IVB disease.

Once comprehensive preoperative staging has occurred, treatment can be planned. Standard treatment approaches for ovarian cancer include either primary cytoreductive surgery followed by adjuvant chemotherapy or neoadjuvant chemotherapy followed by interval debulking surgery and further chemotherapy. Cytoreductive surgery has been shown to increase overall survival if no residual tumour is visible at completion of surgery. The role of imaging is therefore to aid in triage patients to the most appropriate therapeutic pathway and also to guide surgeons regarding 'difficult to resect' lesions prior to surgery and to anticipate requirements for bowel resection or splenectomy. Features shown to predict suboptimal cytoreductive surgery include small bowel and mesenteric disease greater than 1 cm, perisplenic and lesser sac lesions greater than 1 cm and enlarged retroperitoneal nodes above the renal hilum.

CT is also helpful in detecting disease-associated complications including bowel obstruction and hydronephrosis.

There is no role for US in the staging of ovarian cancer. However, on the initial diagnostic US, hydronephrosis, ascites, pleural effusion and peritoneal deposits are often identified.

The role of MRI in staging ovarian cancer and its added value in treatment decision-making is currently undergoing evaluation in several research studies. Peritoneal deposits demonstrate high signal intensity on DWI, which may be shown to improve the identification of small peritoneal lesions.

Recurrence

Even with optimal debulking surgery for advanced ovarian cancer, patients have a significant risk of recurrence. Identifying recurrent disease enables the gynaecology–oncology team to decide upon further surgical or chemotherapy options. CT is commonly used in the surveillance of patients treated for ovarian cancer, in combination with serial CA125 blood testing. CT readily identifies the recurrence of ascites and most peritoneal deposits. However, CT has limited sensitivity in the detection of small peritoneal implants and is particularly challenging in cachectic patients with paucity of intra-abdominal fat.

PET CT readily demonstrates tumour recurrence as avid FDG uptake. However, this modality is too expensive to use in routine surveillance. Several studies have shown that PET CT is best employed in patients with rising CA125 levels than normal CT examination. In addition, when suspected localised recurrence is detected within the pelvis on CT, PET CT is invaluable in the detection of distant disease prior to the consideration of surgery.

In summary:

- US is primarily used for detection and characterisation of adnexal masses.
- MRI has a role in the small minority of adnexal masses that remain indeterminate following US imaging.
- CT is primarily used to aid in preoperative staging, and hence treatment planning, and in surveillance and identifying complications such as hydronephrosis and bowel obstruction.
- MRI imaging for ovarian cancer staging is not routinely utilised, but research is ongoing.

- PET/CT can be helpful in the setting of recurrent disease.

Further Reading

Forstner R, Thomassin-Naggara I, Cunha TM, et al. ESUR Recommendations for MR Imaging of the Sonographically Indeterminate Adnexal Mass: An Update. *Eur Radiol*, 2017, 27, 2248–57.

Management of Suspected Ovarian Masses in Premenopausal Women (Green-top Guideline No. 62) 2011. RCOG.

Management of Suspected Ovarian Masses in Postmenopausal Women (Green-top Guideline No. 34) 2016. RCOG.

Sala E, Rockall A, Freeman S, Mitchell D, Reinhold C. *The Royal College of Radiologists. Recommendations for Cross-Sectional Imaging in Cancer Management, Second edition. Carcinoma of the Cervix, Vagina and Vulva*. London: RCR, 2014.

The Added Role of MR Imaging in Treatment Stratification of Patients with Gynecologic Malignancies: What the Radiologist Needs to Know. *Radiology*, 2013, 266(3), 717–40.

Chapter 4

Concepts of Treatment Approaches in Gynaecological Oncology

Mohamed Khairy Mehasseb

Introduction

While the focus of gynaecological oncology training programmes has long been on the technical surgical aspects when teaching trainees, one of the most difficult aspects of practice remains the complex decision-making skills of offering a particular treatment to a woman. Since treatment must be tailored for the individual woman depending on her overall medical status and comorbidities, preoperative and postoperative management can also be demanding. Clinicians have the duty to apply their specialist knowledge, experience and clinical judgement to identify the treatment – or combination of treatments – that is likely to result in the greatest overall benefit for the individual woman. The delivery and organisation of cancer services in the United Kingdom have undergone an overhaul following the *Calman-Hine report* in 1995 that was written in response to unaddressed variation in cancer care across the United Kingdom. Multidisciplinary teams (MDTs) were introduced, and team decision-making is currently the standard of care in cancer treatment. All women with cancer should have their management plan discussed in a specialty-specific MDT. There is also an increasing weight of evidence suggesting that those women treated in specialist cancer centres have better outcomes than those who are not.

Working in multiprofessional teams is one of the key recommendations of the Improving Outcomes Guidance by Department of Health. The guidance provides detailed information about the membership, structure, organisation and responsibilities of gynaecological cancer MDTs (Box 4.1). For gynaecological cancers, the teams should ideally comprise Consultants or senior members within groups including: Gynaecological surgery, Clinical and Medical Oncology, Radiology, Pathology, Palliative Care, Clinical Nurse Specialist (CNS) and Support Nurses, Research personnel, Audit personnel, Radiography and Pharmacy.

TIP
There is increasing evidence of improved outcome for women treated in specialist cancer centres.

Working effectively in multi-professional teams has several potential benefits:

- **Safer**: because a team creates additional defences against error by monitoring and double-checking decisions

Box 4.1 Responsibilities of the gynaecological oncology MDT

Diagnosis	Establish, record and review diagnoses for all new/registered women
	Assess the extent and verify the stage of each patient's disease
	Discuss the probable course of disease
Treatment	Recommendation for treatment for all new women taking into account womens' own views
	Consideration of adjuvant chemotherapy, adjuvant radiotherapy, surgery and brachytherapy in light of pathology results
	Consider other requirements such as palliative care or referral to other services
Research	Ensure that mechanisms are in place to support entry of eligible women into clinical trials and other research studies
Education	Forum for discussion of complex cases
	Multi-professional educational forum ensuring continuous professional development
Governance	Ensure registration of the required minimum dataset for all the cases of the relevant cancer within a specified area
	Ensure proposed treatments are to agreed national/local guidelines and protocols
	Ensure effective and quality management of the care pathways
	Ensure prompt, effective multidisciplinary decision-making, thus preventing delays in the woman's journey

- **Reduction of patient's anxiety**: with the knowledge that their treatment is based upon the opinion of several experts
- **Continuity of care**: may enhance the implementation of protocols
- **Improving team communication**: because of greater opportunities to talk at weekly meetings
- **Improving cancer care**: through improved staging accuracy, recruitment to clinical trials, adherence to quality-of-care indicators, patient satisfaction and time to treatment

The Role of MDTs in Decision-Making

Despite these perceived benefits, the introduction of MDT working has not resulted in a demonstrable improvement in cancer *survival* in the United Kingdom. Although a treatment plan devised by an MDT may differ from that of a single clinician, whether or not it is a superior or better decision is unclear. MDTs are also resource intensive: the meeting and the time taken to prepare for it are time-consuming. The estimated cost of all MDT meetings in the United Kingdom is around £50 million per year for preparation and the same amount again for attendance, including staff salaries.

Research and evidence showing the effectiveness of MDTs are scarce. Effective MDT working is influenced by a number of factors including the amount of cohesion or conflict that exists, the style of leadership and the level and type of member participation in the group decision-making process. Factors that have been found to influence the decision-making process of MDTs in particular are effective team-working skills, the dominance of team members with medical knowledge, the importance of compliance with policy initiatives and whether a patient is known to the team.

Nevertheless, three key features characterise the MDT's discussions and decision-making:
1. a differential emphasis on different types of information, with disease-centred information taking precedence over patient-centred factors;
2. variation in the extent and type of participation by the different professionals involved;
3. discussions not always ending with a clear decision due to case complexity and/or disagreement among team members.

Although many members of the MDT have a clear view of which treatment they consider to be 'best' in a given clinical situation, they are not always in agreement with one another. Any discussion of which treatment is 'best' depends on the values of the individual, and thus any disagreements may reflect the differing values of the MDT members. When team members disagree, the MDT faces difficulty in presenting this to the patient. First, many MDT members feel that any disagreement and difference of opinion in the MDT meeting should be concealed from the patient. Second, MDT members recognise that the clinician selected to present the treatment choice to the patient may 'frame' their description of the treatment options to fit their own view of best. This only reinforces the argument for making the values and preferences of the patient central to the decision process.

Patient-Centred Decision-Making

Sharing decisions with women is of paramount importance to good quality and safe healthcare delivery. Women vary considerably, not only in their disease and performance status, but also in their psychosocial makeup and life priorities. Thus, some women may be prepared to accept a treatment with significant morbidity for a small chance of cure whereas for others the avoidance of permanent side effects is a priority. It is important that the clinicians do not make any assumptions about the woman's preferences based on generic factors such as age, social status or cultural background.

Faced with a life-threatening diagnosis of gynaecological cancer, women may be willing to accept any treatment that alleviates the prospect of death, even if the chance of success is remote. Although some early gynaecological cancers can be cured or treated by surgery alone, the optimal treatment for the majority of gynaecological malignancies requires multimodal therapy (i.e. surgery combined with chemotherapy and/or radiotherapy).

Well-informed women make different decisions than those who are less well informed, may perceive risk in a different way and adhere better to treatment. Teams who do not effectively involve women in decisions about their health may feel that they are working in the best interests of the woman, but in fact may not arrive at a decision that is right for that particular woman.

Patient-reported outcomes are now widely considered an excellent methodology to evaluate the utility of treatment. Quality of life is now an increasingly

Box 4.2 Elements of quality of life

Physical	Daily activities, appearance, appetite, comorbidities, fatigue, sleep, rest, mobility, pain, side effects, symptoms of disease
Psychological	Body image, anger, anxiety, fear, control, coping, depression, enjoyment, perception and interpretation, prior experience, optimism
Demographic	Age, ethnicity, education, employment, income
Spiritual	Hope, meaning, purpose, religion, spirituality
Social	Family, life events, relationships, roles, sexuality, support

important endpoint in the decision-making process, and reflects the patient's experiences with disease, treatment and accompanying long-term sequelae. It is no longer acceptable to pursue curative treatment with the hope of improving mortality without consideration of treatment morbidity, and without including patient-centred decision-making and quality-of-life implications (Box 4.2).

Although the introduction of MDTs has increased the opportunity for professionals to be included in cancer treatment decisions, opportunities for the patient to be involved have diminished. CNS are in a unique position to ascertain patient preferences, and their participation in the MDT provides a way in which patient-related factors could be systematically incorporated into discussions. However, it is likely that patient-centred information is best considered at multiple points along the treatment journey, as specific issues may affect treatment decisions at different stages, and the individual's preferences and comorbidity may well change over time. It is ethically important to make good, individualised healthcare decisions that respond effectively to the needs of the patient.

Decision-Making Approaches in Gynaecological Oncology

1. Purpose/intent of management (radical/curative vs adjuvant vs palliative)

   The first step in the decision-making process is to decide on the aim of proposed management. There are three main lines of treatment in gynaecological oncology:

   - *Radical/curative* – where the proposed management has a curative intent and the primary treatment is aimed at achieving cure.

   - *Adjuvant* – this additional line of management is aimed at improving the success of the primary or initial treatment, increasing the chance of cure and/or reducing the risk recurrence (local or systemic). Adjuvant treatments could be given before the primary treatment (*neoadjuvant*) to down-stage the disease, at the same time as the primary treatment (*concomitant*) to increase its efficacy or more commonly after the primary treatment (*adjuvant*).

   - *Palliative* – when there is no realistic prospect of cure, and treatment is being offered for symptom relief to improve the quality of life.

TIP

Treatment intent is an important concept and is an important first step in the MDT process and subsequent management.

2. The extent of treatment (local vs regional vs systemic)

   The next consideration is how to treat the local disease, the regional draining lymph nodes and the presence of (or risk of) systemic metastatic disease. Any treatment modality offered could be either loco-regional or systemic. Examples of local treatment are surgery or radiotherapy. The treatment is mainly aimed at control of the local disease in the primary organ of origin. Chemotherapy, hormonal therapy and newer treatments such as immunotherapy, monoclonal antibodies, vascular epidermal growth factor inhibitors and tyrosine kinase inhibitors are all examples of systemic therapy. These modalities of treatment are aimed at control of systemic disease.

   - **Local disease in primary site**: In general, the primary site of tumour is usually treated with radical local treatment such as surgery or radiotherapy. Adverse prognostic factors associated with local spread (e.g. large tumours or close surgical margins) predict the risk of local recurrence, and adjuvant radiotherapy may be recommended.

   - **Regional lymph nodes**: Addressing the regional draining lymph nodes is more challenging. Nodal involvement can be a risk factor for both local recurrence and metastatic disease. Some tumours have a predictable lymphatic drainage pattern (e.g. vulval cancer and inguinofemoral lymph nodes). Surgery to remove the pool of lymph nodes is usually advisable. Alternatively, radiotherapy may be given to eradicate subclinical disease in the next echelon of nodes beyond known disease. Other tumours have a less predictable or wider pool of lymphatic drainage (e.g. endometrial cancer where lymphatic spread could be to the pelvic, inguinal or para-aortic nodes). In these tumours, adjuvant systemic therapy such as chemotherapy may be indicated.

- **Systemic part of the disease**: In cancers with adverse prognostic factors associated with haematogenous spread or risk of distant metastases (e.g. high-grade tumours or lymphovascular invasion), systemic therapy is indicated.

3. The therapeutic ratio (benefit vs side effects) of intended treatment:

   The clinician has to be aware of the acute and/or long-term side effects of any proposed treatment, whether it is radical or adjuvant or palliative in intent. The therapeutic ratio (benefit vs side effects) of treatment is therefore highly dependent on the aim of treatment.

   - **For radical treatments**, most women would be prepared to accept some degree of transient/permanent side effects to achieve a potential cure from an otherwise inevitable death.
   - **For adjuvant treatments**, women may vary in how much toxicity they would be willing to accept for an additional increase of chance of cure or reduction in the risk of recurrence. Counselling and informed consent are particularly important in this context.
   - **For palliative treatments**, side effects and adverse events may reduce any perceived benefit in terms of improved quality of life. Hence any offered treatment has to have benefit profile that would outweigh the side effects. Women faced with inevitable death from their cancer – or their relatives – may be desperate for any treatment and the clinician may be faced with difficult decisions.

4. Other considerations

   Other variables to be considered are tumour, treatment, as well as patient factors.

- **Tumour factors**: The impact of tumour factors on prognosis is usually well documented in the published literature and is rarely the subject of debate among clinicians. The chance of cure of a particular cancer is determined by the tumour type, its grade and histology (affecting prognosis) and the disease stage (affecting prognosis and possibility of cure). For instance, melanomas and small cell tumours are more aggressive than squamous cell carcinoma and more radio-resistant.

- **Treatment factors**: Consideration should be given to the therapeutic ratio, benefit and side effects of any standard treatment and any alternative modalities of treatment. This is not always straightforward as a treatment with a lower chance of cure but less morbidity may have a similar therapeutic ratio to another treatment with a higher chance of cure but with more side effects.

- **Patient factors**: These are less well documented and assessment of patient factors is highly subjective. The clinician has to assess whether there are any treatment options that the woman is unable to tolerate, taking into account any expressed woman's preferences.

Box 4.3 Decision-making approaches in gynaecological oncology

What is the intention of treatment? Why am I offering the treatment?

    Radical curative intent?
    Adjuvant intent? (neoadjuvant, concomitant, adjuvant)
    Palliative intent?

How am I going to address each component of the cancer?

    Local disease in primary site
    Regional draining lymph nodes
    Systemic part of the cancer: metastases or risk of metastatic disease

What are the benefits/side effects of proposed treatment? Is there any alternative?

    Therapeutic ratio of any proposed radical curative, adjuvant or palliative treatment

Are there any other factors to consider?

    Tumour factors
    Treatment factors
    Patient factors

Principles of Treatment of Gynaecological Cancers

The next section will summarise the management strategies for various gynaecological cancers. Details of individual disease treatments are presented in Chapters 10 to 15 of this book.

Ovarian Cancer

Specialist gynaecological surgery and the management by the MDT are associated with a significantly longer survival in women treated for ovarian cancer. The standard management of ovarian cancer is a surgical approach combined with chemotherapy. Primary surgery followed by adjuvant chemotherapy with platinum or platinum/taxane combination should be the mainstay of treatment for advanced ovarian cancer. However, primary surgery may not be appropriate for some women and neoadjuvant (primary) chemotherapy should be considered. Histological confirmation (or cytology when histology is not obtainable) should be available prior to considering neoadjuvant chemotherapy. Response to neoadjuvant chemotherapy should be assessed after three cycles using a combination of radiological methods (CT scan) and tumour markers. Cytoreductive surgery should be arranged for women with stable disease or disease that responded to neoadjuvant chemotherapy. Primary treatment may include entry into clinical trials where appropriate.

The aim of ovarian cancer surgery is to perform staging in women with early-stage disease and to resect all macroscopic disease in women with advanced stage disease. All women should be assessed for the likelihood of bowel surgery and bowel preparation given as required. While laparoscopic surgery is an option for women with early-stage disease, all other women should undergo surgery through a midline incision. Women with suspected stage IA disease, who want to preserve their fertility, may be eligible for conservative surgery. The role of radical surgery in women with stage IV disease and/or extra-abdominal disease remains controversial, as is the role of full pelvic and para-aortic lymph nodes dissection. It is recommended that any enlarged nodal disease be removed; however, there is no role for routine selective lymph node sampling.

The use of radiotherapy in the management of ovarian cancer has a very limited role. It has no place in the primary treatment of ovarian cancer outside the trial setting.

Generally, secondary cytoreductive surgery for recurrent disease after primary treatment has not been shown to improve survival. However, secondary cytoreductive surgery can be considered for women with good response to first-line chemotherapy, good performance status, localised single site recurrence and assessment that all disease can be resected. Palliative chemotherapy should be considered in all cases if appropriate, and occasionally palliative radiotherapy could be delivered for control of local symptoms. Bowel obstruction is a very common problem in advanced or recurrent carcinoma of the ovary and this may be managed medically rather than surgically. Specialist palliative care advice should be sought for the management of bowel obstruction in the context of end-stage disease.

Endometrial Cancer

An MRI scan of the pelvis and/or CT chest, abdomen and pelvis is usually carried out prior to treatment of women with endometrial cancer. Chest imaging is not necessary in low risk (grades 1 and 2) type 1 endometrial cancers. Surgery is the preferred primary modality for treatment as this is the most effective way of controlling symptoms of bleeding as well as establishing the accurate stage. The uterus, cervix, fallopian tubes and ovaries should be removed. Laparoscopic surgery should be considered for all women. The role of lymphadenectomy in endometrial cancer management is controversial. It should not be undertaken in low risk cases (G1–G2, stage IA), but may be considered with G3, IB or type 2 cancer. The extent of lymphadenectomy is usually restricted to the pelvis but para-aortic dissection can be considered in type 2 cancers. There is limited evidence of a therapeutic role for lymphadenectomy; hence its use must be closely linked to plans for adjuvant therapy. Suspicious nodes should be removed if identified preoperatively on MRI or identified intra-operatively. Lymphadenectomy should be performed laparoscopically where possible. Washing of the pelvis for cytology may be taken for prognostication, although it is no longer part of the staging. If uterine serous carcinoma is suspected, then an omentectomy/omental biopsy should be performed. Morbidly obese and high morbidity women could be candidates for vaginal hysterectomy alone, with removal of the tubes and ovaries only if surgically accessible. Stage II disease is usually managed by simple total hysterectomy and adjuvant radiotherapy. There may be cases which benefit from radical hysterectomy. Management of patients with stages III and IV disease should be individualised.

Adjuvant radiotherapy reduces local recurrence but does not affect survival. Adjuvant chemotherapy may be considered for uterine serous carcinoma and carcinosarcomas regardless of stage. Chemotherapy may be useful for treatment of advanced disease. In the palliative setting, high-dose progestagens may be beneficial (e.g. megestrol acetate 160 mg o.d. orally) for control of symptoms. Other hormone manipulation such as aromatase inhibitors may be considered.

Women with recurrent and advanced disease can be considered for radiotherapy/chemotherapy or palliative care treatment. The most common problems requiring symptom control are due to distant metastases to bone, brain or retroperitoneal lymph nodes. Local recurrence of disease can also cause significant issues with bleeding, pain and lymphoedema. Women will need individual management plans to deal with symptoms such as bleeding, recurrent ascites, breathlessness, cough or bone pain.

Cervical Cancer

Any woman with a confirmed diagnosis of cervical cancer greater than stage IA1 carcinoma should have an MRI of the pelvis as a minimum to assess the extent of the primary tumour and to detect lymphadenopathy. MRI is now considered to be the staging investigation of choice. Women with stages 1B1 and higher should have a CT of the chest and abdomen in addition to the MRI, and positron emission tomography–CT (PET-CT) scan is recommended for stage 1B2 and above.

Primary management eventually depends on the stage. Women with a diagnosis of stage IA1 disease can be treated with a large loop excision of transformation zone (LLETZ) or a simple hysterectomy. For women with stage IA2, a pelvic lymphadenectomy is added to the LLETZ or simple hysterectomy. Bilateral salpingectomy is advisable at the time of hysterectomy.

For higher stages, as a principle, radical surgery and radiotherapy are equally effective as curative treatment for squamous cell carcinoma or adenocarcinoma of the cervix. The combination of radical surgery and radiotherapy is not more effect than either single modality given alone but morbidity is significantly increased when both are used in combination. Stage IB1 (and some cases of non-bulky stage IIA) disease is treated with radical hysterectomy and pelvic lymph nodes dissection (open or laparoscopic). If fertility preservation is desired, radical trachelectomy and pelvic lymph node dissection may be considered. Although age is not related to outcome, consideration should be given for older women (>60 years) to undergo radical radiotherapy in preference to surgery. Radical radiotherapy with or without chemotherapy will be considered for all women with stages IB2, bulky IIA and above. Adjuvant radiotherapy with or without chemotherapy is advised for women with node positive disease, or involved surgical margins. Adjuvant radiotherapy should be considered for those with intermediate risk factors for recurrence which include close vaginal surgical margins, bulky tumours, lymphovascular space invasion and/or deep stromal invasion. The addition of chemotherapy with radiotherapy significantly improves survival. However, the risk of late toxicity is unknown.

Exenterative surgery may be indicated in selected women with central pelvic recurrence and radiotherapy can be considered for women who have not previously received this treatment modality. Palliative care measures are considered for common problem symptoms such as bleeding, discharge and pelvic pain. Psychosexual counselling for dyspareunia and sexual dysfunction is also important.

Vulval Cancer

Diagnosis should be established by biopsy of lesion, preferably by a punch biopsy or incisional wedge biopsy from the lesion edge, rather than an excisional biopsy (except for small lesions). Photographic documentation of the extent and location of the lesion is important. Fine-needle biopsy of any clinically suspicious nodes or other metastases should be considered as a positive result may alter the management.

The size and depth of invasion of the tumour, its location and how lateral it is will influence the surgical approach. Wherever possible, surgery to the primary tumour should be radical to remove the tumour and to avoid unnecessary surgical and psychological morbidity. Radical wide local excision (WLE) with the minimum margin of 15 mm disease-free tissue is often sufficient, which should ensure the measured pathological margins are adequate (8 mm or more). Reconstructive surgical techniques should be employed to enable primary surgical closure and to reduce morbidity due to scarring.

Squamous cell carcinoma lesions of less than 2 cm diameter with less than 1 mm invasion (FIGO stage IA) are rarely associated with lymph node metastases. They can be treated with WLE alone, and groin node dissection is unnecessary. Women with truly lateralised (>2 cm from midline) squamous lesions, FIGO stages I and II, initially only require WLE and ipsilateral sentinel node dissection or lymphadenectomy. Sentinel node dissection is suitable for unifocal tumours <4 cm diameter. Centrally located early tumours where excision is possible without sphincter compromise require WLE and bilateral sentinel node dissection or lymphadenectomy. If surgery is likely to result in sphincter damage leading to urinary or faecal incontinence, radiotherapy should be considered either with curative intent or to reduce tumour volume to permit less destructive surgery. Adjuvant postoperative radiotherapy should be considered when two or more lymph nodes are involved with metastatic disease, or when there is extra-capsular spread in any node.

For advanced vulval cancer, the use of preoperative radiotherapy with or without chemotherapy may allow for sphincter preserving surgery. Alternatively, primary radiotherapy to the vulva with groin node dissection may be used. Clinically involved nodes are treated by excision and/or chemoradiotherapy. For metastatic vulval disease, palliation may still require surgery to the primary vulval tumour.

For malignant melanoma, WLE is preferred, as this group of tumours has not been shown to benefit from block dissection of the groin. Relapse in this group is high and correlates with the depth of invasion. Currently no treatment is available to reduce the risk of relapse. Sentinel node dissection should be considered.

For local recurrences, radiotherapy should be considered in preference to surgery if excision would compromise sphincter function. However, if the woman has received treatment with maximum dose with radiotherapy then surgical resection should be considered. The management of groin recurrences is more difficult. Women who have not received radiation and who have histologically confirmed recurrence should be offered radiotherapy. If response to radiotherapy is not complete, resection should be considered. Women who have already received radiotherapy should be offered palliative resection when possible.

Specialist palliative care advice may be needed for pain management with advanced carcinoma of the vulva. Psychosexual referral should be arranged for sexual dysfunction symptoms.

Further Reading

A policy framework for commissioning cancer services: A report by the Expert Advisory Group on Cancer to the Chief Medical Officers of England and Wales. *The Calman-Hine report*, 1995.

Hamilton DW, Heaven B, Thomson RG, et al. Multidisciplinary team decision-making in cancer and the absent patient: a qualitative study. *BMJ Open* 2016; 6: e012559.

Kidger J, Murdoch J, Donovan J, Blazeby J. Clinical decision-making in a multidisciplinary gynaecological cancer team: a qualitative study. *BJOG* 2009; 116: 511–17.

NHS Executive, Department of Health. Guidance on commissioning cancer services. *Improving outcomes in gynaecological cancers*, 1999.

Chapter 5

Radiation Therapy for Gynaecological Malignancies

Christopher Stephen Kent and Paul Symonds

Nothing in life is to be feared, it is only to be understood. Now is the time to understand more, so that we may fear less.

– *Marie Curie*

Introduction

The focus of this chapter is on the application of radiotherapy in gynaecological cancers and its relative merits to maximise tumour control within the pelvis. Radiotherapy is the process of directing ionising radiation towards a target comprising usually of a tumour or area of high risk of tumour recurrence, while minimising collateral damage to surrounding normal tissues. Modern radiotherapy techniques primarily utilise artificially generated high-energy X-rays. Most radiotherapy centres in the United Kingdom use a Linear Accelerator (or Linac) which accelerates a beam of electrons in a straight line towards a material of high atomic number resulting in the generation of X-rays. This produces a useful beam of radiation filtered to a specific energy and then shaped by lead collimators (devices which produce a parallel beam of radiation) to precisely fit the volume required to treat the target tissue. Recent developments in radiotherapy include the introduction of intensity-modulated radiotherapy (IMRT) which allows for sophisticated computer-controlled dynamic variation in the intensity of radiation (fluence) as well as dynamic variation in the shape of the radiation beam by the use of small multi-leaf collimators. IMRT allows clinicians to treat difficult-shaped volumes such as concave structures wrapped around potentially delicate normal structures, for example, the spinal cord. The cost of such a development has been met by the exponential increase in complexity of radiotherapy planning and delivery (Figures 5.1 and 5.2).

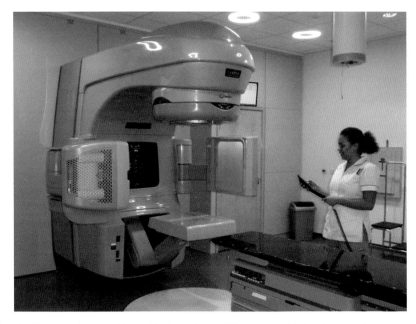

Figure 5.1 Linac. 'A typical linear accelerator with an added cone beam CT for image-guided radiotherapy'

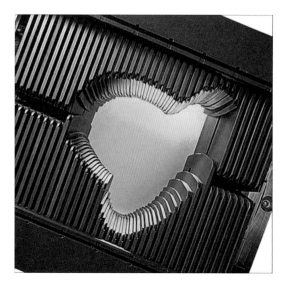

Figure 5.2 MLCs. Small lead multi-leaf collimators are used to shape the radiotherapy beam to fit the target volume

---

TIP
Radiotherapy is the process of directing ionising radiation towards a target comprising usually of a tumour or area of high risk of tumour recurrence, while minimising collateral damage to surrounding normal tissues.

The Biological Basis of Radiotherapy Treatment

The mechanism behind how radiotherapy destroys tumour cells while allowing normal tissues to recover is incompletely understood. Radiation exposure primarily leads to cell death through DNA damage via both the *direct and indirect effects*. Radiation directly damages the individual DNA strands. In contrast, radiation causes indirect effects on the water within the cell causing hydrolysis and generation of free oxygen and hydroxyl radicals which then require the presence of oxygen to lead to fixed and irreparable damage. The direct effect of radiation leads to approximately one third of the damage sustained by the cellular DNA while the indirect effect accounts for the remaining two thirds. This cellular lethality is directly proportional to the number of double-stranded DNA breaks which occur. Double-stranded DNA breaks are usually a lethal event for a cell.

The intrinsic radiosensitivity of such cells therefore depends on several factors such as:

- The rate of cellular turn over (repopulation) – which can accelerate after multiple doses of radiation
- Relative hypoxia (reoxygenation)
- Repair of sublethal cellular damage
- The phase of cell cycle that the target was in while being irradiated (with cells in mitosis being most sensitive and cells in late S-phase being most radioresistant).

Clinical oncologists can exploit these various mechanisms of potential radioresistance by a number of strategies:

- **Accelerated repopulation** can be addressed by reducing temporal gaps between daily treatments, and ensuring that the overall treatment time is not compromised by anticipating (and preventing) acute side effects and planning for public holidays.
- **Hypoxic areas of tumour** are extremely radioresistant, but by splitting the overall radiation dose into smaller daily fractions, the better-oxygenated peripheral cells will be killed and thus there will be improved oxygenation for more central hypoxic cells, consequently increasing their radiosensitivity.
- **Repair of sublethal damage** can be influenced by the use of radiosensitisers (such as concurrent chemotherapy) to increase the radiosensitivity of tumours. This is often at the expense of unpredictable systemic side effects, and exponentially increased acute side effects.
- **Redistribution of cells around the cell cycle** is also influenced by daily fractionation with cells allowed to cycle from a more radioresistant phase to a more radiosensitive phase.

Units of Radiation and Dose-Limiting Effects

Radiation interaction with tissues is measured as an absorbed dose equivalent to the energy absorbed per unit mass and is measured in joules per kilogram (J/kg) (1 J/kg = 1 Gray (Gy)).

Theoretically it is possible to eradicate any tumour by exposing it to a high enough total dose of radiation. However, it is the risk of damage to the adjacent normal tissues that limits the actual amount of radiation that can be delivered to a particular area of the body. Certain tissues react more than others, producing predictable acute side effects and these tend to be those tissues that comprise of rapidly proliferating cells such as the skin and bowel mucosa. Most radiotherapy for gynaecological malignancies will tend to be directed towards the pelvis and thus the most common acute side effects would include moist desquamation of the skin (particularly in skin folds such as the inguinal region), mucositis of the genitals and diarrhoea caused by damage to the jejunal crypt cells. While these side effects are unpleasant for the patient, they are typically short-lived and resolve quickly after completion of the course of treatment. However the risk of long-term late damage is of greater concern, and this occurs from 9 months to 5 years after treatment. These long-term side effects are typically due to damage of the slowly proliferating tissues such as the vascular endothelium. This damage usually leads to progressive fibrosis, arteritis which may then result in necrosis, fistulae or stricture formation. The risk of such complications is approximately 5% but can be even higher in patients with preexisting autoimmune disorders such as inflammatory bowel disease. The increasing use of IMRT has the potential to minimise damage to normal tissues and consequently reduce the intensity of these side effects. However, all patients must be warned of the potential risks and consequences of their treatment.

Radiotherapy Machines

Most modern radiotherapy units utilise a Linac. This produces X-ray energies of 6–20 million electron volts (MeV), which provide several advantages over lower-energy kilovoltage machines in the treatment of pelvic tumours. Mega-voltage X-rays deliver their energy from 1.5 cm below the skin's surface and as a result the skin itself receives a relatively reduced dose. This helps to reduce the side effects to the skin and subcutaneous tissues. Multiple beams are then used to tightly conform the dose around a deep tumour or target structure. Older kilovoltage machines typically generate X-rays with 2–3 times more energy than diagnostic X-ray machines and consequently tend to deposit most of their energy at the skin's surface. While this is undesirable for treating tumours within the pelvis, it can be successfully employed for treating metastatic skin deposits where the clinician can avoid delivering a high dose to the underlying structures.

Brachytherapy (Greek: *brachys therapeia*, short treatment)

Brachytherapy involves the implantation or insertion of radioactive sources near to or within the target volume. The use of specific sources that emit radiation mainly through beta decay (releasing electrons) limits the effective range of the radiation to just a few centimetres with a rapid fall off of dose deeper than this. Consequently, this enables a higher-dose radiation to be delivered to a relatively small volume by selective boosting with brachytherapy. This increases the ability to kill the tumour cells, while sparing nearby tissues, and thus improves the chances of curative treatment.

Modern high-dose rate (HDR) brachytherapy typically comprises of an 'after-loading' technique. This is where the patient has a plastic or metal applicator inserted into or close to the target volume. The applicator is then loaded with a radioactive source (Iridium-192) for a designated amount of time, usually via a computer-controlled machine that is operated by the specialist radiographers. Typical treatments last around 10–15 minutes per fraction. Cervical cancer brachytherapy is employed directly after the completion of a course of external beam radiotherapy and usually involves three or four fractions delivered with a minimum of 6 hours between fractions to allow for normal tissue recovery. Older low- or medium-dose rate units using caesium sources are now almost completely obsolete in the United Kingdom but most clinical trials demonstrating the benefit of brachytherapy were conducted using these techniques. Recent retrospective studies have indicated that HDR brachytherapy is at least as effective as low or intermediate rate and may be more efficacious.

The primary use of brachytherapy in the radical treatment of gynaecological malignancies is in the treatment of cervical cancer where it plays a pivotal role in boosting the dose of radiation to the cervix and parametria to a much higher dose than is possible with external beam radiotherapy alone. Brachytherapy can also be used in the adjuvant setting, the most common use being in the treatment of early-stage endometrial cancer. The PORTEC-2 study demonstrated that brachytherapy was not inferior to external beam radiotherapy in reducing the risk of local vaginal vault recurrence of stage 1 endometrial cancer but had significantly fewer side effects.

Cervical Cancer

Treatment by Stage

Stage Ia1 disease is typically diagnosed incidentally or treated with large loop excision of transformation zone (LLETZ) in younger patients who are keen to preserve fertility. In those who have completed fertility, hysterectomy can be done. Stages Ia2 and Ib1 are treated with either radical hysterectomy and bilateral pelvic lymphadenectomy (risk of nodal metastasis is approximately 7.4%) or radical radiotherapy for those unfit for surgery. Selected patients may be offered a trachelectomy with pelvic lymphadenectomy in an attempt to preserve fertility.

Stage Ib1 and small volume IIa (<4 cm in size) may be treated surgically with radical hysterectomy and lymphadenectomy or with combined external beam radiotherapy and brachytherapy, both treatments resulting in 80–90% 5-year survival rates. Post-surgical chemoradiotherapy is indicated in cases where there are involved surgical resection margins, occult stage IIb disease (parametrial involvement) or where positive lymph nodes are found; however, late morbidity is significantly increased.

Stages Ib2 to IVa (or locally advanced disease) is almost exclusively treated with primary radiotherapy and now usually with concurrent chemotherapy. Multiple trials of concurrent platinum-based chemotherapy have demonstrated an overall survival benefit in patients with stages Ib2 to IVa disease with the risk of death from cervical cancer being decreased by 30–50% compared with radiotherapy alone with the majority of benefits in stages Ib2 and II patients. The 5-year survival rates with radiotherapy alone are approximately 65–75% for stage IIb, 35–50% for stage IIIb and 15–20% for stage IVa which are improved 10%, 7% and 3%, respectively, by concurrent chemotherapy with weekly cisplatin. If a vesico- or recto-vaginal fistula is also present, then urinary diversion or defunctioning colostomy should be considered prior to commencing chemoradiotherapy.

Para-Aortic Radiotherapy

Women with known para-aortic lymph node involvement have a particularly poor prognosis with 5-year survival rates of approximately 40%. Most clinicians will offer para-aortic radiotherapy, although evidence supporting this practice is limited. The largest study to date was conducted by the Gynaecologic Oncology Group (GOG) who enrolled 95 women with biopsy-proven para-aortic nodal involvement and reported 3-year survival rate of 39%. This was at the expense of 19% of patients experiencing severe acute gastrointestinal toxicity and 14% experiencing late gastrointestinal side effects. There are no data to suggest that irradiating the para-aortic region prophylactically improves outcomes and therefore given the toxicity of this treatment it cannot be justified.

The Importance of Time to Completion

All women undergoing radical chemoradiotherapy should aim to complete all of their treatment within 56 days as studies have shown an increased rate of disease progression within the pelvis if the total treatment time exceeds 56 days (26% vs 9%). This may be explained by the phenomenon of accelerated repopulation as described above. Some radiotherapy centres attempt to complete all treatment within 50 days aspiring to further improve pelvic control. With these regimes, the brachytherapy component may overlap with the last few fractions of external beam radiotherapy which can provide significant logistical challenges for certain centres. Care must also be taken to ensure that the patient's haemoglobin is maintained at 120 g/l or above, as it is established that locoregional recurrence rates are higher in anaemic patients. This may be due to the presence of cellular hypoxia.

Radiotherapy Planning Technique

The finer detail of radiotherapy planning, especially IMRT planning, is beyond the scope of this book; however, traditional conformal field borders for cervical cancer are as follows:

- Superior border – L5/S1 interspace
- Inferior border – 2 cm below inferior extent of disease (no more superior than the lower border of the obturator foramen)
- Lateral borders – 1.5 cm outside the bony pelvis
- Posterior border – lower margin of S2 vertebral body
- Anterior border – through the symphysis pubis.

Acceptable dose fractionations include 40 Gy in 20 fractions over 4 weeks, 45 Gy in 25 fractions over 5 weeks and 50.4 Gy in 28 fractions over 5.5 weeks followed by brachytherapy. Brachytherapy applicators are inserted under general or regional anaesthesia in the patient in the lithotomy position. The patient is catheterised and the bladder emptied. An examination under anaesthetic is performed to assess the residual tumour before a uterine sound is placed to assess the length of the uterine cavity. A central intrauterine tube is then placed followed by a ring and the two applicators are secured together before being packed in place.

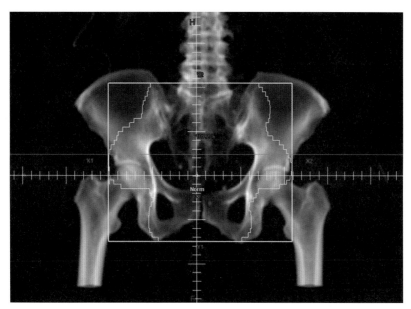

Figure 5.3 Traditional pelvic field. This demonstrates a traditional pelvic field with suggested field borders for an anterior beam arrangement

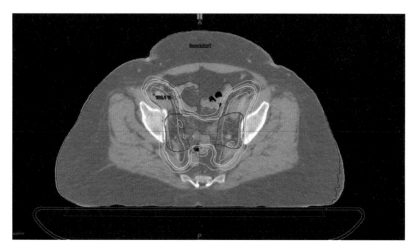

Figure 5.4 IMRT pelvis. This demonstrates the superior technique of IMRT allowing the dose prescribed to be tightly conformed to the target volume and thus sparing the organs at risk

The patient is then recovered from anaesthetic before undergoing a planning CT scan and in some centres a planning MR scan, which are then fused together in the radiotherapy planning suite (Figures 5.3 to 5.5).

Adjuvant Therapy Indications

Adjuvant radiotherapy or chemoradiotherapy may also be considered for women with evidence of high-risk pathological features suggestive of a higher risk of recurrence. Such patients can be categorised into either intermediate or high risk of recurrence.

Intermediate risk patients are defined by Sedlis criteria:

- Presence of lymphovascular space invasion (LVSI) and deep one third cervical stromal invasion in a tumour of any size
- Presence of LVSI and middle one third stromal invasion in a tumour ≥2 cm

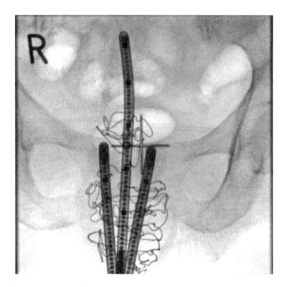

Figure 5.5 Cervix brachytherapy. A patient with cervical brachytherapy applicators in situ

- Presence of LVSI and superficial one third stromal invasion in a tumour ≥5 cm
- Absence of LVSI but deep or middle one third stromal invasion in a tumour ≥4 cm.

Presence of these factors suggests a risk of recurrence and death of approximately 30% following surgery alone. Treatment is with radiotherapy alone as chemoradiotherapy has not been shown to improve overall survival and is associated with a significantly increased risk of haematological and gastrointestinal toxicity.

High-risk patients are defined by Peters's criteria:

- Positive surgical margins
- Pathologically involved pelvic lymph nodes
- Occult parametrial involvement.

Presence of these factors suggest a risk of recurrence and death of approximately 40–50% following surgery alone. Treatment is with chemoradiotherapy as a number of trials and series have demonstrated a significantly reduced risk of relapse and of death at the expense of increased haematological and gastrointestinal toxicity.

Quality of Life

Women treated with radiotherapy have been shown to have significantly lower quality of life scores than those treated with surgery or surgery and chemotherapy with the lowest scores being reported by patients treated with surgery followed by adjuvant radiotherapy.

It is therefore paramount to avoid adjuvant radiotherapy after surgery, unless adverse pathological features are discovered on histology. The main long-term toxicities experienced by these patients are pelvic pain, sexual dysfunction, bowel dysfunction and urinary incontinence. Patients under the age of 45 will almost all develop symptoms of ovarian failure which may be alleviated by the use of hormone replacement therapy. There are few data available as to the safety of HRT in cervical cancer patients but what is available suggests that there is no increased risk of recurrence with its use.

Vagina, bowel and bladder are the major sites of serious late toxicity. These tend to occur within 3 years of completion of treatment by radiotherapy. However in patients treated with chemoradiotherapy approximately 50% of the bowel toxicity and 60% of the bladder toxicity were late effects, occurring up to 7 years after treatment. Interestingly stage and node positivity did not independently affect the probability of developing late side effects, however increasing age did.

Endometrial Cancer

The overall cure rate for endometrial cancer is as high as 77%, as most patients present with stage I disease which carries the best overall prognosis. Radiotherapy has a significant role in the management of endometrial cancer; however there are conflicting views on defining those patients who would benefit from adjuvant treatment. Inevitably this leads to some discrepancy and clinical variation between individual clinicians and treatment guidelines. More recently there has been an appreciation that categorising patients based on their histology alone may not be the optimal way to identify those who will benefit most from adjuvant treatments and a better approach may be to divide tumours by their genomic or molecular subtype. The Cancer Genome Atlas (TCGA) project classifies endometrial cancers into one of four major subtypes:

1. *POLE* ultramutated group – tended to confer a better prognosis than other subtypes.
2. Hypermutated/microsatellite instability group – this group was not associated with clinical outcome.
3. Microsatellite stable/copy number low group – clinical outcome was not linked to this group.
4. Copy number high (serous like) group – the survival of these patients was significantly lower than the other three groups.

Of note the presence of low-grade endometrial cancer within all four of these genomic subtypes suggests that the natural history of low-grade tumours characterised solely by histology can be very different. Also the presence of nearly 20% of high-grade tumours within the serous-like group raises the obvious question as to whether these tumours should routinely be considered a type-1 tumour or classified with other type-2 tumours. It is hoped that further classification may lead to more precise targeting of adjuvant therapy for endometrial cancers but until that time adjuvant treatments will continue to evoke debate in multidisciplinary team meetings.

A total hysterectomy with bilateral salpingo-oopherectomy is the preferred treatment of endometrial cancer, the most common subtype of tumour being an endometrioid adenocarcinoma. Following surgical staging, and until genomic classification becomes validated, certain histological prognostic factors are then used to determine adjuvant treatment options depending on their clinical risk:

- **Low risk** – comprises of patients with grade 1 or 2 endometrioid histology with stage 1A disease which remains confined to the endometrium.
- **Intermediate risk** – includes patients with grade 1 or 2 endometrioid histology and stage 1B disease or cervical stromal involvement (stage II). The presence of LVSI can be used to further sub-stratify patients into higher-intermediate risk.
- **High risk** – includes patients with grade 3 endometrioid disease and all non-endometrioid histology; those with serous or clear cell carcinoma being at high risk of recurrence.

Age is also associated with an increased risk of recurrence and therefore reduced chance of survival. The best illustration of this is from the GOG protocol 33 where 5-year survival with stage I or II endometrial cancer was shown to be

- <40 years old – 96%
- 41 to 50 years old – 94%
- 51 to 60 years old – 87%
- 61 to 70 years old – 78%
- 71 to 80 years old – 71%
- >80 years old – 54%.

Whether age definitely represents an independent prognostic factor remains a matter of some debate given that women aged >65 tend to present with tumours of higher grade, higher stage and deeper myometrial invasion with correspondingly more medical comorbidities which may preclude more radical attempts at cure.

Treatment of Low-Risk Disease

Surgery is the recommended standard treatment for low-risk patients. Routine pelvic lymphadenectomy is not recommended in low-risk patients, as their risk of nodal spread is <5%. Postoperative adjuvant therapy in these patients is generally not warranted as their risk of local recurrence is less than 5%. Furthermore, a 2012 meta-analysis of eight trials of adjuvant radiotherapy demonstrated an increased risk of death compared to observation alone (RR 2.64, 95% CI 1.05–6.66).

Treatment of Intermediate Risk Disease

Following surgical treatment, these patients are further subdivided into those at low-intermediate risk and high-intermediate risk of recurrence by pathological criteria.

The GOG definition of high-intermediate risk is a patient of age >70 with one risk factor, 50–69 with two risk factors and >18 with any of the following three pathological factors:

1. Deep myometrial invasion
2. Grade 2 or 3 histology
3. Presence of LVSI.

The Post-Operative Radiation Therapy in Endometrial Cancer (PORTEC) trials however use a different set of criteria focusing on two of the following three prognostic factors:

1. Age >60 years
2. Stage IB disease
3. Grade 3 histology – N.B. these patients were not eligible for treatment within this trial.

Adjuvant radiotherapy is usually recommended for patients who fulfil the criteria for high-intermediate risk disease. Those with low-intermediate risk disease are better served by observation alone. This approach is based on the GOG trial 99 that demonstrated a statistically significant increase in treatment toxicity without any significant decrease in recurrence risk. The same GOG 99 trial did however demonstrate a reduction in the risk of local recurrence in the high-intermediate risk patient group (2% vs 9%), although there was no decrease in the risk of death, but the trial was not sufficiently powered to evaluate this end point.

Adjuvant radiotherapy usually comprises of vaginal brachytherapy alone for stage IB disease and external beam radiotherapy with a brachytherapy boost for stage II disease. Stage IB disease with grade 3 histology are often treated with adjuvant chemotherapy followed by radiotherapy. Vaginal brachytherapy alone is sufficient for most stage IB patients as demonstrated in the PORTEC-2 study which showed equivalent locoregional control rates (5% vs 3% for vaginal brachytherapy and pelvic RT, respectively) and 5-year disease-free survival (83% vs 78%) as well as overall survival (85% vs 80%). Vaginal brachytherapy also resulted in a significantly lower rate of significant bowel toxicity (13% vs 54%). Adjuvant chemotherapy given during and after pelvic radiotherapy in women with high-risk endometrial cancer provided no significant 5-year failure-free or overall survival benefit, compared with pelvic radiotherapy alone, in the randomized PORTEC-3 intergroup trial. It did, however, show a trend toward improved 5-year failure-free survival (FFS). Radiotherapy techniques are described below.

Treatment of High-Risk Disease

Patients are classified as high risk if they present with stage III or IV disease, or have high-grade serous or clear cell histology. Unfortunately, there is a lack of high-quality data regarding the best approach to manage these patients. The following recommendations based on cancer stage and histological cell type can guide management:

- High-grade serous carcinoma stage IA without myometrial invasion – observation is reasonable although most patients will be offered vaginal brachytherapy.
- High-grade serous carcinoma stage IA or IB – adjuvant chemotherapy (usually carboplatin and paclitaxel) followed by radiotherapy.
- High-grade serous carcinoma stage II – chemotherapy followed by radiotherapy.
- Clear cell cancer stages IA to II – there is limited data to inform the correct treatment choice. Significant variations in practice occur although most clinicians would advocate the use of radiotherapy in such patients.
- Stage III disease regardless of histology – despite limited data the phase 2 RTOG trial 9708 demonstrated a very low pelvic failure rate of 2% in patients treated with external beam radiotherapy and concurrent chemotherapy with single agent for two cycles followed by vaginal brachytherapy and four cycles of combination

chemotherapy after completion of radiotherapy. This can be contrasted to the 18% pelvic failure rate seen in GOG-122 where patients received chemotherapy alone. GOG-258 is awaited which randomised patients to chemotherapy alone vs chemotherapy with pelvic radiotherapy.

- Stages IVA and B patients have a poor prognosis of 25% with a 5-year survival. Limited disease in the pelvis can sometimes be amenable to surgical resection, and there are retrospective case series demonstrating improved outcomes with optimal surgical debulking regardless of histology. Due to the high risk of relapse, adjuvant treatments in this setting are not usually discussed but rather early vs delayed chemotherapy with decisions taken on an individual basis.

Radiotherapy Techniques in Endometrial Cancer

Typically patients will be treated with adjuvant radiotherapy after surgery. Occasionally patients may be considered for primary radical radiotherapy for more advanced or inoperable cases, or if the patient is unfit for surgery. The 5-year survival rates of 70–75% for stage II, 50% for stage III and 25% for stage IV are typically achieved. Traditional field borders for conformal radiotherapy treatment are

- Superior border – L5/S1 interspace unless external or internal nodal involvement in which case it is the lower border of L4
- Inferior border – the upper ½ of the vagina for adjuvant treatment or 3 cm below the most inferior edge of palpable disease for radical treatment
- Lateral border – 2 cm outside pelvic bone sidewalls
- Anterior border – anterior third of symphysis pubis
- Posterior border – 0.5 cm posterior to the anterior border of S2/3 interspace.

Vaginal brachytherapy may be used as a primary adjuvant treatment or selected cervical boost for patients undergoing external beam radiotherapy. Typically this is accomplished with HDR brachytherapy utilising an Iridium-192 source. Treatment begins 3–6 weeks after surgery and consists of 3–5 weekly fractions of radiotherapy treating the upper third of the vagina to a depth of 0.5 cm. A vaginal cylinder applicator is typically used and after-loaded with the Iridium source.

Typical dose fractionations are as follows:

- Adjuvant external beam radiotherapy – 45 to 50.4 Gy in 25 to 28 daily fractions. Vaginal vault brachytherapy boost for stage II patients of 8–10 Gy in two fractions separated by at least 2 days prescribed to 0.5 cm from the surface of the applicator.
- Vaginal vault brachytherapy as a sole adjuvant treatment – 21 Gy in three weekly fractions prescribed to 0.5 cm from surface of the applicator.
- Primary radiotherapy – 45 Gy in 25 fractions followed by vaginal brachytherapy 12 Gy in 3 fractions for stages I and II disease. The 50.4 Gy in 28 fractions followed by vaginal brachytherapy 14 Gy in 2 fractions for stage III disease.
- Para-aortic radiotherapy – 45 Gy in 25 fractions.

Vaginal Cancer

Vaginal cancer is rare and only compromises approximately 3% of all neoplasms of the female genital tract. Eighty per cent occur in women over 60 years of age and are usually squamous cell cancers, although rarer histologies include melanoma, adenocarcinoma, sarcoma, lymphoma and small cell tumours. However, the most common vaginal malignancy is secondary to metastatic spread from another tumour such as cervical, endometrial, vulval, ovarian, lung, kidney and rectal cancers. Clear cell adenocarcinomas of the vagina are most commonly seen in young women exposed to oestrogen therapy *in utero*. Vaginal intraepithelial neoplasia is frequently treated with laser ablation although radiotherapy can achieve very good results albeit with the risk of radiation-induced menopause and vaginal fibrotic changes. Most cases of vaginal cancer are likely to be influenced by HPV infection with studies demonstrating approximately 50% of patients being positive for HPV subtypes 16 and 18.

Radiotherapy is generally considered to be the treatment of choice as radical surgery may lead to impairment of bowel or bladder function. Surgery can be considered if there is a vesico-vaginal or recto-vaginal fistula present. There are, however, no randomised trials to help guide the optimal treatment due to its relative rarity. Therefore most clinicians extrapolate data from other tumour sites including anal and cervical cancers, but the lack of data inevitably results in highly individualised treatment plans that usually depend on the size, location and extent of the tumour. Treatment can be divided into stage I tumours and stage II to IV

tumours with radiotherapy giving overall survival rates of 44–77%, 34–48%, 14–42% and 0–18% for stages I–IV, respectively.

Stage I Tumours

Most patients with stage I tumours will be offered either surgical excision or radiotherapy. Radiotherapy may be more appropriate where tumours are large (greater than 2 cm) as these require extensive surgery with node dissections with the goal of achieving negative surgical margins.

A total radiation dose of 70–75 Gy is the standard recommended dose with 45–50 Gy delivered via external beam radiotherapy and a further boost given via brachytherapy. The technical details of external beam planning especially IMRT are beyond the scope of this book but the radiotherapy volume should include the pelvic lymph nodes, vaginal tumour and whole vagina, paravaginal tissues and inguinal nodes if the tumour is in the lower half of the vaginal canal. When vaginal tumours involve the posterior wall, the sacral and para-rectal nodes are also included. Once external beam radiotherapy is complete, the brachytherapy boost should commence immediately afterwards with tumours of <5 mm in thickness being treated with a vaginal applicator and those of >5 mm deep requiring interstitial implants. Rarely an external beam boost may be required if brachytherapy is not feasible of 15–20 Gy in 8–11 daily fractions.

Stages II to IV Tumours

These cases are usually not suitable for surgery, and instead are offered radical radiotherapy. Given the lack of data to inform as to the correct treatment, most clinicians would offer concurrent chemoradiotherapy with cisplatin ±5-FU as data extrapolated from other tumour sites such as cervical and anal cancer supports its use. There are some small retrospective case series demonstrating a consistently improved locoregional control rate than would be expected with radiotherapy alone. This is to be interpreted with caution however as most patients in these case series have stage I or limited stage II disease and the data is nonrandomised. Radiation volumes and doses are as described above.

Common Side Effects

Premenopausal women invariably develop a radiation-induced menopause. Surgical oophoropexy (surgical elevation of the ovaries to outside of the radiation field) can be successful in preserving ovarian function, but it may lead to a delay in commencing radiotherapy. HRT use may be recommended after a radiation-induced menopause, unless there are contraindications. The most common local side effects after radiotherapy are vaginal stenosis and dryness. The daily use of vaginal dilators after completion of radiotherapy will decrease the risk of developing stenosis, and vaginal lubricating creams or gels containing oestrogen can help with dryness. Women who are sexually active may need to use their dilators less frequently. Rarer complications include recto-vaginal or vesico-vaginal fistulas or vaginal necrosis. In selected cases, these complications may be managed surgically provided local recurrence has been ruled out as a cause. Pelvic exenteration for such patients may be curative but is a major undertaking with significant associated morbidity and mortality and requires careful patient selection.

Vulval Cancer

Vulval cancer is the fourth most common gynaecological cancer with most cases being early-stage T1 or T2 N0 squamous cell cancers in patients with a mean age of 70. Most medically fit patients will receive surgery followed by adjuvant therapy if needed. Some patients will present late, with tumours fixed to vital structures such as the femoral vessels, bone or other pelvic organs and in these patients chemoradiotherapy may be preferred. Overall 5-year survival of 95% for stage I and 85% for stage II are expected; however, if inguinal and/or femoral lymph nodes are involved survival drops to 25–41%.

Radical surgical treatment ranges from a wide local excision for early-stage disease to a radical vulvectomy for larger or multicentric lesions. The aim of surgery is to achieve clear surgical margins (ideally 8 mm clearance in the fixed specimen). Inguino-femoral lymph node dissection (LND) is also recommended in cases of >1 mm stromal invasion and is selected depending on the size and laterality of the tumour. There is an increasing role for sentinel lymph node assessment in the management of vulval cancer.

Neoadjuvant chemoradiotherapy followed by surgery may be considered in patients with locally advanced disease involving the urethra or anus and primary radiotherapy with or without chemotherapy is a reasonable option for patients unfit to undergo radical surgery with weekly cisplatin 40 mg/m^2 administered concurrently.

Indications for Adjuvant Treatment in Vulval Cancer

Node-Negative Disease

Not all patients with early-stage disease require adjuvant therapy; however, data are lacking in early stage I or II disease. Adjuvant radiotherapy is indicated where there are involved surgical resection margins. There is insufficient evidence to routinely advocate radiotherapy in those cases with close (<8 mm) surgical resection margins; however close clinical follow-up in these patients is essential. Most clinicians would advocate adjuvant radiotherapy for tumours with a close resection margin of ≤8 mm. If however macroscopic disease is seen after wide local excision, then a radical local excision or vulvectomy is recommended to gain sufficient clearance. In cases where this is not possible, then radiotherapy is given with or without chemotherapy. This is supported by retrospective data demonstrating improved overall survival compared to no adjuvant radiotherapy (68% vs 29%). Patients with close or involved margins who received radiotherapy had similar survival compared to those who had negative margins (68% vs 66%).

Node-Positive Disease

Adjuvant radiotherapy with or without chemotherapy is indicated where there is one or more macroscopically involved lymph nodes, two or more microscopically involved nodes (after full surgical lymphadenectomy) or evidence of extracapsular spread. The decision between radiotherapy and chemoradiotherapy depends on the health of the patient and risk factors such as multiple or pelvic nodal involvement. This approach is supported by retrospective data demonstrating an improved progression-free survival of 40% vs 26% in node-positive patients who underwent adjuvant treatment. The results of the GROINS-V-II trial are currently awaited to indicate the safety and efficacy of sentinel node biopsy with adjuvant radiotherapy.

Radiotherapy Technique in Vulval Cancer

The finer details of planning radiotherapy especially with IMRT are beyond the scope of this book. In selected cases, radiotherapy can be given to the vulva alone. This is traditionally delivered to the patient in lithotomy position.

When groin node irradiation is indicated, the target volume includes the remaining vulva, inguino-femoral nodes and the pelvic nodes. This is traditionally administered via anterior–posterior opposed fields with the following field borders:

- Superior border – above acetabulum to cover external and internal iliac nodes
- Inferior border – 2 cm inferior to vulval marker
- Lateral border – 1.5 cm outside the bony pelvis to cover the femoral heads.

The use of IMRT is especially advantageous in this situation as it minimises the morbidity associated with the traditional field which delivers significant doses to the femoral head and neck, small bowel, rectum and bladder. IMRT especially limits the haematological toxicity of irradiating large volumes of bone marrow and may therefore increase the patient's concordance with concurrent chemotherapy.

Prescribed doses include

- Adjuvant treatment to vulva alone – 45 Gy in 25 fractions
- Adjuvant treatment to vulva alone, residual microscopic disease present – 45 Gy in 25 fractions with boost 15 Gy in 8 fractions
- Adjuvant treatment to vulva and nodes – 45–50.4 Gy in 25–28 fractions with boost to involved nodal areas 15 Gy in 8 fractions.
- Primary treatment to tumour and nodes – 45–50.4 Gy in 25–28 fractions with boost to primary tumour and nodes of 15–20 Gy in 8–11 fractions.

Common Side Effects of Vulval and Groin Irradiation

Vulval skin is thin and fragile leading to frequent, and sometimes severe, acute skin reactions. Topical hydrocortisone cream can be useful in early reactions, but once moist desquamation occurs additional specialist measures may be required, including adequate analgesia. Urinary frequency, dysuria and proctitis are common side effects and are treated medically. Late effects such as vulval fibrosis and atrophy can occur and are typically treated with vaginal gels. Significant lymphoedema affects up to 30% of patients treated with radiotherapy and surgery. Rare late effects include urethral stenosis or necrosis of the femoral heads.

Palliative Radiotherapy

Palliative radiotherapy is always considered for patients unfit for radical treatments either as a primary treatment or after a recurrence. Symptomatic relief is usually obtained after short intensive radiotherapy treatments and typical doses include

- 20 Gy in 5 fractions
- 30 Gy in 10 fractions
- 8 Gy single fraction (for example haemostasis).

Generally the higher the total dose, the more durable the regression of the tumour. However, higher doses result in greater side effects and the patient will have to attend the radiotherapy department on multiple occasions. Thus there is a balance to be struck for each individual patient between risks, benefits and the opportunity cost of treatment.

More recent developments in radiotherapy have been in Stereotactic Body Radiotherapy (SBRT). Other terms are Stereotactic Ablative Radiotherapy (SABR) or Cyberknife, all of which essentially mean that large doses of radiation are directed very precisely at a tumour and delivered in small numbers of fractions. Such advances have the potential to treat oligometastatic (≤3 metastasis) disease at multiple sites throughout the body even in previously difficult-to-treat areas such as the liver or brain. Some centres are currently commissioned to gain experience in this new radiotherapy technique with the hope that it will be more widely available in the future.

Further Reading

Barnes EA, Thomas G. Integrating radiation into the management of vulvar cancer. *Semin Radiat Oncol.* 2006; 16(3): 168–76.

Churn M, Jones B. Primary radiotherapy for carcinoma of the endometrium using external beam radiotherapy and single line source brachytherapy. *Clin Oncol (R Coll Radiol).* 1999; 11(4): 255–62.

Chyle V, Zagars GK, Wheeler JA, Wharton JT, Delclos L. Definitive radiotherapy for carcinoma of the vagina: outcome and prognostic factors. *Int J Radiat Oncol Biol Phys.* 1996; 35(5): 891–905.

Green J, Kirwan J, Tierney J, et al. Concomitant chemotherapy and radiation therapy for cancer of the uterine cervix. *Cochrane Database Syst Rev.* 2005; (3): CD002225.

Shrivastava SK, Mahantshetty U, Narayan K. Principles of radiation therapy in low-resource and well-developed settings, with particular reference to cervical cancer. *Int J Gynaecol Obstet.* 2015; 131(Suppl 2): S153–8.

Chapter 6

Systemic Therapy in Gynaecological Cancers

Benjamin Masters and Anjana Anand

Introduction

The role, availability and efficacy of systemic therapies in the treatment of cancer is continually evolving. A broad range of systemic treatments are known to be effective in treating gynaecological cancers. These include cytotoxic chemotherapy, biological agents and hormonal therapies. These treatments are used in different clinical settings: neoadjuvant, adjuvant and in the palliative setting.

This chapter outlines how these therapies exert their cytotoxic effects, how they are administered and their associated side effects. It also discusses how to decide which treatments are most appropriate for individual patients and when they should be given in relation to surgery. We also discuss the importance of clinical trials and how the response of novel therapies is compared to current treatments.

Cytotoxic Chemotherapy

Basic Principles

Chemotherapy drugs are designed to target rapidly dividing cells by interfering with normal DNA replication. Cancer cells generally have a rapid cell turnover and therefore constantly need to accurately replicate their DNA prior to each cell division. This renders them more sensitive to chemotherapy agents than the slower dividing cells of the body. However, rapid cellular division also occurs in populations of normal cells within the body such as those of the bone marrow, gut mucosa and hair follicles. These cells are therefore sensitive to DNA damage from chemotherapy drugs and this leads to unwanted side effects.

The majority of chemotherapy agents are administered intravenously on a dedicated cancer chemotherapy day unit. Some chemotherapy agents such as etoposide are active and available as oral formulations, and although normally administered intravenously, bleomycin can be given by intramuscular injection.

Specifically trained chemotherapy nurses administer the drugs, and patients can spend as short as a few hours to almost the whole day on the unit. This depends on the requirement of premedication to prevent side effects, the rate of administration of the drug and pre- and post-administration monitoring. Each treatment is generally referred to as a 'cycle' of treatment and most are given every 3 to 4 weeks. This cycle length allows time for the recovery of normal cells, in particular the patient's bone marrow prior to further treatment. Every patient is reviewed prior to each cycle of chemotherapy to assess their response to treatment and to identify any potential side effects they may have developed.

General Toxicities of Chemotherapy

Most chemotherapy agents cause fatigue, malaise and nausea. Some side effects can be life threatening (in particular neutropenic sepsis and pancytopenia) and therefore not all patients are suitable for chemotherapy. Deciding which patients may not be fit enough for chemotherapy can be complex. The severity of drug-induced adverse effects can be graded using the Common Toxicity Criteria (CTC), a measure developed by the National Cancer Institute. This is a clearly defined scale used to assess the severity of side effects caused by all systemic treatments. It is particularly useful in clinical trials when comparing toxicity profiles of existing drugs with novel therapeutic agents. Adverse effects are graded from 0 to 5:

- 0 – no effect
- 1 – mild
- 2 – moderate
- 3 – severe
- 4 – life-threatening
- 5 – causes death.

Supportive medications such as antiemetics, prophylactic antibiotics, short courses of steroids and also use of granulocyte colony-stimulating factor (GCSF) can be very effective in reducing some of these side effects.

However, despite supportive medications patients may continue to develop severe side effects and these patients may require a dose reduction, delay in their treatment, omission or change of chemotherapy drug.

Specific Chemotherapy Agents

Platinum Agents – Carboplatin and Cisplatin
Mode of Action
Platinum agents exert their cytotoxic effect by forming DNA adducts. These are molecules that insert into replicating DNA strands in place of normal nucleoside bases. This leads to errors in DNA replication and thus results in programmed cell death. In some situations, cisplatin may be used concurrently with radiotherapy as a radiosensitiser. The DNA damage caused by the combination of these two treatment modalities known as chemoradiotherapy has been shown to be more effective than radiotherapy alone in treating some cancers such as cervical, vulva and vaginal cancers.

Administration
Both carboplatin and cisplatin are given intravenously. Cisplatin, like most other chemotherapy agents, is dosed according to the patient's body surface area (BSA), which depends on the patient's height and weight. Carboplatin is different than other chemotherapy agents as its dose is calculated using the Calvert's formula. This is a simple formula based on a patient's glomerular filtration rate (GFR) and the target carboplatin area under the plasma concentration versus time curve (AUC). Both drugs are usually administered every 3 weeks, but cisplatin is given weekly (at a lower dose) when used concurrently with radiotherapy. Both are renally excreted and therefore dose modification is often not needed if liver function is impaired.

Important Adverse Effects
Cisplatin is highly emetogenic and can also cause nephrotoxicity, ototoxicity (high tone hearing loss) and peripheral neuropathy. Due to the nephrotoxic effect of cisplatin, patients require pre-hydration prior to treatment and spend most of the day on the chemotherapy unit. Carboplatin generally has a milder side-effect profile than cisplatin but often causes greater myelosuppression, particularly anaemia and thrombocytopenia. Pre-hydration is not required for carboplatin and therefore treatment time is much shorter. Neither platinum drug causes hair loss. Allergic reactions to carboplatin occur more frequently when patients have received multiple courses of carboplatin treatment and usually patients are successfully switched to cisplatin to complete the course of chemotherapy.

Therapeutic Uses
For epithelial ovarian, fallopian tube and primary peritoneal cancers, carboplatin is used in combination with paclitaxel or as a single agent, in the adjuvant and neoadjuvant setting. It is also used in combination or as monotherapy for recurrent platinum-sensitive disease. Its further use in gynaecological cancers includes treatment of uterine cancers in the adjuvant and metastatic setting either as a single agent or in combination with paclitaxel.

Cisplatin is used in combination with bleomycin and etoposide as part of BEP (bleomycin, etoposide and cisplatin) chemotherapy to treat germ cell tumours of the ovary. Cisplatin is given weekly concurrently with radiotherapy for the treatment of cervical, vaginal and vulval cancers. Carboplatin, paclitaxel and bevacizumab is used to treat metastatic cervical cancer.

Anti-microtubule Agents (Taxanes) – Paclitaxel and Docetaxel
Mode of Action
Microtubules are required for the normal action of the mitotic spindle, which is required for the separation of the paired chromosomes during cell division. For separation to occur, the microtubule structure must undergo polymerisation followed by depolymerisation. Both paclitaxel and docetaxel promote microtubule assembly and then stabilise the microtubule structure, preventing it from undergoing depolymerisation. This prevents chromosome separation and the cell is unable to divide and will undergo programmed cell death.

Administration
Both medications are given intravenously and dosed according to BSA. Docetaxel is given every three

weeks, whereas paclitaxel can be given either weekly or every 3 weeks.

Adverse Effects

Both agents are administered with high-dose steroids and antihistamines to prevent hypersensitivity reactions. Although desensitisation programmes have been shown to be successful in some patients, they are time-consuming and may lead to treatment delay. Both agents can cause hair loss, arthralgia and myalgia. Docetaxel tends to cause more myelosuppression than paclitaxel, whereas paclitaxel tends to cause more peripheral neurotoxicity. This effect is thought to be due to its effect on β-tubulin, a neuro-transport protein found in peripheral nerves. Although the neuropathy can be temporary and improves following treatment completion, many patients can develop long-term loss of sensation in their fingers and toes.

Therapeutic Uses

Paclitaxel is frequently used in combination with carboplatin in the treatment of epithelial ovarian, fallopian tube and primary peritoneal cancers. Paclitaxel alone (monotherapy) is used in platinum-refractory disease and also has activity in uterine cancers. Docetaxel is used in combination with gemcitabine in metastatic leiomyosarcomas.

Anthracyclines – Doxorubicin (Adriamycin) and Pegylated Liposomal Doxorubicin

Mode of Action

Anthracyclines have multiple mechanisms of cytotoxic activity. They intercalate into the DNA structure, which inhibits DNA, RNA and protein synthesis. They also inhibit the topoisomerase II enzyme (see topoisomerase inhibitors) by stabilising the topoisomerase II complex preventing uncoiling and repair of supercoiled DNA, which prevents the DNA from being replicated. They can also induce free radical production causing further DNA damage. Pegylated liposomal doxorubicin (PLD) is encapsulated doxorubicin in polyethylene-coated liposomes. This converts the drug into a slow-release preparation, which alters its activity and side-effect profile.

Administration

Both doxorubicin and PLD are given intravenously and dosed according to BSA. Doxorubicin is generally given three weekly whereas PLD is given every 4 weeks for a total of six cycles.

Adverse Effects

Doxorubicin is cardiotoxic. Cardiotoxicity is dose-dependent and lifetime dose is generally aimed to be less than 450 mg/m^2. In patients with cardiac disease or previous mediastinal radiotherapy, a lower maximum lifetime dose is advised. Doxorubicin tends to cause more myelosuppression, nausea and hair loss than PLD. It is also a vesicant, which means that it can cause tissue inflammation, blistering and necrosis if it extravasates (leaks from the vein into surrounding tissues). Although PLD is less cardiotoxic and causes less alopecia, it can cause painful inflammation of the skin in the hands and feet (palmoplantar erythrodysesthesia), generalised oral mucositis, and rarely a severe painful rash related to pressure areas.

Therapeutic Uses

PLD is an important treatment option in platinum-resistant epithelial ovarian, fallopian tube and primary peritoneal cancers. It can be used in combination with carboplatin or given as monotherapy, and is currently being investigated in a trial in combination with a PD-L1 inhibitor. Doxorubicin is mainly used as a single agent in relapsed uterine cancers and in metastatic leiomyosarcoma of the uterus.

Topoisomerase Inhibitors – Topotecan and Etoposide

Mode of Action

For cells to undergo replication, supercoiled DNA must be unwound to allow formation of two complimentary strands. Topoisomerase enzymes facilitate this process by creating and then repairing small breaks in the supercoiled DNA strand to allow DNA replication. Topoisomerase I is only able to bind to a single DNA strand whereas topoisomerase II can bind to both. Topotecan inhibits the action of topoisomerase I by binding to the topoisomerase enzyme complex after it has cleaved the DNA thus preventing repair of the broken DNA strand. Similarly etoposide forms a complex between topoisomerase II and the DNA strand, which also prevents repair of the DNA strand. These unrepaired breaks cause DNA fragmentation and prevent further DNA replication leading to cell death.

Administration

Topotecan is given intravenously once daily over five consecutive days in three weekly cycles. It is also given as a weekly regimen, which is less toxic and better tolerated. Etoposide can be given orally or intravenously and dosing depends on the route of administration and the indication. Both are dosed according to BSA.

Adverse Effects

Both drugs can cause myelosuppression, alopecia, diarrhoea and liver toxicity. Rarely etoposide can cause myocardial infarction, cardiac arrhythmias and acute leukaemia.

Therapeutic Uses

Etoposide is used as part of the BEP combination regime in the treatment of ovarian germ cell tumours. It can also be given orally for relapsed epithelial ovarian, fallopian tube and primary peritoneal cancers, however response rates can be variable as the bioavailability is different in different patients.

Anti-metabolites – Gemcitabine

Mode of Action

Gemcitabine is a nucleoside analogue which can prevent DNA synthesis by two mechanisms. It mimics the nucleotide base cytosine and is incorporated into newly forming DNA strands in the place of cytosine. Once incorporated into the DNA, it prevents further DNA replication leading to cell death. It also inhibits ribonucleotide reductase, which synthesises deoxynucleosides for DNA replication, therefore also preventing DNA replication.

Administration

Gemcitabine is given intravenously on days 1 and 8 of each three-week cycle and is dosed according to BSA.

Adverse Effects

The most significant side effect of gemcitabine is myelosuppression, predominantly affecting the production of platelets and granulocytes. This is particularly evident when given in combination with platinum agents. Hepatotoxicity is also relatively common.

Therapeutic Uses

Gemcitabine is used in combination with carboplatin in the treatment of relapsed epithelial ovarian, fallopian tube and primary peritoneal cancers. It is also used in combination with docetaxel in the treatment of metastatic leiomyosarcoma.

Antitumour Antibiotics – Bleomycin

Mode of Action

Bleomycin forms an activated bleomycin complex in the presence of metal ions and oxygen. The bleomycin complex interacts with DNA molecules forming free radicals, which damage the DNA strand causing single-strand breaks. It also interacts with RNA molecules, forming free radicals, which cause RNA strand breaks preventing cellular protein synthesis.

Administration

Bleomycin is most commonly given intravenously but can also be given intramuscularly. It is dosed according to BSA in units (rather than in milligrams).

Adverse Effects

The most significant side effect of bleomycin is pulmonary toxicity. Bleomycin pneumonitis is dose- and age-related, with smokers and patients on oxygen therapy most at risk. Other common side effects include skin and nail changes.

Therapeutic Uses

Bleomycin is used as part of the BEP combination regime for the treatment of ovarian germ cell tumours.

Biological Agents

Basic Principles

Cancer research is continually identifying novel mechanisms by which cancers can be targeted to prevent their growth and spread. Tumour angiogenesis and DNA repair are two mechanisms that have been shown to be effective in preventing cancer growth in some gynaecological cancers.

Angiogenesis Inhibitors – Bevacizumab

Mode of Action

Cancer cells require a blood supply to maintain rapid cellular growth. Vascular endothelial growth factor (VEGF) is a molecule, which is involved in initiating new blood vessel formation. VEGF is overexpressed in many tumours including those of gynaecological origin. Bevacizumab is a monoclonal antibody that directly binds to the VEGF molecule and acts to prevent it binding with the VEGF receptor and therefore inhibiting VEGF-induced angiogenesis.

Administration

Bevacizumab is given intravenously and dosed according to body weight. It is administered at three weekly intervals.

Adverse Effects

Bevacizumab increases the risk of hypertension, arterial and venous thromboembolic events, haemorrhage, gastrointestinal perforation, fistulae formation and also delays wound healing. Due to these effects bevacizumab should be avoided 28 days before and after surgery, and not re-commenced until the wound has fully healed. It can also affect the kidneys causing proteinuria and nephrotic syndrome.

Therapeutic Uses

It is used as maintenance treatment following first-line combination chemotherapy for high-risk epithelial ovarian, fallopian tube and primary peritoneal cancers including stages 3 and 4 disease with macroscopic residual disease of >1 cm after debulking surgery. It is also used in the first-line treatment of metastatic cervical cancer in combination with carboplatin and paclitaxel.

PARP Inhibitors – Olaparib and Niraparib

Mode of Action

Olaparib is a poly(ADP-ribose) polymerase 1 (PARP1) inhibitor and niraparib inhibits PARP1 and 2. BRCA and PARP are proteins that are required for DNA repair. Patients with BRCA mutations have defective BRCA proteins and therefore depend on other DNA repair proteins such as PARP to repair damaged DNA. These patients are at increased risk of having incorrectly repaired DNA leading to DNA mutations, which increases their risk of developing certain cancers. Some cancer cells (particularly in patients with BRCA mutations) also have defective BRCA proteins. These cells therefore rely on other DNA repair proteins such as PARP1 and 2 to repair their DNA following damage from cytotoxic chemotherapy. Olaparib and niraparib are able to inhibit these PARP proteins, preventing the cancer cell from repairing its DNA, which leads to cell death.

Administration

Olaparib is given orally at a dose of 400 mg twice a day as maintenance therapy after platinum-based chemotherapy. Niraparib is also given orally 300 mg once daily.

Adverse Effects

Olaparib can cause diarrhoea and bone marrow suppression. Cases of myelodysplastic syndrome, acute myeloid leukaemia and pneumonitis have also been reported, and although relatively rare they can be fatal. Niraparib also causes myelosuppression in particular thrombocytopenia and anaemia.

Therapeutic Uses

Olaparib is used as a maintenance treatment for relapsed, platinum-sensitive, BRCA mutation-positive epithelial ovarian, fallopian tube and primary peritoneal cancer after response to second line or subsequent platinum-based chemotherapy.

Niraparib has shown improvement in progression-free survival (PFS) regardless of BRCA mutation status in patients with platinum-sensitive, recurrent epithelial ovarian cancer. NICE guidance and recommendations for usage of this drug are currently in development and are due to be published in March 2018.

Hormonal Therapies

Basic Principles

Some types of cancer express hormone receptors (oestrogen and progesterone receptors). These can act as growth factors in the presence of the hormone activating the hormone receptor resulting in cancer cell growth and multiplication. By reducing the hormone circulating in the body or by blocking the receptor, cancer growth can be prevented. In premenopausal women the main site of oestrogen synthesis is the ovary, whereas in postmenopausal women oestrogen synthesis occurs in the adipose tissue through the action of the enzyme aromatase.

Oestrogen Receptor Modulators – Tamoxifen

Mode of Action

Tamoxifen binds to oestrogen receptors, which alters (modulates) the shape of the receptor preventing oestradiol from binding to it. This prevents the activation of oestrogen-dependent genes, thus preventing oestrogen-dependent cell growth.

Dosing

Tamoxifen is given orally at a daily dose of 20 mg.

Adverse Effects

Common adverse effects include hot flushes, vaginal discharge and irregular vaginal bleeding. Tamoxifen increases the risk of venous thromboembolic disease. It is also associated with an increased risk of endometrial pathology, including a small increased risk of endometrial cancer.

Therapeutic Uses

Tamoxifen is generally limited to use in asymptomatic patients with low volume, relapsed epithelial ovarian, fallopian tube and primary peritoneal cancers.

Aromatase Inhibitors – Anastrazole and Letrozole

Mode of Action

Anastrazole and letrozole are non-steroidal competitive inhibitors of aromatase. By inhibiting the action of the P450 aromatase enzyme in adipose tissue circulating levels of oestrogen are reduced, which prevents oestrogen-dependent cancer growth.

Administration

Anastrazole is given orally at a dose of 1 mg per day and letrozole is also taken orally at 2.5 mg once per day.

Adverse Effects

Aromatase inhibitors can cause fatigue, arthralgia and reduced bone mineral density. They should only be given in premenopausal women after suppression of ovarian function, as low serum levels of oestrogen leads to activation of the hypothalamic–pituitary–gonadal axis leading to gonadal stimulation.

Therapeutic Uses

Aromatase inhibitors can be used in recurrent oestrogen receptor-positive epithelial ovarian, fallopian tube and primary peritoneal cancers with low volume, asymptomatic disease.

Progestogens – Medroxyprogesterone Acetate and Megestrol Acetate

Mode of Action

Progestogens act systemically on the hypothalamic–pituitary–gonadal axis, leading to inhibition of gonadotrophin production, which leads to a reduction in circulating levels of oestrogen in premenopausal women.

They also inhibit oestrogen-mediated cell proliferation, as progesterone can inhibit oestrogen receptor gene expression and increase oestrogen receptor degradation.

Administration

Medroxyprogesterone acetate is usually given orally at a dose of 200 mg once a day. Megestrol acetate is given orally at a dose of 160 mg per day.

Adverse Effects

Common side effects include weight gain, hot flushes, peripheral oedema, irregular menstruation and deranged liver function. Long-term use can cause Cushing's syndrome or a Cushing's type effect on the body and can reduce bone mineral density. Progestogens can also increase the risk of thromboembolic events including venous thromboembolism, myocardial infarction and stroke.

Therapeutic Uses

Progestogens are used in the treatment of metastatic endometrial cancers where response rates of up to 30% are seen.

Planning Systemic Therapy

A diagnosis of cancer should always be confirmed on histology before commencing chemotherapy. This can be obtained at the time of definitive surgery or by biopsy depending on the clinical circumstances. The histology report provides important information about the origin of the cancer, its natural history and will therefore guide the clinician to decide which drugs can be used to treat each particular tumour type. Imaging is frequently helpful in determining the likely stage of the cancer at the time of diagnosis (early/localised versus advanced/metastatic) and in deciding on the treatment intent (curative or palliative). Other factors to consider before embarking on chemotherapy are the patient's age, performance status (PS), comorbidities, severity of symptoms and nutritional state. When deciding on specific chemotherapy regimens, it is essential to set realistic treatment goals. These tend to be the aim of cure, for disease control or to alleviate symptoms. These goals will influence the choice of chemotherapy agents and the intensity of treatment.

Single Agent versus Combination Chemotherapy

Combination chemotherapy is generally used in the neoadjuvant or adjuvant setting where the ultimate goal of treatment is to cure the cancer. Drugs used in combination regimens have independent activity against a specific tumour type, varied modes of action and different dose-limiting toxicities. An excellent example of combination chemotherapy is BEP chemotherapy used in the treatment of ovarian germ cell tumours. All three drugs are active against germ cell tumours as monotherapies. They all also have slightly different cytotoxic effects; as bleomycin causes free radical-induced DNA damage, etoposide inhibits the topoisomerase II enzyme and cisplatin forms DNA adducts. The toxicity profiles of each drug are very different. Bleomycin can cause pulmonary toxicity but is not usually myelosuppressive. Cisplatin is nephrotoxic but not myelosuppressive, whereas etoposide is very myelosuppressive but does not affect the lungs or kidneys. As there are no overlapping toxicities, the full dose of each drug can be given and this regime is very successful in the treatment of germ cell tumours, with cure rates of over 90%.

Single-agent chemotherapy usually forms the basis of palliative chemotherapy. These drugs are used intermittently to palliate symptoms and to achieve some degree of disease control. An example of this is carboplatin, doxorubicin and paclitaxel chemotherapy, which can be used as single agents for treatment of recurrent metastatic endometrial cancers with response rates of over 20% with manageable toxicities.

Assessment of Response

After systemic therapy is administered, it is important that the response is assessed, so that continuing management can be planned. This can be evaluated in a variety of domains, including clinical, biochemical (via tumour markers) and radiological assessment.

Clinical Assessment

Tumours can cause local symptoms such as pain or ascites. Resolution of these symptoms may reflect reduction in the size or activity of the tumour.

Tumour Markers

Some tumours release specific molecules which can be measured serologically. Reductions in circulating levels of these molecules suggest a reduction in the size and activity of the tumour. This is particularly useful in ovarian cancer, as CA 125 can be measured.

Radiological Assessment

The most reliable measurement of tumour burden is through radiological assessment. Most patients will have baseline scans prior to commencing systemic treatment. A further scan is usually carried out following a course of treatment or at set intervals.

Standardising the Assessment of Tumour Response

The assessment of change in tumour burden is essential in evaluating the cytotoxic effect of novel systemic therapies. However, the change in tumour size needs to be standardised so that response to specific treatments can be compared within and across separate trials. The World Health Organisation (WHO) criteria were used for assessing tumour response, but this has now been superseded by the Response Evaluation Criteria in Solid Tumours (RECIST) criteria which is now the internationally recognised method of assessing tumour response. Tumour burden is separated into measurable and non-measurable disease. Non-measurable disease includes lymphangitis, pleural effusions and ascites. The RECIST criteria has superseded the WHO criteria for several reasons. First it simplifies measurements of lesions into unidimensional measurements rather than bi-dimensional. It also incorporates lymph node involvement and does not classify an isolated increase in a single lesion as disease progression. Table 6.1 summarises the WHO and the RECIST 1.1 criteria for tumour response. It also includes specific guidelines for CA 125 progression in ovarian cancer developed by the Gynaecologic Cancer Intergroup.

Patient-Centred Care

No two cancer patients are exactly identical. Clinical trials help identify which treatments can be the most effective when treating younger patients with fewer comorbidities, but they are often not representative of patients attending oncology clinics. Frail patients have been found to gain less benefit and develop greater toxicity from more intensive treatments. Knowing which treatments are right for each patient is not always an easy decision. The PS score can be used to help identify patients who may be able to tolerate and benefit from more intensive treatments. It can also help to identify patients where intensive treatments may cause more harm than benefit. This is particularly important in patients with advanced, incurable disease in whom quality of life is one of the most important factors in deciding on systemic treatment.

Performance Status

PS is an estimate of the patient's ability to perform activities of daily living (ADLs) without the help of

Table 6.1 Summary of the WHO and RECIST 1.1 response criterias

	WHO	RECIST 1.1
Method	Bidimensional measurements (sum of the two longest diameters in perpendicular dimensions)	Unidimensional measurements (longest diameter of lesions and shortest axis of lymph nodes)
Classification of lesions	Measurable and non-measurable	Measurable (lesions ≥10 mm in longest diameter, lymph nodes ≥15 mm in short axis) and non-measurable
Lesions included	All lesions (lymph nodes not included)	Target lesions: maximum of 5 lesions (2/organ) and all pathological lymph nodes Non-target lesions: all other lesions and borderline lymph nodes (≥10 mm to <15 mm)
Objective response		
Complete response (CR)	Disappearance of all known lesions; confirmed at 4 weeks	Disappearance of all known lesions and all lymph nodes <10 mm
Partial response (PR)	≥50% decrease in size; confirmed at 4 weeks	≥30% decrease in sum of diameters of target lesions Reduction in CA 125 level by ≥50%; confirmed at 4 weeks
Stable disease (SD)	Neither PR or PD criteria met	
Progressive disease (PD)	≥25% increase, no CR, PR or SD documented before increased disease, new lesion(s) or ≥25% increase in 1 lesion	≥20% increase baseline sum of measurements (must be >5 mm) or new lesion(s) Rise in CA 125 to ≥2× UNL (upper normal limit)[a] or rise in CA 125 to ≥2× nadir value; confirmed at 4 weeks[b]

[a]Patients with elevated CA 125 pretreatment and normalisation of CA 125 following first-line treatment.
[b]Patients with elevated CA 125 pretreatment, which never normalises following first line treatment.

others. ADLs include getting dressed, washing and eating as well as more complex activities including being able to continue with their job if they are employed. PS is one of the most important factors when deciding the most appropriate cancer management for individual patients. It has a role in both predicting a patient's prognosis and determining the best treatment for that patient. The most widely used scale is the Eastern Cooperative Oncology Group (ECOG) scale, also known as the Zubrod scale. The ECOG scale ranges from 0 (fully functional, asymptomatic patient) to 4 (bedridden, fully dependent patient). These are summarised in the Appendix.

Cytotoxic chemotherapy, in particular, has been associated with lower response rates, higher rates of toxic effects and shorter survival in patients with a poor PS. Many clinical trials are restricted to fitter patients such as those with PS of 0 to 1. Consequently, there is limited evidence available for treatment effects in frail patients. A patient's PS will also change over time and will decline as the cancer progresses due to the spread of the cancer and the cumulative effect of treatments. Chemotherapy is generally considered in patients with a PS of 0 to 1 and should usually be avoided in patients with a PS of 3 to 4. However, less toxic and

less intensive treatments such as hormone therapies can be considered in all patients. However, there will be some patients who initially present with a poor PS due to a combination of rapid progression of the cancer and a delay in presentation. This frequently occurs in patients with ovarian and small cell cancers. Despite presenting with a low PS, cytotoxic platinum-based chemotherapy is often administered as these cancers are generally platinum-sensitive and in many of these patients, chemotherapy can dramatically improve symptoms, PS and quality of life.

Quality of Life

Quality of life is a widely used term that conveys an overall sense of well-being that encompasses aspects of happiness and satisfaction with life in general. It is one of the most important factors when considering systemic treatment in patients with incurable disease. In patients with advanced incurable cancer, treatment should aim to improve quality of life by palliating troublesome symptoms and prolong life if possible. Quality of life is also becoming increasingly important for patients with potentially curable cancer. Treatments are becoming increasingly effective and therefore more patients are cured with many more experiencing longer remission periods. Consequently the long-term effects of their treatments need to be considered. For example, an uncommon side effect of paclitaxel is chronic, disabling neuropathic pain. Although the importance of curing the cancer greatly outweighs the concerns of long-term adverse effects, long-term effects are becoming more prevalent and should be considered when planning treatment and ongoing care.

Measuring the impact of individual treatments on a patient's quality of life can be difficult. Health Related Quality of Life (HRQoL) is a measure of the individual's physical and mental well-being. Nowadays, quality of life is assessed as an integral part of clinical trials and several tools have been developed to measure quality of life. They are usually generic questionnaires such as SF-36 (Short Form with 36 questions) and FACT scale (Functional Assessment of Cancer Therapy). These questionnaires are simple and can be completed easily within minutes. They have a scoring system and the results can be quantified. Disease-specific measures of HRQoL have also been developed. The European Organisation for Research and Treatment of Cancer (EORTC) has developed a generic cancer-related questionnaire called EORTC QLQ-30 and also gynaecology cancer-specific quality-of-life questionnaires – EORTC QLQ-CX24 (cervical), QLQ-EN24 (endometrial) and QLQ-OV28 (ovarian).

Surgery and Systemic Therapy

Surgery is the standard of care for the majority of gynaecological cancers and forms an integral part of the management plan for ovarian, fallopian tube, primary peritoneal and uterine cancers. When chemotherapy is indicated after surgical treatment, it should be commenced as soon as possible to prevent regrowth of any residual cancer cells. In practical terms the timing of this will depend upon the extent and type of surgery, postoperative complications, healing of the surgical wound and the patient's general recovery from the operation.

Surgical planning and systemic therapy has become particularly important in the treatment of advanced epithelial ovarian, fallopian tube and primary peritoneal cancers. A standard treatment approach for these patients has been primary debulking surgery (PDS) with the aim of removing all visible tumours (complete debulking) followed by adjuvant combination chemotherapy with carboplatin and paclitaxel. However, in a

substantial proportion of patients complete debulking is not achieved. This may be due to extensive preoperative disease with severe morbidity associated with poor nutritional state, hypoalbuminaemia, ascites, pleural effusions and risk of thromboembolism. Patients may be slow to recover, or experience perioperative complications. In such patients, adjuvant chemotherapy is frequently delayed due to significant postoperative morbidity. Ideally chemotherapy should be started as soon as possible following surgery (preferably within 4–6 weeks). Delay in starting chemotherapy is associated with early disease recurrence and reduced overall survival (OS).

An alternative approach is to administer a short course of adjuvant chemotherapy (NACT) first with the aim of shrinking the tumour and improving the patient's fitness prior to interval debulking surgery (IDS). After IDS, the patient then completes the full course of chemotherapy. The EORTC 55971 trial randomised patients with advanced-stage epithelial ovarian, fallopian tube and primary peritoneal cancer to PDS or NACT-IDS and it showed that outcomes in terms of PFS and OS were similar in both treatment groups. However, postoperative rates of adverse effects and mortality tended to be higher following PS rather than IDS. The CHemotherapy OR Upfront Surgery (CHORUS) trial with a similar trial design also concluded that NACT-IDS is non-inferior to PDS. Furthermore, patients in the NACT arm had a better quality of life, less chemotherapy-associated side effects, shorter stay in hospital after surgery and the tumour was more likely to be optimally debulked. Since publication of the above trial results, IDS after a short course (three cycles) of neoadjuvant carboplatin and paclitaxel chemotherapy has become an acceptable and widely used treatment option for patients with extensive disease.

If surgery is planned to take place after a course of chemotherapy, it is necessary for the surgical and anaesthetic team to be aware of the potential impact of chemotherapy on the patient's perioperative course. This requires careful preoperative assessment and planning. Myelosuppression is a common side effect of chemotherapy, and rapid deterioration with life-threatening sepsis can occur with neutropenia. Although most patients have had recovery in their bone-marrow function by the time their surgery is planned, the medical team should confirm this prior to proceeding with elective surgery. A haematology consultation may be advisable if there are significant abnormalities that have not resolved spontaneously.

Bevacizumab is an anti-angiogenic agent that may be indicated in selected patients with advanced-stage epithelial ovarian, fallopian tube and primary peritoneal cancers. Patients taking bevacizumab require careful surgical planning because it has been associated with multiple surgical complications, including delayed wound healing, wound dehiscence, surgical site bleeding, bowel perforation, venous thromboembolic disease and wound infection. Where elective surgery is planned, bevacizumab must be withheld for a minimum of 28 days prior to surgery and reintroduced into the chemotherapy regime at least 28 days after surgery, and only after the surgical incisions have fully healed. Patients who require emergency surgery while taking bevacizumab pose significant management challenges. Bowel perforation is a rare but serious complication of bevacizumab treatment. If emergency surgery is necessary, then re-anastomosis of bowel must be avoided in these patients.

TIPS
Surgeons and anaesthetists should be aware of the potential complications presented by chemotherapy drugs and have an appropriate management plan for their patients. Specialist advice should be sought in complex cases.

Clinical Trials

The process of developing a new drug is complex and takes many years for a new idea or concept to become a successful treatment option. When a new drug is being developed, it initially undergoes preclinical testing in the laboratory on human tumour cell lines and if they show promise further testing is conducted in animal models. This process itself can take several years and when the new drug is finally available for use in humans, rigorous testing through clinical trials are conducted in humans to evaluate efficacy, toxicity and response rates. Most of the chemotherapy treatment protocols that are being used currently are based on successful trials which have shown benefits in terms of response rates, disease-free survival and OS. Clinical trials are classified into Phases I to III:

- Phase I – this is the first attempt in evaluating a novel drug in humans. The primary objective is to determine the maximum tolerated dose as defined by acceptable toxicity. The secondary objectives are to study pharmacokinetics and to describe any tumour response.
- Phase II – when the drug is tested in patients with a specific diagnosis. The objective is to determine if a particular drug has antitumour activity against the tumour type in question. The primary end point for most phase 2 trials is response rate.
- Phase III – a trial designed to compare novel treatments with standard therapy. These trials have objective end points such as disease-free survival, OS and symptom control. Phase III trials are also known as randomised controlled trials.

Summary

- Systemic therapies include cytotoxic chemotherapy, biological agents and hormonal therapies.
- A confirmed histological diagnosis of cancer is essential prior to commencing systemic treatment.
- Planning appropriate treatment requires a highly individualised approach that considers both the disease and patient factors.
- Factors that must be taken into account when planning systemic therapy include the disease itself, goals of treatment, PS, comorbidities and quality of life.
- Careful surgical planning is required for patients receiving systemic therapies, as these pose specific perioperative risks. Surgeons and anaesthetists must be familiar with these risks in order to provide optimal surgical management.
- Clinical trials are essential to develop new therapies and to guide clinicians in advising the most suitable treatments for their patients.

Further Reading

Eisenhauer EA, Therasse P, Bogaerts J, Schwartz LH. New Response Evaluation Criteria in Solid Tumours: Revised RECIST guideline (version 1.1). *Eur J Cancer* 2009; 45: 228–47.
ESMO. *ESMO Clinical Practice Guidelines: Gynaecological Cancers.* Available from: www.esmo.org/Guidelines/Gynaecological-Cancers. Accessed on 20 April 2017.
Lundqvist EA, Fujiwara K, Seoud M. Principles of chemotherapy. *Int J Gynaecol Obstet.* 2015; 131 (Suppl 2): S146–9.
Seoud M, Lundqvist EA, Fujiwara K. Targeted therapy in gynecologic cancers: Ready for prime time? *Int J Gynaecol Obstet.* 2015; 131(Suppl 2): S150–2.
West H, Jin JO. Performance status in patients with cancer. *JAMA Oncol.* 2015; 1(7): 998.

Preinvasive Disease, Screening and Hereditary Cancer

Dhivya Chandrasekaran, Faiza Gaba and Ranjit Manchanda

Preinvasive Disease

Malignant lesions for most epithelial organs are thought to arise from specific 'preinvasive neoplastic lesions'. The histopathological characteristics of these lesions have been well described. A number of other terminologies have been used to describe these lesions, including incipient, precancerous, pre-neoplasia, or commonly intraepithelial neoplasia, as well as at times epithelial dysplasia or preinvasive neoplasia.

Cervical Intraepithelial Neoplasia

Cervical intraepithelial neoplasia (CIN) is a histological term that refers to precancerous transformation of squamous cells of the cervical transformation zone. Typically graded as I–III in the United Kingdom, CIN I represents mild dysplasia confined to the basal third of the epithelium, CIN II represents moderate dysplasia confined to the basal two thirds of the epithelium and CIN III represents severe dysplasia involving more than two thirds of the epithelium or even full thickness. Risk factors associated with CIN include: early age of first intercourse, multiple sexual partners, presence of high-risk subtypes of human papillomavirus (HPV), smoking and immunodeficiency (e.g. HIV, transplant patients on immunosuppressant medication).

> **TIP**
> Persistent infection with high-risk (oncogenic) subtypes of HPV is the cause of virtually all premalignant and malignant epithelial lesions of the cervix.

Classification

The terminology used to classify preinvasive disease of the cervix has been modified to reflect changes in our understanding of underlying biology and disease management. In the United Kingdom, the CIN I–III system has been the standard classification and is still used in the current guidelines for histopathology reporting. However, the World Health Organisation has endorsed the findings of the Lower Anogenital Squamous Terminology (LAST) project and recommends the use of an alternative system, the Bethesda classification, for reporting of low-grade and high-grade squamous intraepithelial lesions (SIL). This is now the most widely used terminology worldwide.

There are important conceptual differences between the two classification systems. The CIN system requires the identification of a lesion followed by determination of its grade on a continuum of CIN I–III. However, the SIL classification is based on the histological changes seen as a result of two different groups of HPV infection, with productive HPV leading to low-grade SIL (LSIL) and transforming HPV to high-grade SIL (HSIL). Generally, LSIL equates to CIN I and/or HPV-related changes, and HSIL equates to CIN II–III.

The two-tiered SIL classification is in keeping with our current understanding of the biology of HPV-associated preinvasive cervical disease. It also reduces diagnostic variability. Even though the histological features on CIN are well described, there is considerable inter-observer variability in the grading of CIN. However as the SIL classification is dependent on the type of HPV that is present (i.e. productive or transforming), the problem of inter-observer discrepancy of CIN grading is significantly minimised.

An important argument in favour of the continued use of the three-tier CIN grading system in the NHS Cervical Screening Programme (NHSCSP) is to ensure continuity in the recording, transfer and storage of coded data on current databases. Collection and analysis of this data is paramount in assessing the effectiveness of the screening programme. Arguments against persisting with the three-tier system include a change from a three- to a two-tier system for classifying the cytological grade of dyskaryosis (low and high grade), which in turn makes correlation of a three-tier CIN classification system with cytology harder. Also for practicality, patient management is based on a two-tier grading system of low-(CIN I) and high-(CIN II–III) grade abnormality.

Screening for Cervical Cancer

The NHSCSP has led to a significant decrease in cervical cancer incidence in the United Kingdom. Protection against cervical cancer incidence offered by cervical screening ranges approximately from 60% to 85%. It is slightly lower in the age group under 40 than above 40. The coverage of the NHSCSP in England is above 70%. Of the 4.4 million women invited, 3.6 million underwent screening. It has been suggested that an overall coverage of 80% can potentially decrease associated mortality rates by 95%. Although cytological screening may be less effective against cervical adenocarcinoma (which account for 15% of cervical cancers), it does have a substantial impact even in this subgroup. Sensitivity and specificity of cervical cytology have been reported to range between 30% to 87% and 86% to 100%, respectively.

Liquid-based cytology (LBC) is now the method of choice for obtaining and preparing cervical cells for cytological assessment. This has replaced the 'pap-smear' test. LBC results in homogeneous, easy to read slides and a more efficient automated laboratory sample handling process and thus increased productivity. However, LBC lacks formal criteria used for defining smear adequacy.

HPV Testing and Cervical Cytology

There is firm evidence to show that HPV DNA testing may exceed the performance of traditional cervical cytology tests. High-risk (HR) HPV DNA testing has been shown to have a higher sensitivity but slightly lower specificity (of the order of 8–12%) than cytology alone for detecting high-grade disease. A combination of HPV testing and cytology is associated with an even higher sensitivity, and may save additional years of life at reasonable costs compared with cytology testing alone. Women who test negative for HR HPV DNA and have a normal cytology are extremely unlikely to develop CIN/cancer in the next 5–10 years. HR HPV DNA negative women with a borderline/atypical cells of undetermined significance (ASCUS) smear have a

<2% risk of high-grade CIN/cancer in the next 2 years, which is similar to women with a negative smear. A positive HR HPV DNA test in the presence of a severely dyskaryotic smear and high-grade disease at colposcopy suggests a 60–80% risk of CIN III or worse in the next 2 years.

According to the NHSCSP Colposcopy and Programme management guidelines, HPV DNA testing is recommended in triaging borderline or low-grade cytology, follow-up of untreated histologically confirmed CIN I, follow-up of treated CIN I–III and follow-up of CGIN after treatment. HPV triage helps identify women who are more likely to develop high-grade CIN/cancer. Thus, compared to cytology alone HR HPV testing can improve risk stratification and increase the efficiency of cervical cancer screening. In January 2016, the UK National Screening Committee issued its recommendation to adopt primary HPV testing in place of cytology for cervical screening.

NHS Cervical Screening Programme

The NHSCSP offers women screening depending on their age. The current programme is as follows:

- First cervical cytology test by age 25 (women are invited 6 months prior to their 25th birthday).
- Three yearly screening between the ages of 25 and 49 years.
- Five yearly screening between the ages of 50 and 64 years.
- Women over the age of 65 years are only invited for screening if they have had a recent abnormal test or they are invited upon request if they have not had an adequate screening test reported since the age of 50.

While most experts agree that cervical screening is effective, discussion continues over the most appropriate screening interval. Shortening the interval between screening tests does improve protection against cervical cancer, especially in younger women, but only modestly. Any gain in protection has to be considered against the considerable cost of the screening programme. The ideal age for starting routine cervical screening has been a matter of debate for some time. This is reflected by variances in practices across the countries of the United Kingdom. For women under 25, prevalence of HPV infection after coitarche is high, and consequently women in this age group are likely to have HPV-related cellular changes. However, HPV infection is less likely to persist in younger women and most low-grade abnormalities identified in cytology samples regress spontaneously with time. Consequently screening in women 20–24 years leads to the detection of many cytological abnormalities (most of which would resolve of their own accord) resulting in unnecessary referrals to colposcopy and subsequent over treatment. Screening has not been shown to reduce the incidence of, or mortality from, cervical cancer in women under the age of 25.

Routine cervical screening in the United Kingdom ceases at the age of 65. The prevalence of CIN III and invasive cancer in women over 50 is low: 11/100,000 in well-screened women compared to a prevalence rate of 59/100,000 women in the population as a whole. Most women diagnosed with invasive cancer after the age of 50 have not participated fully in the cervical screening programme.

Human Papilloma Virus and Vaccine

HPV is a sexually transmitted infection. It is a ubiquitous organism, and consequently both men and women are likely to contract this infection at some point, most commonly at around the time of coitarche. Most infections will regress in <2 years, but persistence of infection is necessary for the development of CIN. The causal relationship between HPV, the development of CIN and cervical cancer is well established. HPV DNA has been found in 99.7% of cervical tumours. Cancer is usually a late consequence of HPV infection, often developing 5–30 years after the primary infection. The virus is also responsible for other anogenital preinvasive diseases and cancers. To date, over 100 HPV types have been identified. There is considerable worldwide variation in the distribution of HR viral types, but around 70% cancers have been linked to HPV types 16 and 18 with another 10–20 serotypes accounting for majority of the other cases.

> **TIPS**
> HPV viral infection causes cervical cancer. The most common 'high risk' subtypes are HPV 16 and 18.
> Women who smoke are more likely to have persistent HPV infection, and should be advised of this and encouraged to stop.

Several determinants have been found to promote progression of oncogenic HPV infection to CIN, including smoking, multiple sexual partners, use of the oral contraceptive pill, having children, immunodeficiency (e.g. HIV) and infection with other sexually transmitted pathogens.

The vast majority of HPV infections resolve spontaneously. There are several commercially available subtypes of HPV vaccines in the market at present:

- Cervarix – bivalent vaccine targeting HPV 16 and 18, which account for over 70% of cervical cancer cases worldwide
- Gardasil – quadrivalent vaccine targeting HPV 16, 18 and the subtypes responsible for anogenital warts (6 and 11)
- Gardasil9 – nonavalent HPV vaccine targeting high-risk HPV types 16, 18, 31, 33, 45, 52 and 58 in addition to the low-risk HPV types 6 and 11.

Clinical trial data have indicated that the vaccines are highly effective in preventing new cases of HPV16- and 18-associated diseases, with significantly lower rates of high-grade CIN. Cervarix and Gardasil protect against 50% of CIN II–III and 70% of cervical cancer. Nonavalent HPV is expected to increase the protection against cervical cancer to approximately 90% and for CIN I, CIN II and CIN III lesions, the increases are 20%, 30% and 30%, respectively. Prevention of cancer is more likely in women who receive the HPV vaccination prior to exposure to the virus.

> **TIPS**
> In the United Kingdom, a national HPV vaccination programme using Cervarix was introduced in September 2008 in schools, with a recommended three doses administered to girls aged 12–13 years. A catch-up programme was also implemented for older girls up to 18 years of age from 2009 to 2011. Gardasil is the vaccine currently used in the UK vaccination programme.

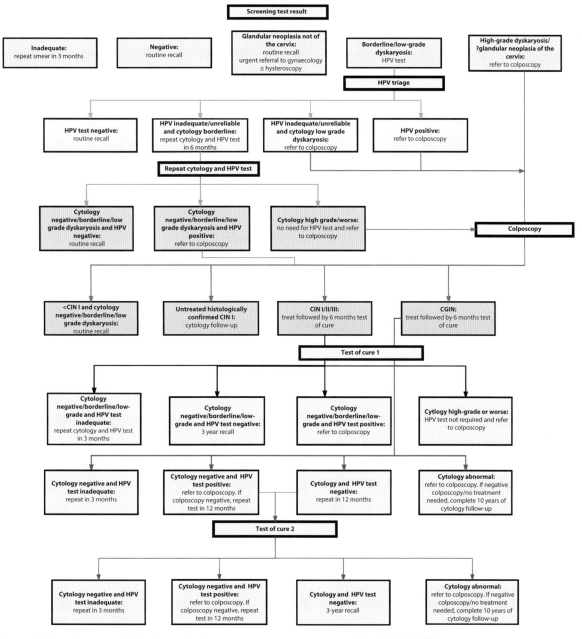

Figure 7.1 Screening protocol algorithm and colposcopy management recommendations for CIN/CGIN
Adapted from the NHSCSP.

Management of Preinvasive Cervical Disease

Figure 7.1 is adapted from the NHSCSP and summarises the current screening protocol algorithm and colposcopy management recommendations.

Women with abnormal cytology results are referred to colposcopy clinic. Current standards for the NHSCCP programme are as follows:

- Three consecutive inadequate cytology samples – offer colposcopy within 6 weeks

- HPV-positive borderline or low-grade cytology – offer colposcopy within 6 weeks
- High-grade/suspected invasive disease – offer colposcopy within 2 weeks.

Colposcopy involves inspection of the cervix under high magnification. A range of different solutions (including acetic acid and iodine) are painted onto the surface of the cervix to help the colposcopist assess for changes indicating the presence of CIN. Depending on the combination of the cytology result and colposcopic assessment, the following management options are usually considered:

- Conservative management with repeat cytology at prescribed interval
- Punch biopsies of small areas of a lesion, to aid in diagnosis and to facilitate management planning
- Excisional biopsy of abnormal transformation zone.

Low-grade disease, such as CIN I, is usually managed conservatively by observation and planned follow-up with repeat cytology as it often regresses spontaneously. Persistent or progressive CIN may require excisional treatment. In most circumstances, the recommended treatment for high-grade lesions (CIN II and III) is excision.

Most lesions are treated by large loop excision of the transformation zone (LLETZ). When excision is used, the specimen should be removed as a single sample wherever possible. Removing the transformation zone in multiple fragments can increase the difficulties in histopathological assessment and if microinvasive disease is present, it may be difficult to stage or define completeness of excision.

- The majority of treatments can take place in the outpatient setting under local anaesthesia.
- Excisional techniques are recommended for treatment of high-grade disease.
- LLETZ is the most commonly used excisional technique.
- Ablative techniques are not routinely recommended as there will be no histological evaluation of the specimen.
- Repeated LLETZ, and those with a depth of 10 mm or more, may increase the risk of preterm birth.

Box 7.1 outlines the NHSCSP management in special circumstances.

Cervical Glandular Intraepithelial Neoplasia

Cervical glandular intraepithelial neoplasia (CGIN) is a preinvasive endocervical glandular lesion of the cervix that is less common than CIN. It is a precursor to usual-type cervical adenocarcinoma. The prevalence of CGIN is increasing due to better recognition by pathologists, higher prevalence of HPV and/or a change in the distribution of HPV types. Cervical screening with cytology and HPV can predict the presence of CGIN abnormalities. Colposcopic assessment of CGIN is challenging as the lesion is within the endocervical cells, and it is difficult to visualise the full extent of the lesion (i.e. the endocervical margin).

Treatment

As high-grade CGIN often occurs in young women conservative management in the form of excision biopsy is recommended for those desiring to retain fertility, provided the margins of the excisional specimen are negative and invasion is excluded. A punch biopsy may be inadequate for diagnosis in cases of abnormal high-grade glandular cytology. The endocervical excision margin must be shown to be clear of disease after treatment. If not, or if there is uncertainty, then a repeat procedure should be performed to obtain this. Management by simple hysterectomy may be an option for those cases where fertility is not required, there are positive margins after an adequate excisional procedure or treatment by cone biopsy is followed by further high-grade CGIN.

> **TIPS**
> Each unit has a colposcopy MDT. All cases of invasive cervical cancer, complex cases and those where there is diagnostic uncertainty or treatment dilemma should be discussed at the MDT.

Vulval Intraepithelial Neoplasia

SIL of the vulva, known as vulvar intraepithelial neoplasia (VIN), are considered to be precursors of invasive squamous cell carcinoma of the vulva.

Classification

In 1986, the International Society for the Study of Vulvovaginal Disease (ISSVD) created a classification system for VIN: VIN I, VIN II, VIN III. It is now widely believed that VIN I is not a precursor of VIN II

Box 7.1 Management of preinvasive disease of the cervix in special circumstances

Post hysterectomy	• Women on routine recall and with no CIN in their hysterectomy specimen do not require vaginal vault cytology
	• Women not on routine recall and with no CIN in their hysterectomy specimen should have vaginal vault cytology at 6 months following their hysterectomy and no further samples if cytology is negative
	• Women who undergo hysterectomy and have completely excised CIN should have vaginal vault cytology at 6 and 18 months
	• Women who undergo hysterectomy and have incompletely excised CIN (or uncertain excision), follow-up should be as if their cervix remained in situ:
	– CIN I: vault cytology at 6, 12, 24 months
	– CIN II–III: vault cytology at 6 and 12 months, followed by nine annual vault cytology samples
	– Follow-up for incompletely excised CIN continues to 65 years or until 10 years after surgery (whichever is later)
Pregnancy	• Routine screening should be deferred until after pregnancy
	• Abnormal cytology should undergo colposcopy in late first or early second trimester unless there is a clinical contraindication. However for low-grade changes triaged to colposcopy on the basis of a positive HPV test, assessment may be delayed until after delivery
	• If a previous colposcopy was abnormal and in the interim the woman becomes pregnant, colposcopy should not be delayed
	• If a pregnant woman requires colposcopy or cytology after treatment (or follow-up of untreated CIN I), assessment may be delayed until after delivery unless there is an obstetric contraindication. However, assessment should not be delayed if the first appointment for follow-up cytology or colposcopy is due following treatment for CGIN. The 'test of cure' appointment should not be delayed after treatment for CIN II–III with involved/uncertain margin status
Immunocompromised states	• Women 25–64 with renal failure requiring dialysis, who have never been screened, must have cervical cytology performed at or shortly after diagnosis
	• All women with HIV should have annual cytology and initial colposcopy if resources permit. Subsequent colposcopy for screening abnormality should follow national guidelines. The age range screened should be the same as for HIV-negative women. Despite the higher cervical treatment failure rate, high-grade CIN should be managed according to national guidelines. Lesions < CIN II should probably not be treated as these are likely to represent persistent HPV infection of the cervix which responds poorly to treatment and may clear spontaneously
	• Women with multifocal disease should be assessed by cytology, HPV testing (within the context of the NHSCSP), colposcopy, vulvoscopy and biopsy where indicated at least every six months
Repeat excision for high-grade CIN	• Should be considered in women over 50, with high-grade lesions, especially if satisfactory cytology/colposcopy cannot be guaranteed
	• Is not essential in women <50 if there is no glandular abnormality or invasive disease

or III and that it has low malignant potential, unlike VIN II–III. VIN is now classified as follows:

• VIN usual type – associated with HPV infection
• VIN differentiated type – accounts for 5% of cases, and is associated with lichen sclerosus and lichen simplex chronicus

Epidemiology

VIN is an uncommon condition. VIN usual type is regarded as a disease of younger women mainly in their thirties and forties. Several studies report that the mean age of women diagnosed with VIN III has decreased in the last 50 years, which coincides with an increased incidence of VIN III. This may be related to an increase in sexual promiscuity, HPV, smoking and greater awareness of the disease in clinical practice. The peak incidence of VIN occurs in the 30–50 years age group, but there is often a second peak among 60–80 year olds, which may reflect the peak incidence of differentiated-type VIN.

Usual-type VIN, especially the warty subtype, accounts for the majority of VIN. Between 32% and 84% of women with VIN are current smokers and even higher numbers have a history of smoking: in some studies approaching 100%. Therefore it is generally believed that cigarette smoking is strongly associated with VIN, usual type. This type, like other forms of lower genital tract preinvasive disease, is more frequent among immunocompromised women. The percentage of women with VIN who are immunosuppressed has been reported as 5%. Development of squamous cell carcinoma in women with VIN has been reported to occur in 9–18.5% of cases.

Treatment

The UK National Guideline on the Management of Vulval Conditions (British Association for Sexual Health and HIV) include:

- Local excision – the most effective and the treatment of choice for small well-circumscribed lesions
- Imiquimod cream 5% – unlicensed, with significant side effects, with possibility of partial or complete response
- Vulvectomy – for those with extensive lesions or background field change.

Alternative treatments include local destruction (e.g. laser), 5-fluorouracil cream or surveillance and close follow-up of the lesion. The recurrence rates at follow-up tend to be higher than for excision, but cosmesis is usually good. The 5-fluorouracil cream is unlicensed in its use to treat VIN but may lead to resolution of some lesions but results are variable and side effects are common. There is currently no consensus on usefulness or regimen.

With supervision, some lesions will spontaneously regress. This may be the best policy for partial thickness VIN. However, there is a risk of progression and patients should be made aware of this. Multifocal lesions can be treated in the same manner as single lesions, but may have a higher recurrence rate.

Vaginal Intraepithelial Neoplasia

Vaginal intraepithelial neoplasia (VaIN) is a rare preinvasive condition of the vaginal epithelium that is now more widely recognised with improved colposcopic training and cytologic screening. Incidence is 0.2 per 100,000 women, and it accounts for 0.4% of all intraepithelial diseases of the lower genital tract. The lifetime risk of malignant transformation from VaIN to invasive vaginal carcinoma is 9–10%. VaIN is frequently diagnosed at colposcopy as a result of concurrent CIN. Coexisting VaIN is seen in 1–6% of women with CIN. The main etiological factor is high-risk HPV. Other risk factors include smoking, immunosuppression and pelvic radiotherapy. VaIN most commonly affects the upper one third of the vagina, although multifocal involvement may also be seen, making treatment challenging. Diagnosis is histological, and adequate biopsy is vital to exclude invasion and to plan appropriate management. VaIN is classified as low grade (VaIN I) or high grade (VaIN II–III).

Treatment

VaIN is best treated in a specialist centre with appropriate expertise. Many factors must be considered: age, comorbidities, site of disease specifically proximity of the bladder and rectum under the vaginal mucosa, multifocality, preservation of sexual function and risk of recurrence. Treatment modalities include surgery, brachytherapy and medical management. Excision and radiotherapy used to be more common, but conservative approaches have now been adopted.

Endometrial Hyperplasia

Endometrial hyperplasia is defined as irregular proliferation of the endometrial glands with increased gland to stroma ratio when compared with proliferative endometrium. Risk factors include obesity, polycystic ovarian syndrome, unopposed oestrogen in the form of hormone replacement therapy (HRT) in postmenopausal women, long-term tamoxifen use and oestrogen secreting ovarian tumours (e.g. granulosa cell tumours).

Classification

The current and most widely used classification system for endometrial hyperplasia is based on cellular atypia and is as follows:

- Endometrial hyperplasia without atypia
- Atypical endometrial hyperplasia.

Previous categories referred to the complexity of histological architecture, but this is no longer part of the classification.

Epidemiology

Endometrioid-type endometrial carcinoma is the most common form of endometrial cancer, and endometrial

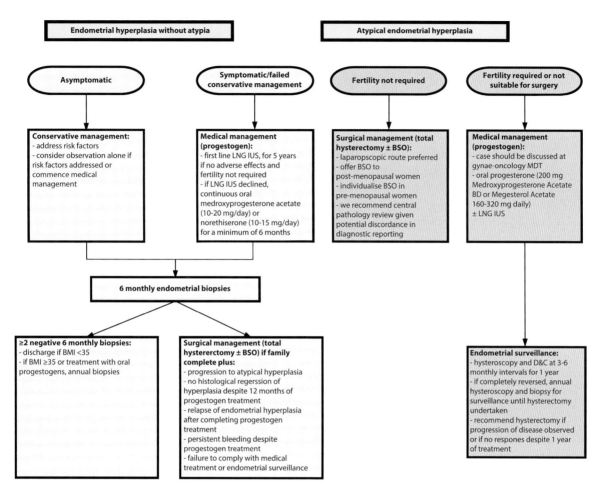

Figure 7.2 Management of endometrial hyperplasia 76, 87

hyperplasia is its precursor lesion. If left untreated, endometrial hyperplasia with atypia can progress to cancer. The commonest presentation of endometrial hyperplasia is abnormal uterine bleeding including heavy menstrual bleeding, intermenstrual bleeding, irregular bleeding, unscheduled bleeding on HRT and postmenopausal bleeding.

Management

The management of endometrial hyperplasia is summarised in Figure 7.2.

The management of endometrial hyperplasia depends upon a number of factors including:

- the risk of developing malignancy
- current symptoms
- fertility issues.

Endometrial hyperplasia without atypia – has a low risk of progression to malignancy, with rates reported as less than 5% over 20 years. The majority of cases regress spontaneously during follow-up. Treatment is commonly in the form of progestogens, which can be administered locally using the intra-uterine Levonorgestrel (LNG) IUS, or oral progestogens. Progestogen treatment is associated with higher regression rates (89–96%) compared with observation alone (74.2–81%). Hysterectomy may be indicated for women who do not wish to preserve their fertility if there is persistence despite 12 months of progestogenic treatment, persistent symptoms or progression to atypical hyperplasia.

Endometrial hyperplasia with atypia – is associated with a higher risk of developing cancer. Approximately 40% of women may already have an

69

underlying malignancy at the time of diagnosis (identified at subsequent hysterectomy). The risk of developing malignancy if left untreated approaches 30% after several years. Due to the risk of underlying malignancy or progression to cancer, a total hysterectomy is advised, preferably laparoscopically where possible.

Those women with atypical hyperplasia who wish to preserve their fertility or who are not fit for surgery can be offered medical management with close surveillance. Pretreatment investigations must be targeted at ruling out malignancy. Management includes the following:

- Adequate histological assessment on hysteroscopy, imaging to assess for malignancy.
- Counselling on the risks of underlying malignancy and progression to cancer
- Treat and optimise risk factors and coexisting morbidity for patients unfit for surgery
- Modify risk factors – weight loss programmes when there is obesity
- Once fertility is no longer required, offer hysterectomy.

First-line medical treatment is with LNG-IUS (Mirena) and/or with oral progestogens. There is limited cohort evidence available regarding regression rates with medical treatment, or as a guide for duration of treatment. Response rates of around 66–74% have been reported. Conservative management should be discontinued in favour of surgery (where possible) if there is no response over 1 year or in those in whom progression is observed. Follow-up is therefore highly individualised, and should include 3 to 6 monthly reviews, including endometrial biopsy, until two consecutive negative biopsies are obtained. Even for women with biopsy-proven regression, long-term follow-up with biopsy at 6–12 monthly intervals is recommended. The indication for hysterectomy should be reviewed at regular intervals.

Serous Tubal Intraepithelial Carcinoma

Pelvic high-grade serous carcinomas (HGSCs) including ovarian, tubal and primary peritoneal carcinomas are presenting at advanced stage, have rapid progression, poor prognosis and high mortality rate. Accumulating evidence suggests that a significant proportion of HGSC arise in the distal end of the fallopian tube and serous tubal intraepithelial carcinomas (STICs) are potential preinvasive or precursor lesions of HGSCs.

Definition of STIC

STIC lesions are limited to the epithelium of the fallopian tube. The histological diagnostic criteria of STIC are as following: a discretely different population of malignant cells replacing the normal tubal epithelium; disorganised growth pattern and lack of cell polarity without ciliated cells; in malignant cells, elevated nuclear-to-cytoplasm ratio with more rounded nuclei; marked nuclear pleomorphism with prominent nucleoli and a high mitotic index and occasionally abnormal mitotic figures.

STIC lesions were first observed in the fimbria of tubes that had been prophylactically removed from women at high risk of developing ovarian cancer due to BRCA1/2 mutations. Approximately 5% of these women undergoing risk-reducing salpingo-oophorectomy (RRSO) have occult STIC and/or invasive lesions and 70% of these lesions occur in the tube but not in the ovary. Also, STICs have been reported in 50–60% of cases of sporadic pelvic HGSCs.

Unlike most other gynaecological preinvasive disease, STIC in itself has no clinical manifestations and is not detectable on imaging. STIC is different from other preinvasive gynaecological disease, as abnormal cells can be shed from the fallopian tube directly onto the ovarian or peritoneal surfaces.

Fallopian Tube Histological Assessment

Thorough examination of the fallopian tubes is vital to maximise identification of STIC lesions. Laboratory protocols have been devised to increase the detection of STIC lesions by pathologists. STIC lesions are located predominantly in the fimbrial end of the tube. Serial sectioning and examination of tubal specimens aims to maximise the proportion of the fallopian tube mucosa that is accessible for microscopic examination.

The classic method is the 'Sectioning and Extensively Examining the Fimbrial End' (SEE-FIM) protocol which is a meticulous protocol mandating that the ampullary portion of the tube is sectioned at 2–3 mm intervals, and the infundibulum separated and sectioned longitudinally to maximise exposure of fimbrial mucosa. The latter increases longitudinal surface area of the fimbria that is examined by approximately 60% versus conventional serial cross-sectioning. The SEE-FIM protocol significantly increases the detection of STIC lesions and occult microinvasive cancers.

Screening for Ovarian Cancer

Ovarian cancer is the fifth most common cause of cancer deaths in women and the commonest cause of deaths from gynaecological cancer in the United Kingdom. Despite recent advances in treatment, long-term survival rates remain disappointing. Screening for ovarian cancer is not currently recommended outside the context of a clinical trial. A couple of randomised-controlled trials (RCTs) have investigated the mortality impact of screening for ovarian cancer in the general (low-risk) population. Following a RCT showing survival benefit from screening, the *Prostate Lung Colorectal and Ovarian Cancer Screening* (PLCO) trial in the United States and the United Kingdom Collaborative Trial on Ovarian Cancer Screening (UKCTOCS) national UK study evaluated the mortality impact of screening low-risk women for ovarian cancer. The PLCO trial recruited 78,216 postmenopausal women and used absolute CA 125 levels and ultrasound scan as their screening tool. This study found no mortality benefit from screening, with only 28% of cancers detected being Stage 1 or 2. Additionally they reported a significantly high complication rate of 15% in women undergoing surgery for abnormalities that had been detected as a result of screening. The UKCTOCS study was a very large RCT of over 200,000 postmenopausal women. This trial evaluated two different screening protocols in a 1:1:2 randomised design compared to controls. The two different screening strategies investigated were (a) annual ultrasound alone and (b) multimodal screening which involved serial CA 125 levels that assessed the change in CA 125 level over time using a customised algorithm called risk of ovarian cancer algorithm (ROCA).

The results of the ROCA-driven multimodal screening appeared encouraging, with 1 in 3 operations per ovarian cancer detected and a much lower complication rate of 3% compared to the PLCO study. Additionally ROCA-based screening led to significantly more ovarian cancers being detected at an earlier stage (40%) compared to controls (26%). Although the primary analysis did not show a significant mortality reduction from screening, statistical modelling provided initial evidence of a potential delayed mortality benefit from multimodal screening.

The UKCTOCS cohort is therefore being followed up till 2020 to establish whether there is a delayed benefit on mortality from ovarian cancer screening.

TIP

There is currently insufficient evidence to recommend a national screening programme for ovarian cancer in low-risk women in the general population.

Hereditary Gynaecological Cancers

Most women with gynaecological malignancy will have a sporadic, rather than an inherited cancer. However, approximately 10% ovarian and 5% endometrial cancers are hereditary. The commonest cancer syndromes encountered in gynaecological practice include:

- Hereditary breast and ovarian cancer (HBOC) syndromes
- Hereditary ovarian cancer (HOC) syndromes
- Lynch syndrome (LS)
- Rarer syndromes including Cowden, Peutz–Jeghers and Li Fraumeni.

Table 7.1 is the summary of hereditary gynaecological cancers.

It is important to identify individuals who may be at risk of gynaecological malignancy through an inherited genetic abnormality, so that measures can be taken to minimise or manage their risk. Traditionally, women at higher risk have been identified by obtaining a detailed family history, usually going back three generations. This should include both maternal and paternal sides of the family, ethnicity, type of cancer, age of onset and age of death. A number of family history-based risk models and clinical criteria have been used to predict mutation probability and detect women at increased risk who would be eligible and should be referred for genetic testing. This approach is entirely dependent on the availability and accuracy of family history.

Genetic testing based on family history alone can miss up to half of all mutations. More recently, strategies such as offering genetic testing at the time of cancer diagnosis have been introduced. Next generation sequencing technologies, coupled with advances in bioinformatics, and computational analysis which incorporate epidemiological and genetic factors are likely to drive significant future developments in risk assessment, prediction and identification of women at higher risk of gynaecological malignancies. This may shift practice towards more population-based approaches of genetic testing, therefore enabling greater access to screening/preventative methods for those at higher risk.

Table 7.1 Summary of syndromes that increase risk of gynaecological cancers

Syndrome	Endometrium	Ovary	Cervix	Breast	Other
Hereditary breast and ovarian cancer (BRCA1, BRCA2)		✓		✓	
Moderate risk ovarian cancer genes: RAD51C, RAD51D, BRIP1		✓			
Lynch	✓		✓		Colon, gastric, ureteral, biliary, pancreatic, glioblastoma
Cowden	✓			✓	Colon, thyroid, benign hamartomas
Peutz–Jeghers		✓	✓	✓	Bowel hamartomas, gastric, pancreatic

Hereditary Breast and/or Ovarian Cancer Syndromes

The most common HOC are associated with mutations in *BRCA1* and *BRCA2* genes, and these are inherited in an autosomal dominant fashion. The prevalence of BRCA1 and BRCA2 mutations in the general population was reported to be around 1 in 400, but recent data suggest even higher estimates than initially suspected of around 1 in 200. These mutations are more common in Ashkenazi Jews. Around 1-in-40 Ashkenazi Jewish individuals carry one of three commonly found Jewish BRCA1/2 mutations called founder mutations. Together BRCA mutations account for approximately 8% to 22% of all non-mucinous high-grade epithelial ovarian cancers. BRCA mutations are associated predominantly with an increased risk of breast and ovarian cancer as follows:

- BRCA1 mutation – approximately 30–50% cumulative risk by age of 70 of ovarian cancer, and 65% risk of breast cancer
- BRCA2 mutation – approximately 10% cumulative risk by age of 70 of ovarian cancer, and 45% risk of breast cancer.

In addition they are also associated with an increased risk of prostate, pancreatic and male breast cancer (the latter two being linked mainly with BRCA2).

The National Institute of Health and Care Excellence (NICE) currently recommends that BRCA1/BRCA2 testing should be offered to men/women who are estimated to have a 10% combined probability of carrying a BRCA1/BRCA2 mutation.

Various scoring systems are available to estimate an individual's chance of carrying a BRCA mutation, based on family history of female/male breast cancers, ovarian cancers, prostate and pancreatic cancers on the same side of the family. Box 7.2 shows an example of risk assessment criteria that is currently used to identify high-risk women in the London familial gynaecological cancer MDT. Different family history criteria exist for the Jewish population due to the higher prevalence of BRCA1/2 mutations in them.

It is also important to differentiate between diagnostic and predictive genetic testing:

- **Diagnostic genetic testing** is a test carried out to identify a mutation in the family for the first time and is usually carried out on the individual affected with cancer.
- **Predictive genetic testing** is offered to unaffected family members and is a targeted test for a specific pathogenic mutation, which has been identified in another family member.

> **TIP**
> This unselected cancer case series-based genetic testing in epithelial ovarian cancer is now advocated by NHS England and a number of international bodies such as the Society of Gynaecological Oncology and American College of Obstetricians & Gynaecologists.

Population testing: The Ashkenazi Jewish population is the first population for whom population testing (irrespective of family history) for BRCA1/BRCA2 mutations may become a future reality. This has been evaluated in three large studies including a UK randomised trial. This can identify >50% more carriers, does not detrimentally effect quality-of-life or psychological health and is cost-effective for the NHS. This approach is supported and advocated by many experts and patient groups.

Box 7.2 Criteria to identify high-risk families (London Cancer MDT)

Volunteer/proband should either have been affected by cancer or be a first-degree relative (FDR) of an affected family member. Affected relatives should be on the same side of the family (i.e. maternal or paternal)

Families with ovarian[a] or ovarian[a] and breast cancer

>2 individuals with ovarian cancer (any age) who are FDR

1 ovarian cancer (any age) and 1 breast cancer <50 who are FDR

1 ovarian cancer (any age) and 2 breast cancers <60 who are FDR

Breast cancer in volunteer/proband and FDR with both breast and ovarian cancer (in the same person)

Woman with both breast and ovarian cancer (in the same person)

The first three criteria can be modified where paternal transmission is occurring, i.e. families where affected relatives are related by second through an unaffected intervening male relative and there is an affected sister eligible

Families with a known gene mutation

The family contains an affected individual with a mutation in one of the known ovarian/endometrial cancer predisposing genes, e.g. BRCA1, BRCA2, MLH1, MSH2, MSH6, PMS2, PTEN, STK11/LKB1

LS/HNPCC Families

The family contains three or more individuals with a LS or HNPCC-related cancer,[b] who are FDR and >1 case is diagnosed before 50 years and the cancers affect >1 generation (Amsterdam Criteria-II)

Molecular (IHC/MSI) analysis of unselected colorectal and endometrial cancer cases is recommended to identify those who can have MMR gene testing[c]

Families with only breast cancer

4 breast cancers in the family (any ages)

3 breast cancers related by FDR:

(i) 1 <30 years or
(ii) 2 <40 years or
(iii) All <60 years or
(iv) 1 male breast cancer (MBC) and 2 breast cancers <60 years

Breast cancer in volunteer/proband (<50 years) and:

(i) Breast cancer in mother (age of onset being <30 years) or
(ii) Bilateral breast cancer in mother (<40 years onset) or
(iii) 1 FDR with MBC

MBC in the family and proband is a FDR of one of them

Families with Ashkenazi Jewish (AJ) or Polish ancestry[d]

Female breast cancer diagnosed <50

FDR with female breast cancer diagnosed <50

Male BRCA-related cancer (breast/prostate/pancreas) any age

FDR with male breast cancer

Women with non-mucinous invasive high-grade epithelial ovarian cancer (EOC)

Women with invasive non-mucinous high-grade EOC regardless of family history/ethnicity

Women with triple negative (TN) breast cancer <50 years

Women with TN breast cancer <50 years

Manchester Scoring System

Manchester Score ≥15

---

[a]History of tubal/primary peritoneal cancers may be considered equivalent to ovarian cancer.
[b]LS or HNPCC related cancers include colorectal, endometrial, small bowel, ureteric and renal pelvic cancers.
[c]While this is recommended, practice varies with centres offering testing in cases under 50, under 60 or at all ages. In practice, testing is more well established in colorectal cancers than endometrial cancers.
[d]BRCA Founder mutation testing only.

Moderate-Risk Genetic Mutations for HOC

In addition to BRCA1/2, newer moderate risk genes have been identified that are associated with an increased risk of ovarian cancer (but not breast cancer). These genes, with their cumulative risk of ovarian cancer by the age of 70 years, are as follows:

- RAD51C – approximately 11%
- RAD51D – approximately 12%
- BRIP1 – approximately 6%.

Testing for these genes is gradually being introduced into clinical practice.

Additionally, a number of lower penetrance or common genetic variants or single nucleotide polymorphisms (SNPs) have been identified and found to

be associated with breast and ovarian cancers in several genome-wide association studies. While the absolute level of risk of cancer with each individual SNP is very small, it is believed that the presence of combinations of SNPs along with other epidemiological factors in any one individual may push up the risk to a high enough level warranting clinical intervention. This is still a matter of ongoing research.

Targeted Therapy for Genetic Cancers

Identification of inherited genetic mutations is also helpful in targeting cancer treatment for those with cancer. For example, studies have shown that women with BRCA-associated ovarian cancers who develop recurrent disease show improved progression-free survival with poly(ADP-ribose) polymerase (PARP) inhibitors such as Olaparib. Therefore, routine testing of all women with high-grade non-mucinous epithelial ovarian cancers for BRCA mutations will guide treatment decisions and potentially enable recruitment into clinical trials.

> **TIPS**
> Testing for genetic mutations is helpful to inform family members of their risks, to help them access screening or prevention strategies. Additionally it is also beneficial to the affected individual as they may benefit from targeted therapies.

Risk-Reducing Strategies

Genetic testing for hereditary cancers identifies women at significant risk of developing malignancy. These women have the opportunity to reduce their risk of cancer, and should be offered appropriate information and advice. These issues are complex, and are best managed within specialist clinics by multidisciplinary professionals who may be clinical geneticists, gynaecological oncologists, breast surgeons, psychologists and genetic counsellors. The decision-making process is very individual for each woman and her family. Counselling should cover:

- Advice on their personal risk of developing malignancy
- Lifestyle advice to lessen their risks, such as the benefits of the oral contraceptive pill and breast feeding
- Symptom awareness – Department of health ovarian cancer symptom index
- The option of risk-reducing surgery for ovarian cancer and advice on HRT where appropriate
- The current lack of a national screening programme for ovarian cancer
- Screening and risk-reducing mastectomy for breast cancer via specialist or family history breast clinics
- Chemoprevention (tamoxifen or anastrazole) options for women at significant risk of breast cancer
- The possibility of assisted reproduction and preimplantation genetic diagnosis for women planning a family who wish to prevent passing the gene mutation on to their children.

Risk-Reducing Salpingo-Oophorectomy

Women at a high risk of ovarian cancer can opt for RRSO, after they have completed their family. This has been shown to reduce the risk of EOC by 80–96% in BRCA1/2 mutation carriers. However, this approach does not eliminate risk completely, and women must be advised that their residual risk of primary peritoneal cancer is approximately 2–4%. The age at which surgery is offered depends on a woman's fertility aspirations, the type of mutation she has and the age of onset of ovarian cancer in her relatives. A BRCA1 mutation carrier's risk of ovarian cancer increases significantly from the age of 35, and therefore RRSO is offered from age 35 to 40 years, once her family is complete. BRCA2 mutation carriers are offered RRSO later, from the age 40 to 45 years, as their risk begins to rise at the age of 40 years and increases significantly from age 45 years. Surgery may also be offered up to 5 years before the earliest onset of ovarian cancer in the family. However, the timing of RRSO needs to be individualised to the patient, and decision making can be a complex process. Surgery should only be undertaken once women have completed their family. Women should be adequately counselled regarding the effects of iatrogenic menopause and its detrimental effects on cardiovascular, bone, neurological and psychosexual health. HRT should be offered to premenopausal women until the age of 50, unless they have a personal history of breast cancer. For women with a history of breast cancer, HRT is usually contraindicated but this should be discussed on a case-by-case basis with the breast oncology team.

Approximately 5% BRCA women undergoing RRSO are found to have an occult in situ/invasive cancer at histological examination of their tubes or ovaries. These cases should be managed by the MDT, and may need a further surgery for full staging. Approximately 70% of these occult lesions are found in the tube rather than the ovary.

RRSO may also be offered to women with RAD51C, RAD51D, BRIP1 mutations and BRCA-negative women with a very strong family history of 'ovarian' or 'ovarian and breast' cancer but no identified mutation in the family. It may be delayed in women with BRIP1 mutations till 50 years.

> **TIPS**
> Risk reducing salpingo-oophorectomy is the most effective strategy to prevent ovarian cancer in high-risk women. Furthermore, it has been thought to reduce the risk of breast cancer in premenopausal women, but recently conflicting data showing no reduction in risk have also been published.

Risk-Reducing Early Salpingectomy with Delayed Oophorectomy

It is a relatively recent approach that has been proposed due to increasing evidence that the fallopian tube, rather than the ovary, may be the site of origin of a large proportion of epithelial ovarian cancer. Risk-reducing early salpingectomy with delayed oophorectomy (RRESDO) has been proposed as an attractive alternative to RRSO; surgery is performed as a two-stage procedure where the tubes are removed first, then the ovaries are removed at a later date when ovarian function is no longer required. This has the potential advantage of offering some level of risk reduction (by removing the tubes) to those women who still require or desire ovarian function. However, at present there is insufficient data available to support this approach in routine practice. The precise level of risk reduction and long-term consequences on ovarian function are unknown. Therefore, RRESDO should only be offered within the context of a clinical trial. Trials are currently underway in the Netherlands, France, the United States and a UK study is expected to start by the end of 2017.

Screening for Ovarian Cancer in High-Risk Women

A national screening programme for ovarian cancer is currently unavailable for women at high familial risk of ovarian cancer. The United Kingdom Familial Ovarian Cancer Screen Study (UKFOCSS) was a large cohort screening study of ~4,300 high-risk UK women who had declined RRSO. Phase 2 of the study used a ROCA-driven four-monthly CA125 and annual ultrasound scan-based screening strategy. A similar strategy was adopted in the US GOG and CGN trial. Results from the UKFOCSS Phase-2 study published earlier this year showed women who were undergoing screening had significantly lower stage 1–3a disease and were also more likely to achieve complete macroscopic resection of disease (zero residual disease) at surgery. While these data appear promising and suggest potential benefit of four-monthly longitudinal CA 125 algorithm-based screening, more research is awaited.

Lynch Syndrome

LS, formerly known as hereditary nonpolyposis colorectal carcinoma (HNPCC) is an autosomal dominant inheritable condition associated with a broad spectrum of malignancies:

- Approximately 60% risk of colorectal cancer
- Approximately 40–60% risk of endometrial cancer
- Approximately 10% risk of epithelial ovarian cancer
- Other malignancies are less common, but include increased risk of stomach, bowel, hepatobiliary, ureteric, renal pelvic and brain cancers.

LS is caused by germ-line mutations in one of the DNA mismatch repair (MMR) genes including *MSH2*, *MLH1*, *MSH6* and *PMS2*. Unlike *BRCA*-associated ovarian cancers, which are usually high-grade late-stage serous tumours, Lynch-related ovarian carcinomas are often early stage and moderately or well differentiated. LS also has a greater likelihood of synchronous endometrial and ovarian tumours. Cancer risks may vary depending on which gene is impaired. *MLH1* gene mutations are associated with higher risk of colorectal cancer at younger age compared to *MSH2* and *MSH6* carriers. For *MSH6* gene mutation carriers, the risk of endometrial cancer appears to be higher. Overall, there seems to be a lower cancer risk associated with PMS2, with up to 20% for colorectal cancer and 15% for endometrial cancer.

Identification of Individuals at Risk for LS

Family history-based criteria have been developed to help identify individuals at risk for LS, including the Amsterdam Criteria-II (Box 7.2). LS should be suspected in patients with colorectal/endometrial cancer <50 years, lower uterine segment endometrial cancers, synchronous tumours, multiple LS-associated tumours and in cases where there is familial clustering of LS-associated cancers.

Diagnostic Testing

Germline testing for all patients suspected of having LS is currently extremely expensive. Therefore, initial genetic evaluation of the tumour itself is recommended in the first instance. The tumour is evaluated for MMR proteins by immunohistochemistry (IHC) and/or microsatellite instability. Those patients with tumours that show characteristics typical of LS are then selected for germline testing. Direct germline testing may be appropriate in selected high-risk individuals in cases where tumour tissue itself is not available. Bethesda criteria were earlier used to select patients for tumour testing. However, now unselected tumour testing of colorectal cancers is recommended in the NHS for ascertainment of LS. A similar approach is needed for endometrial cancers.

Risk Reduction for Endometrial and Ovarian Cancer in LS

More than 75% of carriers who develop endometrial cancer present with stage I disease, and the 5-year survival rate can be as high as 88%. Although the evidence base is limited, screening may allow for detection of early-stage endometrial cancers in asymptomatic premenopausal women. Annual transvaginal pelvic ultrasound with hysteroscopy and endometrial biopsy from the age of 35 has been recommended in women with LS. Aspirin is recommended for reducing cancer risk in LS. The optimum dose is being evaluated in the CAPP-3 study. Other principles like lifestyle advice and preimplantation genetic diagnosis described earlier should also be considered in LS.

Risk-reducing hysterectomy and bilateral salpingo-oophorectomy surgery is effective for preventing endometrial and ovarian cancers in women with LS. This should be offered after women have completed their family, usually after the age of 40 years. The residual risk of primary peritoneal cancer in this population is extremely low (unlike BRCA1/2 carriers). HRT is recommended in premenopausal women until the age of approximately 50, to minimise the risks of early menopause.

Screening for colorectal cancer should be also offered and arranged through specialist genetic clinics.

Cowden Syndrome

Cowden syndrome (CS) is an autosomal dominant condition secondary to mutations in the tumour suppressor phosphatase and tensin gene *PTEN*. CS is a relatively rare cancer predisposition syndrome characterised by macrocephaly, multiple hamartomas and an increased risk of several benign and malignant tumours, in particular breast, thyroid and endometrial, but also colorectal, melanoma and renal cell carcinoma. The lifetime risk of developing endometrial cancer is around 30%, breast cancer 50% and thyroid cancer 10%. It is not associated with an increased risk of ovarian cancer. Women can be offered prophylactic hysterectomy with ovarian conservation once their family is complete. Annual hysteroscopy-based screening has been offered on an individual basis in women who decline or are unable to undergo risk-reducing surgery.

Peutz–Jeghers Syndrome

Peutz–Jeghers syndrome (PJS) is an autosomal dominant gastrointestinal polyposis disorder caused by a mutation in the *STK11/LKB1*. This leads to an increased risk of breast, gastrointestinal, cervical and sex cord stromal ovarian tumours. Clinical manifestations are characteristic pigmented lesions on the lips and buccal mucosa, which should prompt clinicians to consider the underlying diagnosis. Screening for cervical cancer is offered from the age of 18 with annual cervical smears.

Further Reading

Evans D, Lalloo F, Wallace A. Update on the Manchester Scoring System, *J Med Genet* 2005; 42(7): e39.

Gaba FM, Manchanda R. Genetic testing for gynaecological cancer, *Obstetrics Gynaecol Reprod Med* 2017; 27(1): 29–31.

Manchanda R, Jacobs I. Genetic screening for gynecological cancer: where are we heading? *Future Oncol* 2016; 12(2): 207–20. Review.

NICE. *Familial Breast Cancer: Classification, Care and Managing Breast Cancer and Related Risks in People with a Family History of Breast Cancer*. National Institute for Health and Care Excellence, London, 2013 (CG164).

Public Health England. *NHS Cervical Screening Programme: Colposcopy and programme management*. NHSCSP Publication number 20, London, 2016.

RCOG. *Endometrial Hyperplasia, Management of (Green-top Guideline No. 67)*. Royal College of Obstetrics & Gynaecology, London, 2016.

Surgical Principles in Gynaecological Oncology

Jane Borley and Maria Kyrgiou

Introduction

Gynaecological oncology surgery encompasses a wide range of procedures including open ultra-radical debulking surgery, advanced laparoscopic procedures and reconstructive vulval and groin surgery. There are common underlying principles that are relevant to all surgical procedures within and outside of gynaecology, alongside principles that are more specific to gynaecological cancer operations. This chapter provides a review of surgical principles in the context of gynaecological cancer surgery. Other perioperative principles will be reviewed, including surgical complications, peri- and postoperative care, enhanced recovery (ER) and special issues relating to challenging patients.

Basics of Surgical Principles

Box 8.1 provides a comprehensive summary of basic principles that should be considered when undertaking surgery.

Preoperative, Intraoperative and Postoperative Issues

Preoperative

Preoperative assessment and optimisation are essential in gynaecological oncology patients as they are, in general, likely to be older with more complex comorbidities than the general gynaecological surgical patient. Thorough history-taking is essential to identify significant comorbidities which may have an impact on surgical planning, postoperative care and identification of potential intra- and postoperative complications.

Several preoperative investigations may be necessary to identify risks and to identify those whose clinical condition needs to be optimised prior to surgery.

Preoperative investigations may include
- Routine blood tests
  - Full blood count – to identify anaemia, to ensure recovery of neutrophils in chemotherapy patients, etc.
  - Renal function – especially in those with signs of renal obstruction
  - Clotting – in those malnourished or at risk of bleeding
  - Group and save – to identify those with atypical antibodies which may interfere with availability of cross-matched blood for transfusion
  - LFTs – to assess preoperative albumin reflecting nutritional status in patients undergoing extensive surgery such as ultra-radical surgery for advanced ovarian cancer or exenterative surgery for recurrent cancer
- Chest X-ray – especially for those at risk of pleural effusion
- HbA1c and random glucose – for those with diabetes
- Electrocardiogram
- Lung function tests
- Echocardiogram
- Pregnancy test – in all of those of child-bearing age.

A detailed discussion of the individual patient's needs and expectations preoperatively will help determine an individualised patient approach. For example, a discussion on the impact of treatment on fertility and the availability of fertility-sparing options is vital in young women. The contribution of the Clinical Nurse Specialist from the start of the process cannot be understated. In addition, the opportunity for patients to have access to verbal and written, procedure-specific, patient information has been associated with reduced need for pain relief and improved patient satisfaction.

Box 8.1 Basic surgical principles

Know your patient:

- Understand the patient's oncology diagnosis and presumed stage of disease.
- Appreciate the patient's complexities, comorbidities and anaesthetic challenges.
- Understand the emotional and psychological challenges of living with an oncology diagnosis and the side effects of any treatment they are receiving.

Choose your procedure:

- Several management and surgical approaches may be possible for each individual case. It is important for the surgeon to take into consideration the patient morbidities and the surgical procedure required in order to achieve the optimal outcome with minimal morbidity.
- Understand the aims that the operation is trying to achieve, for example curative versus palliative.
- Consider fertility-sparing approaches when appropriate.
- Use input from the multidisciplinary team, as radiological features and anaesthetic review may change the course of action.

Know your anatomy:

- An excellent understanding of the anatomical structures and individual variations is necessary for all types of surgery.
- In gynaecological oncology surgery further knowledge of lymphatic drainage, retroperitoneal and upper abdominal anatomy is required.
- Anatomical structures can often be distorted because of disease. The ability to define those structures is necessary to avoid complications and inadvertent organ injury.

Know your equipment and energy sources:

- A good understanding of the equipment and energy sources is essential to ensure safety and to minimise the risk of thermal injuries to anatomical structures.
- It is the responsibility of the surgeon to understand the equipment and risks involved.
- The surgeon should have the ability to troubleshoot if malfunctions arise in the equipment.

Apply good surgical techniques:

- Basic surgical techniques apply in all surgical procedures. This includes handling of instruments and tissue, identification of

surgical planes, correct knot tying and the ability to identify anatomical structures. This is especially important in cancer surgery, which can involve major structures such as the aorta and vena cava.

Understand your limitations:

- The ability to recognise personal limitations in skills and to call for help from a more specialised surgeon in the field is essential to optimise safety and achieve good outcomes for the patients.
- Overconfidence may be harmful to patients.
- Multidisciplinary surgical teams may be required for individual cases and may involve hepato-biliary, gastrointestinal (GI), vascular and urology surgeons.
- When learning new techniques it is important to understand the impact of learning curve for new procedures, and to ensure the appropriate governance issues in relation to new procedures have been addressed within the hospital.

Develop a good theatre team:

- A well-functioning theatre team that understands the steps of the procedure is important for good outcomes.
- The surgical team comprises of the surgeon, the assistants, the anaesthetist and the nursing staff.
- The surgeon should give feedback to the anaesthetist and theatre team if a complication, such as severe bleeding, occurs to allow them to prepare the equipment and take appropriate action.

Take appropriate consent:

- The patient needs to understand the proposed procedure, the alternatives (if any), the risks and possible complications, and should have time to reflect on the information received. This may require more than one visit, and is highly individualised to each patient.
- The consent should be taken by someone competent in performing the procedure who understands the risks and recovery to counsel the patient appropriately.

Recognise and treat complications early:

- Complications are inevitable in surgery.
- The ability to recognise and manage complications gives the best outcome to patients.
- A good understanding and raised awareness of the possible complications that can occur is necessary.

Optimisation of the patient prior to surgery may require the following:

- Drainage of pleural effusions – to allow adequate ventilation during surgery, reduction in postoperative hypoxia and lower respiratory tract infections
- Inferior vena caval filter insertion – may be considered in those with a recent diagnosis of venous thromboembolism (VTE)
- Conversion of oral anticoagulation such as warfarin to more controllable injectable low-molecular-weight heparin

- Optimisation of chronic diseases such as diabetes, hypertension and respiratory disease by medication review
- Improving nutritional status of the patient who has been on chemotherapy and is being considered for ultra-radical surgery.

TIP
Detailed discussion of an individual patient's needs and expectations preoperatively can determine a tailored approach to treatment.

Other considerations – Management of the immediate pre-operative period is important to ensure that the patient remains well and enters surgery in an optimal condition. Surgical stress in the presence of fasting worsens the catabolic state, increases insulin resistance and may impair postoperative recovery. Preoperative complex carbohydrate drinks are recommended in those without diabetes and have been shown to significantly improve insulin resistance. Patients also feel more comfortable with a reduction in pre- and postoperative thirst, hunger, anxiety and nausea. Preventing dehydration by allowing the patient to drink free fluids up to 2 hours prior to induction and the use of intravenous fluids when necessary will also improve outcomes.

Bowel preparation – Mechanical bowel preparation to clear the bowel prior to surgery has not been shown to improve patient outcomes in either colorectal or benign gynaecological surgery. There is currently no evidence on the use of bowel preparation in ultra-radical ovarian cancer debulking surgery. Individual surgeons may opt to use bowel preparation in selected cases due to concerns with faecal contamination, infection risk and anastomotic leak. Its use should be at the discretion of the operating team. Polyethylene glycol electrolyte lavage solutions and sodium phosphate are the most commonly used preparations. Adequate fluid resuscitation is important to avoid dehydration caused by its effects.

Intraoperative Issues, Complications and How to Avoid Them

A good surgical technique, together with knowledge of anatomy and experience, will help reduce intraoperative complications. In cancer patients, anatomy is often distorted or adjacent viscera may be involved with disease and partial visceral resection may be a necessary consequence of surgery.

Visceral Injury

Bowel

The large or small bowel may be injured during surgery within the abdominal cavity. Small bowel injury may arise due to adhesions from previous infection or surgery. It may be adherent to the anterior abdominal wall and sustain injury at the time of abdominal opening. Serosal injury can be easily recognised and repaired simply with continuous or interrupted dissolvable sutures. When closing the defect care must be taken to ensure the lumen width is not compromised, therefore sutures should be perpendicular to the length of the bowel. For larger areas of damage, resection and primary anastomosis by use of gastrointestinal stapling devices are recommended.

The large bowel may be damaged by adhesions or disease. For example, the transverse colon itself or vessels within the mesentery may be injured during the dissection of a large omental metastasis. In the pelvis, the rectosigmoid may be adherent to the uterus from adhesions, disease or endometriosis. As the large bowel contains pathogens, healing of the injured large bowel can be less successful than of the small bowel and consequently the risk of bowel leak is higher. Serosal defects can be oversewn but more extensive injuries may require resection and primary anastomosis, with or without defunctioning colostomy or ileostomy. Defunctioning stomas may be reversed in 3 to 6 months depending on overall prognosis and response to adjuvant treatment.

Faecal peritonitis can be fatal, especially if the diagnosis is delayed. Postoperative attention to early identification of any anastomotic leaks is crucial. Signs may include an acute rigid abdomen, fever, tachycardia, rising inflammatory markers, elevated lactate levels and green discolouration of drain contents. Urgent imaging such as CT abdomen and pelvis should be performed if there is concern. A high index of suspicion is essential to prevent delayed diagnosis.

Urinary Tract

The bladder is often adherent to the lower segment of the uterus after previous caesarean section. It may also be necessary to strip the entire pelvic peritoneum from the bladder in women with peritoneal tumour deposits.

A bladder injury which is located away from the ureteric orifices should be repaired in two layers with a continuous absorbable suture. However if the defect is situated close to the ureteric orifices, it may be necessary to stent the ureters first. Continuous drainage of the bladder with a Foley catheter for 10–14 days is required to allow healing and closure. Prior to removing the indwelling catheter, a retrograde cystogram will determine whether full closure has been achieved.

The ureter is at risk of injury during pelvic surgery. It runs close to the infundibular pelvic ligament and then passes underneath the uterine artery midway along its length. The path of the ureter can be distorted by fibrosis, adhesions, endometriosis or tumour and should always be identified and carefully dissected if necessary to prevent injury. Radical hysterectomy requires complete dissection of the ureter, and there is a risk of devascularisation injury in these cases. There may also be situations where the ureter is obstructed by tumour and firmly adherent to a mass that needs removal. In these cases, ureteric resection may be required. Ureteric stents can be placed cystoscopically to help identify the ureter during surgery, or in cases of potential devascularisation they may be placed to prevent stricture and stenosis.

A partially or completely transected ureter can be repaired with 3.0 or 4.0 absorbable suture and insertion of a stent. Spatulation of both ends of a completely transected ureter helps avoid the development of stenosis. If a complete transection occurs close to the bladder, reimplantation of the spatulated ureter may be required. It may be necessary to mobilise the bladder to allow the ureter to reach without tension.

Early identification of a bladder or ureteric leak is necessary in the postoperative period to minimise complications from uraemia. Haematuria, excessive drain output or a rising blood creatinine may be the first signs. Drain fluid can be sent for biochemical analysis. A significantly elevated creatinine level in the fluid will confirm the presence of urine. Definitive confirmation of injury requires imaging such as a CT urogram. Renal obstruction may arise as a consequence of ureteric injury or obstruction and may need to be managed by emergency insertion of a nephrostomy, retrograde ureteric stenting or reimplantation.

Haemorrhage

Haemorrhage can arise from any of the major vessels in the pelvis. Direct haemorrhage can occur from the vascular pedicles as a result of poor surgical technique or inadequate knot tying. When tying pedicles, it is important not to exert too much traction and cause avulsion of the vessel. Damage to the larger vessels can occur because of closely adherent tumour or lymph nodes. Direct damage to a large vein or artery can occur at lymphadenectomy. Veins are more susceptible to injury as they are less robust than the major arteries. Direct suturing with 4.0 (or finer) monofilament nonabsorbable sutures is necessary. If the defect is greater than 2–3 mm in width, it may occasionally be necessary to position a vascular clamp across the defect to allow visualisation and direct suturing. Each suture must pass through the full thickness of the vessel wall.

In a narrow operative field such as obturator fossa, it may not be possible to place a suture. Surgical ligaclips can be applied when the bleeding vessel is clearly identified and isolated.

In addition to stopping the bleeding, adequate resuscitation is necessary in major haemorrhage. Red blood cells and clotting products such as fresh frozen plasma, platelets and cryofibrinogen will be necessary. Various haemostatic products are available to help with general oozing from a surgical bed but they will be ineffective against arterial bleeding.

> **TIP**
> An excellent knowledge of anatomical structures and individual variations is vital for good outcomes of surgery.

Postoperative Issues, Complications and How to Avoid Them

Early mobilisation is key to the immediate postoperative period. It prevents muscle loss and weakness, improves lung function, tissue oxygenation and reduces the risk of VTE disease. Patients should be encouraged to feed early and reduce intravenous fluids when possible.

Infection and Antibiotic Prophylaxis

The development of postoperative surgical infection is the most common complication of gynaecological surgical procedures. Before the advent of routine antimicrobial prophylaxis, the risk of developing a pelvic infection was thought to be as high as 30%. With antibiotic prophylaxis, these rates have decreased to 2.7%.

Gynaecological surgery remains a unique challenge due to the pathogenic microorganisms, which can ascend from the vagina and endocervix. In addition, the frequent need for bowel surgery in ovarian cancer debulking surgery increases this risk. Risk factors for postoperative infection are also common traits in gynaecological oncology patients and procedures (Box 8.2).

Common organisms include the aerobes, *Staphylococcus aureus*, *Staphylococcus epidermidis*, Group B streptococcus, *Enterococcus faecalis*, *Escherichia coli* and the anaerobes *Bacteroides* sp.

Antibiotic prophylaxis at the time of anaesthetic induction, before the incision is made, should be given for all major gynaecology–oncology procedures.

Box 8.2 Risk factors for postoperative complications

- Obesity
- Radical surgery
- Excessive intraoperative blood loss
- Prolonged operative time
- Diabetes mellitus
- Poor nutrition
- Immunosuppression

Box 8.3 Risk factors for VTE

- Surgical pelvic procedures lasting >60 minutes
- Active cancer or cancer treatment
- Age >60 years
- Dehydration
- Critical care admission
- Obesity
- One or more significant comorbidities
- Use of hormone replacement therapy
- Use of oestrogen-containing contraception
- Personal history of first-degree relative with VTE

This has been shown to reduce postoperative surgical site infections. Prophylactic antibiotics should have broad-spectrum cover and the choice of agents will depend on individual unit protocols based on local patient population commensals and resistance patterns. An example would include Cefuroxime 1.5 g and Metronidazole 500 mg, or Clindamycin 600 mg and Gentamicin 5 mg/kg in penicillin allergic patients. Repeated doses should be administered in patients who have a long operative procedure, or who experience major haemorrhage. Preoperative preparation of the skin and vagina with Povidone–Iodine or chlorhexidine gluconate is also crucial to minimise the risk of infection.

Venous Thromboembolism and Prophylaxis

Complex pelvic surgery is a major risk factor for developing VTE. Gynaecological cancer patients frequently have additional risk factors for VTE and thromboprophylaxis is essential in order to reduce risk (Box 8.3).

Thromboprophylaxis with low-molecular-weight heparin and thromboembolic deterrent (TED) stockings is recommended. Wherever there are risk factors for bleeding conditions such as thrombophilias, lumbar puncture/epidural within the last 4 hours or expected in the next 12 hours, thrombocytopenia or active bleeding, other devices such as intermittent pneumatic compression boots may be utilised.

Surgery may need to be postponed for those with a recent diagnosis of VTE, and may be an indication for neoadjuvant chemotherapy over primary debulking surgery in ovarian cancer patients. Use of inferior vena-cava filters can be considered as these have been shown to reduce the risk of pulmonary embolism in those where anticoagulation is contraindicated. However, they do not reduce mortality in the acute cancer-related thrombosis setting. In complex cases, specialist advice from a haematologist and/or interventional radiologist may be helpful.

Postoperative Pain and Analgesia

Adequate control of postoperative pain is essential for patient comfort, to allow early mobilisation, quicker discharge from hospital, a reduction in postoperative atelectasis and subsequent lower respiratory tract infections. Pain relief should be discussed with the patient by the anaesthetic team prior to surgery, and when appropriate be guided by patient's choice. There are a variety of different methods of pain control, including intravenous opioid patient-controlled analgesia (PCA), spinal and epidural analgesia and transversus abdominis plane (TAP) block. Review by the acute pain team in the immediate postoperative period will optimise pain management.

Enhanced recovery (also known as 'fast track', 'rapid' or 'accelerated recovery') is a model which aims to reduce the physical and psychological impact of elective surgery on patients. In doing so, this helps promote a quicker recovery, shortened length of hospital stay and improved return to normal activity and has been demonstrated to be associated with increased patient satisfaction (Box 8.4).

ER is based on three main principles:

1. The patient is in the best possible condition for surgery.
2. The patient has the best possible management during and after her operation.
3. The patient experiences the best postoperative rehabilitation.

Incision Types (Advantages/Disadvantages)

The choice of surgical incision is of major importance in gynaecological oncology surgery. The choice of

Preoperative

- Adequate assessment of comorbidities, previous surgery
- Confirmation of treatment required and possible complications
- Ensure adequate patient information available
- Optimisation of patient – changes to medications, drainage of pleural effusions, etc.

Perioperative

- Avoid dehydration by allowing patients to drink freely up to 2 hours prior to anaesthesia
- Use of complex carbohydrate drinks
- Careful use of bowel preparation
- Avoidance of long-acting sedative premedication
- Use of minimal access techniques whenever possible
- Routine use of nasogastric tubes and abdominal drains should be avoided
- Avoidance of intraoperative hypothermia
- Goal-directed fluid therapy using stroke volume

Postoperative

- Early feeding
- Reduce the volume of routine intravenous fluids
- Early mobilisation
- Remove catheters, drains, vaginal packs to encourage mobilisation

Discharge

- Discharge patients when mobile, pain well-controlled, passed flatus and able to eat and drink
- Consider laxatives
- Consider discharge with catheter in situ when necessary
- Provide written information for emergency contact details and practical postoperative advice

surgical approach (open or laparoscopic) and incision can only be made when the tumour sites, extent of the disease, patient characteristics and the surgical procedure and objective have been clearly defined and assessed carefully (Box 8.5).

Open Abdominal Incisions

The choice of abdominal incision in open gynaecological oncology surgery depends on the tumour site and procedure, the stage and expected extent of disease, the anatomical structures that need to be exposed, the patient's risk factors and characteristics (body mass index (BMI), risk of wound dehiscence, previous abdominal scars, etc.).

Box 8.5 Principles to follow when making the choice of the approach and site of incision

- The incision should allow adequate visualisation of the anatomical structures to allow safe completion of the objectives of the surgery
- The procedure and safety should not be compromised by the surgical approach or site of incision
- The access to the surgical site should be adequate
- The incisions should be based on anatomical principles

The abdominal incisions are broadly divided into (A) vertical, (B) transverse and (C) other incisions (Figure 8.1).

(A) **Vertical incisions** – In gynaecological cancer surgery, a *midline incision* is mainly used, particularly for debulking surgery in ovarian cancer. *Vertical incisions* allow good visualisation of the peritoneal cavity and give flexibility as they can be extended if required to gain access to the upper abdomen. Although a midline incision provides excellent surgical exposure, this incision has an increased risk of postoperative complications when compared to transverse incisions, such as wound infection, dehiscence and incisional hernias. Appropriate skill in closure is necessary to minimise these complications. Upon closure, a delayed absorbable suture such as looped PDS (polydioxanone) should be used. The suture should include at least 1 cm of sheath from the fascial edge with no more than 1 cm distance from each continuous bite. Two or more sutures may be required for large incisions. Mass closure with a slowly absorbable monofilament suture minimises the risk of dehiscence and herniation. The tensile strength of the rectus sheath never fully recovers after a midline incision, with the regained strength being 50–60% at 6 weeks and 93% at 18 months postoperative. In the past, surgeons used the *paramedian incision* to minimise the complications of midline incision (that injures the weakest part of the abdominal wall). The use of modern suture materials and mass closure have more recently minimised this need, and this approach is rarely used.

(B) **Transverse incisions (suprapubic transverse or Pfannenstiel)** – These were used commonly in the past in gynaecological cancer surgery as these incisions are largely strong, at low risk of

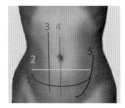

1   Pfannenstiel incision
2   Maylard incision
3   Paramedian incision
4   Midline incision
5   Modified Gibson incision

Figure 8.1 Abdominal incisions used in gynaecological oncology surgery

dehiscence, follow the anatomical dermatomes and heal well within the skin creases, although access to the upper abdomen is limited. Recent advances in minimal access surgery have largely replaced the transverse incision, as the majority of procedures that were previously performed through these incisions are now carried out laparoscopically. Although transverse incisions are relatively uncommon in modern practice of gynaecological oncology surgery, they are still used in obstetrics, benign gynaecology and in cases of endometrial or cervical cancer surgery with large uterine size where intact removal of the uterus is not feasible with laparoscopy and morcellation is contraindicated. A modification of the suprapubic transverse incision, the *Maylard incision*, provides better access when necessary as the rectus muscle is divided and the inferior epigastric vessels are ligated.

(C)   **The modified Gibson incision** – This is used to gain extraperitoneal access to the pelvic sidewall but is not used frequently in gynaecological oncology surgery. Extraperitoneal pelvic and para-aortic lymph node dissections are now commonly performed laparoscopically.

Laparoscopic Incisions

The choice of laparoscopic surgical approach is preferable in certain tumour sites such as cervical and endometrial cancer. Minimal access surgery has been associated with improved recovery, reduced pain, smaller scars and wound complications and better visualisation of the operative field for some cancers, without compromise to the surgical and oncological outcomes (Box 8.6).

(A)   Two different *entry techniques and incisions* for the creation of pneumoperitoneum are mainly used in laparoscopic surgery: the closed (Veress needle) and the open (Hasson) technique. There is no agreement on which approach is superior; however surgeons should be able to use either of these if needed. The open technique is preferable in low BMI patients as this reduces the risk of vascular injury. The intra-umbilical area, where all the deeper tissues are tethered together, and the Palmer's point, 3 cm below the mid-clavicular line, are the most commonly used sites. When using Palmer's point, care should be taken to ensure that there is no hepatosplenomegaly, no previous gastric surgery and the stomach is empty by passing a nasogastric tube (Figure 8.2).

(B)   The choice of the *incisions for the ancillary trocars* depends on the procedure planned (upper or lower abdomen), the size of the uterus, the abdominal shape and BMI and the surgeons' preferences. The majority of surgeons use 5 mm ancillary suprapubic and left lateral ports and an additional 5 mm right lateral port for the assistant when operating in the pelvis. Some surgeons prefer to use two operative ports on the left side, while some use a right and left lateral incision for small procedures.

(C)   *Incisions for extraperitoneal dissections* of para-aortic lymph nodes are increasingly used in gynaecological cancer surgery, particularly for high-risk endometrial tumours. Three ports on the left abdominal wall are required.

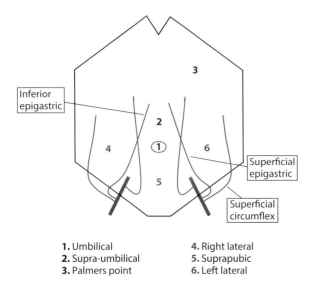

1. Umbilical   **4.** Right lateral
2. Supra-umbilical   **5.** Suprapubic
3. Palmers point   **6.** Left lateral

Figure 8.2 Primary (1–3) and accessory (4–6) port site placement in relation to vessels of anterior abdominal wall

---

TIP

Extremes of BMI are associated with increased risk of complications with laparoscopic surgery, including port insertion.

Principles of Energy Devices

Traditional surgical and haemostatic techniques relied predominantly on the use of scalpel, scissors and haemostatic sutures. These surgical techniques have been largely complimented or replaced by advanced haemostasis and dissecting techniques that use different energy sources. Minimal access surgery relies almost exclusively on energy sources, with increasing use in open surgery.

Types of Energy Device

The energy devices can be broadly categorised into the following groups (Figure 8.3):

(A) **Monopolar electrosurgical diathermy**: The monopolar current runs from the active electrode through the patient and then grounds to the return electrode on the patient. An electrosurgical unit produces the current which flows at high density into the small surface tip (needle, scissors, etc.) and then returns back to a much larger surface area. Monopolar works with desiccation and fulguration. In cutting mode, the waveform uses high-frequency, low-voltage current and cuts with desiccation. With

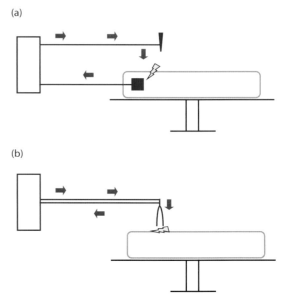

Figure 8.3 Electrosurgery devices. (a) Monopolar diathermy. The monopolar current (red arrows) runs from the active electrode through the patient and grounds to the return electrode (blue square) on the patient. (b) Bipolar diathermy. The current flows (red arrows) only through the tissue that is held between the jaws of the grasper that includes both the active and the passive electrode.

coagulation and fulguration, a low-frequency, high-voltage waveform is required and heating occurs by direct tissue contact.

(B) **Bipolar electrosurgical diathermy**: The bipolar current flows only through the tissue that is held between the jaws of the grasper that includes both the active and the passive electrodes. The tissue damage is therefore more controlled than with monopolar diathermy. The potential tissue damage beyond the point of contact may reach 5 mm. New technologies have feedback sealing properties and integrated dissection capabilities. They use a function of time, pressure and heat generation for sealing and/or cutting.

(C) **Ultrasonic cutting and coagulation**: This technology uses a high-frequency oscillating blade that generates energy by ultrasonic vibration. These devices are precise cutting and haemostatic instruments with minimal smoke and tissue charring. There are new hybrid ultracision instruments that also combine diathermy.

(D) **Laser**: There are several types of lasers (CO_2, ND:YAG, argon/KTP). The laser may be used for cutting, while coagulation properties are limited to small vessels. The CO_2 uses a monochromatic beam and allows precise cutting, while the ND:YAG provides better coagulation. Laser energy is not commonly used in gynaecological oncology surgery but it is a useful tool in the surgical treatment of endometriosis.

(E) **Plasma energy**: Plasma is an ionised gas consisting of positive ions and free electrons, which is electronically neutral. PlasmaJet is a surgical tool which ionises argon gas to provide a plasma–argon beam which releases its energy as light, thermal and kinetic energy. Dependent on the distance of the plasma–argon beam to the tissue, it can cause a variety of effects such as tissue shrinkage and coagulation to vaporisation.

Complications of Energy Devices

Complications related to the use of diathermy can occur. A good understanding of the principles of energy devices is essential. Advanced training of surgeons in the principles of energy sources, the risks and potential complications, as well as advances in the technology have now substantially reduced untoward events. Although novel technologies have introduced energy feedback to alarm for possible problems with the equipment, the surgeons should be aware of these complications. This should be considered when there is a problem with the energy source rather than increasing the power to reach the necessary strength.

Insulation failure occurs when the integrity of the insulated shaft is damaged. Thermal burns can occur throughout the length of the instrument, often outside of the surgeon's view. These injuries are usually not observed at the time of surgery. This is less likely to occur when using disposable instruments.

Direct coupling occurs when the active electrode is in close proximity to, or touching another metal instrument. Current will flow through the pathway of least resistance, and potentially damage adjacent structures that are in direct contact with the secondary instrument.

Capacitive coupling occurs in laparoscopic surgery when current is transferred from an insulated instrument to an uninsulated instrument or tissue through capacitance. Capacitance happens when there is storage of electrical charge, and arises in tissue or metal instruments running parallel to, but not directly in contact with the active electrode. This

current may seek an alternative path, and create a high-density current that may transfer to adjacent tissues or other conductive instruments without direct contact. Inadvertent tissue injury can arise, which is usually unrecognised.

Thermal injury occurs predominantly with the use of monopolar diathermy that produces very high tissue heating. The tissue damage extends far from the point of the contact of the electrode to the tissue. Although thermal spread and tissue damage is much more controlled with bipolar diathermy, the two jaws of the instrument become very hot and care should be taken to protect the surrounding tissues. Unintended activation of the instrument while handling sensitive structures can occur. Unrecognised thermal injuries of the bowel and urinary tract are some of the most common complications. Thermal injury is operator-dependent and not caused by equipment failures. Attention to detail, and cooling the tissue and instruments with irrigation and wash may be necessary.

Other complications include laser- and ultracision-specific complications. When using the laser, care should be taken to ensure that the beam does not affect tissue in front or behind the target. The staff using the laser should be specially trained and wear protective eyewear.

Special Considerations

Body Mass Index

Those with a higher BMI have an increased risk of all major complications following surgery. Difficulties related to surgical access and visualisation, increased risk of VTE and infection make laparoscopic surgery even more advantageous in this population.

Careful consideration is needed in placement of the primary and accessory ports due to the change in surface anatomical landmarks that arise in obesity. The bifurcation of the aorta is cephalad to the umbilicus in morbidly obese women (Figure 8.4). Port placement therefore needs to be perpendicular or directed cranially in relation to the skin at the umbilicus to prevent tunnelling through subcutaneous tissue. If the abdominal pannus is very large, then the umbilicus may hang lower than the pelvis. Entry can be achieved above the umbilicus in the midline in these cases. In order to gain access to the pelvis, the patient will need to be in a steep Trendelenburg tilt and use of supportive equipment such as the 'bean bag' is essential to safely position patients.

Conversely patients who are underweight with a BMI of <18 are also at risk due to the increased chance of major vessel injury. The aorta may lie <2.5 cm below the skin in these women. Use of optical entry ports, open Hasson approach or insertion at Palmer's point is preferable in this situation.

Laparoscopic Surgery

Laparoscopic surgery should be considered in all cases of early-stage endometrial and cervical cancer when the uterus is not grossly enlarged. The benefits of reduced pain, shorter recovery time and hospital stay, reduced VTE and patient preference have been well-recognised for over 20 years. Cochrane review of laparoscopic versus open hysterectomy for early-stage endometrial cancer demonstrated no statistically significant difference in the risk of death or disease recurrence between women who underwent laparoscopy and those who underwent laparotomy. In addition, a meta-analysis reported that the rate of severe postoperative adverse events was significantly lower in the laparoscopy group compared with the laparotomy group.

There are no randomised controlled trials in regards to open versus laparoscopic surgery for early-stage cervical cancer in regards to survival, although retrospective studies suggest that the laparoscopic approach is safe.

Robotic Surgery

Robotic surgery is deemed as having further advantages to laparoscopic surgery as the instruments allow seven degrees of freedom, eliminate surgical tremor and the fulcrum effect (in laparoscopic surgery the end of the instrument moves in the opposite direction to the surgeon's hands). The design is also ergonomically superior to laparoscopic surgery as the surgeon operates sitting down, although the surgery can take longer to perform. Due to higher costs, the use of the robot will depend on individual institutional needs and expertise.

Fertility Sparing Approaches

In some situations, women may present with malignancy before they have completed their family. Where fertility is desired, careful consideration, counselling and an up-to-date view of the latest literature are necessary. Table 8.1 summarises possible situations where a fertility-sparing approach may be acceptable, but individualised risk of recurrence, patients' age, other factors contraindicated to pregnancy should always be considered.

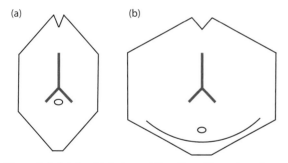

(a)   (b)

Figure 8.4 Relationship between bifurcation of the aorta and umbilicus in (a) normal body weight and (b) obesity

Table 8.1 Fertility-sparing options in gynaecological oncology

Condition	Stage/disease	Management
Cervical cancer	Stage 1A1	LLETZ/cone biopsy
	Stage 1A2–Stage 1B1 (<2 cm tumour)	Trachelectomy or conisation pelvic lymphadenectomy
Endometrial cancer	Stage 1A low-grade endometrioid tumours Complex atypical hyperplasia	High-dose progestogens ± insertion of Mirena IUS
Ovarian cancer	Stage 1A or B fully staged epithelial ovarian borderline or malignant tumours	Unilateral salpingo-oophorectomy with omentectomy with peritoneal biopsy ± pelvic/para-aortic lymphadenectomy
	Early-stage granulosa cell tumours	
	Germ cell tumours	Neoadjuvant chemotherapy in those with extraovarian disease prior to fertility-sparing surgery
Gestational trophoblastic disease (GTD)	Low-risk choriocarcinoma, persistent GTD	Low dose chemotherapy dependent on risk factors
		Resection of lesion if confined to uterus

In some situations, a fertility-sparing approach may be appropriate with a view to completion surgery after childbearing is complete.

Summary

This chapter has highlighted general surgical principals in gynaecology oncology. This encompasses a broad range of tools in order to achieve the goal of ensuring that the patient is optimised for surgery; the surgical procedure is carefully planned and completed and postoperative recovery is successful. The prevention and early recognition of any complication should be prioritised in the high-risk setting.

Further Reading

Enhanced Recovery in Gynaecology. Scientific Impact Paper No. 36. Royal College of Obstetricians and Gynaecologists, 2013.

Obtaining Valid Consent for Complex Gynaecology Surgery. Clinical Governance Advise No. 6b. Royal College of Obstetricians and Gynaecologists, August 2010.

Preventing Entry-related Gynaecological Laparoscopic Injuries. Green Top Guideline No. 49. Royal College of Obstetricians and Gynaecologists, May 2008.

Venous Thromboembolism: Reducing the Risks for Patient in Hospital. NICE guidance CG92. January 2010. Updated June 2015.

Role of Laparoscopic Surgery

Hans Nagar

Introduction

There have been a number of reports demonstrating the feasibility and safety of laparoscopic surgery in gynaecological oncology, and the last decade has seen a significant increase in the use of minimal access surgery (MAS) in managing gynaecological cancers. Most gynaecological oncologists now offer laparoscopic surgery as a standard of care in the surgical management of endometrial and cervical cancers. The survival outcomes in endometrial and cervical cancers appear similar after laparoscopic surgery and laparotomy. There is an increasing interest in the potential role of laparoscopy to aid in the assessment of patients with advanced ovarian cancer, with the aim of determining the likelihood of achieving complete cytoreduction at debulking surgery.

Table 9.1 provides an overview of the potential uses of MAS in the management of gynaecological cancers.

Important factors to consider in complex laparoscopic surgery for gynaecological cancers are in-depth knowledge of anatomy and its variations, the extent of disease by clinical assessment and imaging, surgical techniques and technological innovations. The surgeon must have had adequate training in advanced laparoscopic surgery, and should have acquired proficiency through regular exposure to these procedures.

The potential advantages of laparoscopic surgery are reduced levels of postoperative pain, fewer wound complications, early discharge from hospital and an earlier return to normal activity. Despite the well-reported benefits and safety of laparoscopic surgery in gynaecological cancers, there are a number of limitations to consider. These include availability of the technology, difficult and long learning curve, variable training among surgeons and their experience, perceived and actual longer operative times and patient factors such as prior surgery, extent of disease and obesity.

TIP
The overall objective is to achieve optimal oncological outcomes with improved quality of life by a given surgical approach without compromising patient safety.

Basics of Laparoscopic Surgery

Laparoscopic surgery requires a different set of skills compared with open surgery. These include the development of fine motor skills, depth perception and visuospatial awareness. The complex nature of surgery such as ureteric tunnel dissection and lymph node dissection requires advanced specialist training. This training should include expert supervision by a mentor and work-based assessments. Modern training should involve the use of simulation using box trainers and computer simulators.

The surgeon must have a thorough understanding of the laparoscopic equipment being used. A typical laparoscopic stack incorporates a high-definition camera control unit with a camera head that attaches to the laparoscope. The stack system contains a light source, which is transmitted via a fibre-optic cable to the laparoscope. A carbon dioxide insufflator is used to establish the pneumoperitoneum within the abdominal cavity at the desired pressure. The insufflator has variable flow rate and will have a safety feature that will cut off insufflation when the set level of intra-abdominal pressure has been achieved. A variety of laparoscopes are available. The most common sizes used are 5-mm or 10-mm diameter scopes. Most gynaecologists use a 0° laparoscope, although 30° and 45° angled laparoscopes are available, which are helpful during surgery.

Careful consideration should be given to the ergonomics of the laparoscopic set-up to ensure that the surgical team are as comfortable as possible throughout the procedure. The operating table should be kept at a height that allows for a relaxed position of the surgeons' arms. Standing platforms may be required

Table 9.1 The potential role of laparoscopic surgery in gynaecological cancers

Cancer	Procedure	Indication	Note
Vulval	Laparoscopic defunctioning colostomy	To divert faecal stream for tumour involving or close to anus	Combined with radical vulvectomy and possible rotational flap to improve wound healing
Cervical	Total laparoscopic hysterectomy (TLH)	Optional for patients with stage 1A1 and possibly 1A2 cancer (with bilateral pelvic node dissection)	TLH does not offer any advantage over excisional treatment (LLETZ) in stage 1A1
	Laparoscopic radical hysterectomy and pelvic node dissection; ovaries may be conserved	Stage 1a2 and Ib1	Randomised-controlled trials report lower complications rates
	Laparoscopic extra-peritoneal para-aortic node dissection	Locally advanced cervical cancer; to allow addition of radiotherapy to para-aortic area if node positive	Currently limited evidence for this approach, and is the subject of ongoing LILACS study (a randomised-controlled trial)
Endometrial	TLH and bilateral salpingo-oophorectomy	Apparent stage 1 and 2	LACE and LAP2 studies showed no difference compared with laparotomy, with lower complication rates and better quality of life
	TLH, BSO, pelvic +/− para-aortic node dissection	More aggressive histopathological types such as serous cancer to plan adjuvant therapy	Addition of node dissection is controversial; the ASTEC trial result showed no survival benefit
Ovarian	Laparoscopic staging including TLH, BSO, pelvic and para-aortic node dissection and omentectomy	Apparent stage 1 disease; to determine need for chemotherapy	Limited data with case series report up to 30% will be upstaged to stage 3
	Laparoscopic assessment and biopsy	Stage 3 or 4	To confirm histology and to assess possibility of optimal cytoreductive surgery

where a disparity in height exists between surgeons, or if the operating table cannot be lowered sufficiently for comfort. Audio-visual monitors should be positioned at a slight downward angle of 15° to eye level.

> **TIP**
> A sound understanding of anatomy and familiarity with basic as well as specialised equipment is essential for safe and effective laparoscopic surgery.

Preoperative, Intraoperative and Postoperative Considerations in MAS

Preoperative Considerations

The purpose of preoperative evaluation before MAS is to aid appropriate case selection, assist surgical planning, minimise the risk of anaesthetic and surgical complications and improve surgical outcomes.

Preoperative factors to consider before MAS in gynaecological cancers are as follows:

- Ascites
- Peritoneal disease
- Significant cardiorespiratory compromise
- Morbid obesity or very low body-mass index (BMI)
- Diaphragmatic hernia
- Significant intra-abdominal adhesions from bowel surgery or stoma
- Previous surgical history
- Large pelvic mass
- Haemodynamic instability
- Intestinal obstruction
- Use of anticoagulation
- Hepatomegaly
- Splenomegaly

A complete medical history and examination must be undertaken before surgery. The extent of disease should be assessed clinically and by imaging for its feasibility to carry out a safe laparoscopic surgery. An abdominal examination should be carried out to assess for masses, hernias and scars from previous surgery. It is important to exclude enlarged spleen or liver before placement of supra umbilical or Palmer's point entry.

Risk factors for intra-abdominal adhesions should be assessed as this will increase the risk of complications and chances of conversion to laparotomy. A history of previous bowel surgery or stoma formation should alert clinician of a potentially difficult procedure. Conversion to laparotomy may be necessary either because it is technically difficult to complete the surgery via a laparoscopic approach or due to complications that arise during the procedure that require an open approach to address.

Other important issues include medical problems that impair haemostasis or the ability to tolerate pneumoperitoneum, such as ischaemic heart disease. Patients with restricted respiratory reserve may not be able to withstand the steep Trendelenburg position (head down tilt) and pneumoperitoneum that is required during laparoscopic cases.

Patients should be fully informed of the potential benefits and risk of laparoscopic surgery compared to open surgery and any alternative approaches that are available. Preoperative counselling should also address factors that are specific to the patient, such as any characteristics that increase their risk of complications, in addition to any concerns that are important to that particular individual.

> **TIP**
> All patients undergoing laparoscopic procedures should be made aware of the risk of conversion to laparotomy and the associated longer hospital stay and recovery period.

Intraoperative Considerations

Patient Positioning

Careful positioning is required to maximise ergonomic access for the surgeon, allow adequate access to the vagina and to avoid neurological injury. Usually the patient's arms are tucked by their sides and legs placed in booted stirrups to allow for adjustment of the legs during the procedure. The hips and knees should be moderately flexed, with minimal abduction or external rotation of the hips. Where vaginal access with instruments is required, it is helpful to start with the buttocks several centimetres beyond the edge of the table

to allow full range of movement of the vaginal instruments. Not all procedures require elevation of legs and certain procedures such as laparoscopic tubal/ovarian surgery or biopsies can be carried out in a supine position with straight legs.

Most gynaecological procedures require the patient to be tilted in the Trendelenburg position in order to displace the bowels and aid visualisation and access to the pelvis. The surgical team should be mindful that steep Trendelenburg tilt (30° to 45°) and the use of braces to strap the patient in place may contribute to brachial plexus injury and appropriate precautions should be taken to prevent this. Equipment such as the surgical 'beanbag' can be helpful to mitigate the effects of gravity causing the patient to slip down the operating table.

The bladder should be emptied for all major cases. For minor cases it is not necessary to catheterise the patient; however, the patient should be asked to void just before entering the theatre.

Establishment of a Pneumoperitoneum and Primary Port Placement

Primary trocars are typically placed through or above the umbilicus. Palmer's point (in the left upper quadrant) may be used as the point of entry if the surgeon is concerned about the presence of adhesions. There are various ways of establishing a pneumoperitoneum and inserting the primary port. There is no evidence to suggest one method is superior to the other. A common method used by gynaecologists is insufflation using the Veress needle, i.e. a spring-loaded device. Prior to insertion of the needle the surgeon should palpate the anterior abdominal wall to determine if there is a large mass present underneath, for the presence of hernias and the position of the aorta (in thinner patients). This method involves a small incision in the umbilicus through which the surgeon inserts the Veress needle at right angles to the skin, and two audible clicks are heard as the spring-loaded mechanism passes through the layers of the anterior abdominal wall. Excessive lateral movement of the needle should be avoided. Various tests have been designed to determine whether the needle is in the correct place. Perhaps the most helpful is measuring intra-abdominal pressure, with a level below 8 mmHg being reassuring. Higher pressures may suggest incorrect placement and the surgeon should either re-position the Veress needle or switch to an alternative entry technique. Once the Veress needle is in the correct position the carbon dioxide can be insufflated into the abdominal cavity. The RCOG recommendation is that the intra-abdominal pressure should be at a level of 20–25 mmHg prior to the insertion of the ports. This pressure tents the abdominal wall and reduces the risk of injury to underlying abdominal structures. The surgical and anaesthetic team should be aware that high intra-abdominal pressures may result in cardiac or respiratory compromise in patients with comorbidities. Once the ports have been inserted the pressure should be reduced to between 10 and 15 mmHg for the rest of the procedure.

Alternative techniques include the modified Hasson's open entry method. This is achieved by creating a small incision through abdominal wall, rectus sheath and peritoneum. The sheath may be suspended by lateral or purse-string sutures. A blunt-ended trocar is then inserted into the abdominal cavity under direct vision, and is held in place by sutures, creating an airtight seal. The laparoscope can be used to confirm successful entry into the peritoneal cavity, and the gas insufflated directly through the primary trocar. A more recently developed technique is the optical direct entry approach. This method involves inserting the laparoscope down into the primary trocar to allow vision at the tip of the trocar. This is then inserted through the layers of the anterior abdominal wall under direct vision.

> **TIPS**
> There is no evidence of difference between Veress needle entry and open/direct entry in terms of preventing major vascular or visceral complications. An open technique, however, is associated with reduced incidence of failed entry, extra-peritoneal insufflation and omental injury.

Using Palmer's Point Entry

Previous abdominal surgery increases the risk of bowel injury occurring during laparoscopy especially at time of port insertion. The risk of adhesion formation could be as high as 50% after one previous midline laparotomy and 23% following one lower transverse incision. Other conditions that increase adhesion formation are previous peritonitis, inflammatory bowel disease or bowel surgery. Adhesions are least likely to occur in the left upper quadrant and therefore this site can be used as a site of primary entry. Palmer's point lies in the left mid-clavicular line, 3 cm below the costal margin. The anaesthetist is asked to pass a temporary naso- or orogastric tube to ensure that the stomach is

deflated. A Veress needle is inserted at Palmer's point, and the abdominal cavity insufflated with carbon dioxide. After correct port placement has been confirmed by checking the intra-abdominal pressures, a 5-mm trocar is inserted at Palmer's point, to allow the passage of a smaller 5-mm laparoscope. This can be used to evaluate the abdominal cavity, paying particular attention to the presence and site of any adhesions, and can be used to guide the insertion of further ports under direct vision. Palmer's point entry is contraindicated in women with significant splenomegaly, or a previous history of surgery in the left upper quadrant.

> **TIP**
> A naso- or orogastric tube should be inserted to deflate stomach prior to entry at Palmer's point.

Accessory Port and Placement

The site of secondary port placement depends on both the operation being performed and the individual surgeon's preference. Secondary trocars should be inserted under direct vision, with the intra-abdominal pressure set between 20 and 25 mmHg. When placing lateral ports the inferior epigastric vessels should be visualised so that they can be avoided. These vessels run lateral to the medial umbilical fold. Visualising these vessels can be difficult in obese patients, and if so it is preferable to place the ports lateral to the rectus muscle to avoid the vessels. At the end of surgery all secondary ports should be removed under direct vision, in order to detect any occult bleeding from the port sites. Deep fascial closure should be performed on all lateral ports >7 mm and midline ports >10 mm to prevent port-site hernias. Closure should be carried out under direct vision to avoid picking up bowel or omentum in deep sutures.

Instrumentation

An enormous range of laparoscopic instruments and devices are available for use in MAS and covers the spectrum of instruments that are typically available for use during open surgery. The surgeon must be familiar with their choice of equipment and be prepared to troubleshoot whenever there are technical difficulties. The surgeon will use a range of equipment, which may include some or all of the following: the laparoscope, imaging devices and instruments for tissue dissection, haemostasis, suction/irrigation and tissue removal.

In many cases it is helpful to use a uterine manipulator, with or without a colpotomy cup, depending upon the planned procedure. The manipulator facilitates access to the pelvic structures, and allows traction to be applied to the uterus and adnexal structures. In women who have previously had a hysterectomy, rectal dilators or swab holding forceps may be placed in the vagina to manipulate the vaginal vault. Uterine instrumentation is avoided if there is a possible pregnancy.

A variety of energy sources are available to achieve both cutting and coagulation, including conventional monopolar and bipolar diathermy, advanced bipolar diathermy and ultrasonic energy devices. Harmonic device works on mechanical energy of ultrasound vibrations to achieve tissue cutting while simultaneously providing haemostasis. The ability to perform laparoscopic suturing is important and recent developments include barbed unidirectional sutures that reduce the need for laparoscopic knot tying.

Postoperative Considerations

The majority patients undergoing laparoscopic surgery will be suitable for an enhanced recovery programme approach that involves a combination of early feeding, early mobilisation, avoidance of drains and timely removal of bladder catheter. The majority of patients are suitable for discharge within 24–48 hours of surgery. Patients are advised to avoid heavy lifting/straining while the abdominal incisions are healing and to increase other activities as tolerated. Patients may expect a recovery period of 2–4 weeks before resumption of most daily activities. Vaginal sexual intercourse should be avoided for 4–6 weeks after total hysterectomy.

> **TIPS**
> Patients should recover reasonably quickly after laparoscopic surgery. A delayed postoperative recovery can indicate an underlying postoperative complication and should be investigated promptly for bowel, bladder or ureteric damage.

Anaesthetic Considerations

The cardiorespiratory effects of laparoscopy vary during an operation and may be exacerbated by pre-existing cardiovascular disease, old age and a steep Trendelenburg position. This is important as many of the women in gynaecological oncology are older or obese compared with women undergoing similar procedures in general gynaecology.

The presence of pneumoperitoneum causes a number of effects such as vagal nerve stimulation which can lead to bradycardia, the release of catecholamines and vasopressin with an increase in mean arterial pressure. Splinting of the diaphragm due to the distension of abdominal cavity reduces functional residual capacity and pulmonary compliance, resulting in lung atelectasis and increased peak airway pressures especially in a steep Trendelenburg position. Both splanchnic and renal perfusion is also reduced leading to decreased urine output.

Carbon dioxide is rapidly absorbed into the circulation leading to hypercarbia and associated acidosis. Its absorption appears to reach a peak at around 1 hour after starting laparoscopy. Hyperventilation is required to correct acidosis which otherwise may cause decreased cardiac contractility, sensitisation to arrhythmias, and increased systemic vasodilatation.

Complications of Laparoscopy

Serious complications during laparoscopy are rare. Complications may arise at the time of entry, as a consequence of the pneumoperitoneum, or during the operative procedure itself as a result of tissue dissection or haemostasis. Conversion to an open procedure may be required to manage the complication. While the RCOG Guidelines for laparoscopic injuries quotes the rate of serious complications at about 4 in 1,000, this depends on the type and complexity of the laparoscopic procedure. In the LACE randomised-controlled trial of laparoscopic hysterectomy versus open surgery for endometrial cancer, the intraoperative complication rate was 7.4% (compared with 5.6% in the open arm) and serious adverse incident rate of 7.9% (compared with 19% in the open arm).

Risk factors for complications include:

- Prior surgery
- Extremes of BMI
- Bowel distension
- Large abdominal or pelvic mass
- Complex surgery
- Inexperienced surgeon.

Complications related to abdominal entry – About half of the complications occur at the time of laparoscopic entry. The most serious complications are access-related vascular injuries and injuries of the bowel. Knowledge and experience of safe laparoscopic entry techniques is essential.

Vascular injury – It can usually be managed by a combination of pressure with tonsil swabs, bipolar diathermy and haemostatic agents. Targeted suction is usually helpful in identifying the site of injury. The 'blind' application of diathermy can result in collateral damage to adjacent structures; therefore it is imperative to be aware of surrounding structures to avoid inadvertent injury during attempts at haemostasis. Larger injuries may require open surgery and the help of a vascular surgeon. Urgent assistance from a surgeon experienced in managing vascular injury must be summoned. While waiting for help, simple measures can be instituted including adequate resuscitation by the anaesthetist, Trendelenburg position and direct pressure to the injured vessel. This may require a rapid laparotomy and direct pressure and packing while waiting for the help to arrive. Injury to the inferior epigastric artery is managed by a combination of pressure, suturing and diathermy. The use of a Foley catheter balloon to provide compression has been described.

Bowel injury – It is another serious complication that can occur on entry or during the procedure. Unrecognised bowel injury increases the risk of morbidity and mortality, and surgeons must maintain a high index of suspicion of this during and after surgery. If recognised at the time, most limited bowel injuries can be repaired without recourse to stoma formation, but a specialist opinion should be sought.

Urinary tract injury – Damage to the bladder should be suspected if there is unexplained distension of the urinary catheter bag with air, significant haematuria, or leakage of urine from port sites. Bladder defects that are distal to the ureters can be managed by laparoscopic suturing, an indwelling catheter followed by a postoperative cystogram at 7–14 days to confirm healing. Injuries close to the ureteric ridge require intraoperative insertion of ureteric stents. Postoperatively, the vast majority of patients should improve day by day. Failure to do so should raise the suspicion of a possible complication. Injuries from intraoperative or delayed postoperative ischaemia may lead to devascularisation of ureter and delayed fistula formation. Therefore ureteric perivasculature should be preserved and minimal handling of ureter is encouraged intraoperatively.

Nerve damage – Transient nerve injuries that can occur during laparoscopic surgery include the sciatic, perineal and brachial nerves (over extended arm during surgery). Damage to the genitofemoral nerve during pelvic node dissection is common and results in paraesthesia in the inner upper thigh and anterior

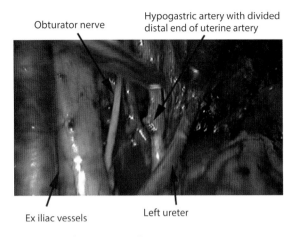

Figure 9.1 Left pelvic side wall

vulva. It is best to safely identify and guard the nerve at the beginning of a node dissection. The obturator nerve can also be damaged within the obturator fossa during a pelvic node dissection (Figure 9.1). The nerve supplies sensory branches to the medial thigh and motor branches to the adductor muscles of the thigh.

Port-site hernias – These are less common than hernias due to open surgery. The incidence is related to the diameter of the port used, body BMI, age and prolonged operating times. The risk is minimised by closing the rectus sheath in all midline ports >10 or 12 mm, lateral ports >7 mm, and certainly in patients with significant risk factors.

Port-site metastases – These are specific complications that can arise after laparoscopic surgery in the presence of intra-peritoneal malignancy. Measures to minimise the risk include the use of wound protectors, specimen extraction bags and excision of port sites. Fortunately they are rare, affecting approximately 1–2% of patients.

Avoiding Complications

Complications are reduced with ongoing training and experience. Surgeons should use the entry technique they are most comfortable and familiar with. They should recognise when this is not working and have a backup plan. Surgeons should only embark upon newer techniques after thorough knowledge, experience and supervised training of such techniques. In keeping with open surgery, morbidity and mortality related to laparoscopic complications can be reduced by prompt intraoperative or early postoperative recognition and treatment of complications.

All side-port insertions should be carried out under direct vision to avoid injury to inferior epigastric vessels. During insertion of ports medial slippage of the trocar towards the vessels should be avoided by appropriately directing the trocar. During port placement, higher intra-abdominal pressure is used to control the depth of trocar insertion. It is a good standard practice to obtain a 360° view of the abdominal cavity following laparoscopic entry to allow early identification of any trauma. Bowel injuries go unrecognised in approximately 15% of cases intra-operatively and then present much later during the postoperative period. Therefore a high index of suspicion is required when patient is not recovering quickly after a laparoscopic surgery.

The distal ureter is vulnerable to injury at the point where the uterine artery crosses superior to it, close to the lateral fornix of vagina. Use of a uterine manipulator and bladder dissection during hysterectomy reduces this risk of ureteric injury. The next most common site of ureteric injury is at the pelvic brim, adjacent to the infundibulopelvic ligament. Avoiding ureteric injury requires visualisation and, where necessary, careful dissection of ureter with minimal traction, so that the periureteric connective tissue and vasculature is preserved. For suspected ischaemic damage to the ureter, a urological surgeon's opinion should be sought and ureteric stents may be inserted.

Uterine perforation can occur during placement of manipulator and this may carry a risk of spillage and upstaging of endometrial cancer. This can be avoided by accurate measurement of uterine size by preoperative imaging and careful placement of uterine manipulator accordingly. In certain circumstances, a hysterectomy can be carried out without using a uterine manipulator. Similarly ovarian masses that are likely to be malignant are at risk of spillage, and this factor should be considered in preoperative planning of the procedure.

Urinary bladder injuries can occur if the patient has bladder adhesions due to caesarean section. A technique to avoid this is intraoperative filling of bladder with blue dye to demarcate bladder edge or aid in the detection of any small leaks. Additionally, approaching the bladder dissection from lateral to medial, to avoid central adherent portion of the bladder, and sharp dissection can also help to avoid bladder damage.

When small bowel injury is suspected, a thorough inspection of whole small bowel is necessary and help from a general surgeon should be summoned so that laparoscopic repair of injury can be considered. If rectal injury is suspected, an air leak test should be carried out by insufflating air into the rectum after filling pelvis with water.

Pelvic lymphadenectomy risks injury to pelvic sidewall vessels, ureter and obturator nerve. Complex pelvic sidewall surgery is only safely feasible with clear views on the monitor and modern equipment such as high-definition screens, and three-dimensional cameras can be of value. To avoid injury to obturator nerve, any diathermy in the obturator fossa should be carried out under direct vision and only after identification and securing of the obturator nerve. Direct handling of the iliac vessels during lymphadenectomy should be avoided to prevent damage to vessel intima. Surgeons should be mindful that the iliac veins are collapsed during laparoscopy, due to a combination of high abdominal pressures and Trendelenburg tilt. Care should be taken not to inadvertently tear or diathermise these veins during lymphadenectomy.

TIPS
Diathermy-related injury can be avoided by thorough understanding of energy sources and the degree of lateral thermal spread from the energy device. Lateral spread of bipolar energy is generally limited to 2 mm, while monopolar spread is related to the power utilised and the duration of application.

Special Considerations

- Suspected adhesions – Consider a non-umbilical entry (e.g. Palmer's point).
- Prior hernia repair – Avoid entry at the site of hernia, especially if mesh has been used.
- Large pelvic mass – Take care to avoid puncture as it may lead to bleeding or spillage of malignant contents which may worsen prognosis.
- Pregnancy – Consider if an open approach is safer. If laparoscopy is appropriate, consider the position of the uterus relative to the umbilicus, and adjust entry and port sites appropriately.
- Low BMI – Women with low BMI are at risk of a vascular injury at time of insertion of Veress needle or primary port entry. Palpation of the abdomen and aorta can guide the entry technique to be used with Palmer's point entry as an option.
- Obesity – The relative position of the umbilicus to the aortic bifurcation is altered in obese patients, and is more likely to be caudad. A supraumbilical approach may be needed for correct positioning of the camera. If a Veress needle is used for

insufflation, a standard needle may be too short, and there is an increased risk of pre-peritoneal insufflation.

Obesity – Women with a high BMI may benefit from laparoscopic surgery with early mobilisation, smaller wounds leading to reduced infections, wound dehiscence and avoidance of potentially fatal venous thromboembolism. A high BMI raises particular challenges for both the surgeon and the anaesthetist. Safe insertion of Veress needle of optical trocar can be difficult often requiring a near vertical insertion to avoid extra-peritoneal insufflation of CO_2. A lower abdominal fat pad or pannus increases the torque effect limiting fine movement of laparoscopic instruments. Obese patients may not tolerate a steep Trendelenburg position and high intra-abdominal gas pressure leading to a poor view of the pelvis obscured by bowel and visceral fat. All these factors increase the cardiorespiratory compromise caused by a pneumoperitoneum. Successful completion of a laparoscopic procedure frequently requires reduced intra-abdominal pressure and limited Trendelenburg position. Occasionally very obese patients may not be considered suitable or safe for laparoscopic surgery.

Robotic Surgery

Robotically assisted laparoscopic surgery is an evolution of MAS rather than a revolution. In current platforms the surgeon may be seated in a separate room and remotely operates laparoscopic robot arms. Perceived benefits include three-dimensional vision, control of the laparoscope by the operating surgeon, more precise instrument movement and a shortened learning curve. Perhaps the biggest advantage is the use of instruments that fully articulate at the end in the manner of a human wrist allowing fine delicate movements and camera view that is not dependent on the assistance.

Disadvantages include the cost of the robotic system and the ongoing cost of instruments with a limited life span and maintenance. Other reported issues include increased operating time, the need for further training and the lack of tactile (haptic) feedback from the instruments. High-level evidence supporting robotic instead of standard laparoscopy in gynaecological cancer surgery is limited. Two RCTs concerning hysterectomies for benign gynaecological indications failed to show any advantage over conventional laparoscopic hysterectomy. A single small RCT of 99 women

with endometrial cancer has been published comparing laparoscopic hysterectomy (including a vaginal component) plus PND with robotic hysterectomy with PND. This reported robotic surgery was associated with a significantly shorter operating time (139 vs 170 minutes) and similar surgical outcomes.

Cancer-Specific Considerations in Laparoscopic Surgery

Cervical Cancer

Most gynaecological cancer centres have adopted the laparoscopic approach for radical hysterectomy and pelvic lymphadenectomy in the surgical management of early cervical cancers. A radical hysterectomy may be performed either as a laparoscopically assisted or a total laparoscopic procedure. The choice of approach depends on the degree of uterovaginal prolapse, vaginal access and the ability of the surgeon to perform dissection of the vesicouterine ligament (ureteric tunnel) via the vagina. Bilateral pelvic lymphadenectomy is usually carried out at the same time. The other role for laparoscopic approach is laparoscopic trachelectomy and placement of cervical suture.

As with most surgical procedures, a learning curve is apparent with complication rates decreasing with experience. Complications are similar to the open procedure and include haemorrhage, damage to bowel, bladder, ureter and autonomic nerve dysfunction. A single randomised-controlled trial has compared laparoscopic vaginal radical hysterectomy with open abdominal radical hysterectomy. This reported on complications but not prognosis, with significantly fewer short-term complications such as bleeding or bladder dysfunction in the laparoscopic group, but with a less radical resection and longer operating time. Several retrospective studies have reported that laparoscopic surgery is safe and offers outcomes equivalent to open surgery. These studies suggest longer operating times, reduced rates of bleeding and similar rates of other complications.

Some very early cervical cancers can be treated with simple total laparoscopic hysterectomy (TLH) and lymphadenectomy. Radical surgery is associated with a significant risk of long-term consequences including lower urinary tract symptoms, sexual dysfunction and colorectal motility disorders, secondary to autonomic nerve dysfunction. Less radical surgery is associated with a lower risk of long-term side effects. There is increasing interest in the potential role for less radical surgery in patients with low-risk early stage disease. The SHAPE trial is one such study that is currently underway to determine safety of simple hysterectomy and pelvic lymphadenectomy in small volume (<2 cm) stage 1B early cervical cancers.

The number of lymph nodes removed by the laparoscopic approach is comparable to open pelvic nodes dissection. The main disadvantage is the increase in the operating time required, although this decreases with the experience of the surgeon. Advantages include a reduction in bleeding from small vessels due to tamponade effect of the pneumoperitoneum. The rate of blood transfusion is lower for laparoscopic surgery than open dissection. The superior view afforded by the laparoscope should decrease the risk of injury to vessels in the obturator fossa. The rates of other complications such as injury to the ureter, nerves and the formation of lymphocele are similar to open surgery. Laparoscopic removal of enlarged lymph nodes is also considered before treating a large volume cervical cancer with chemoradiotherapy. There is also an emerging role of sentinel node identification and biopsy with technetium-99 or indocyanine green (ICG) so that full lymphadenectomy can be avoided with a view to reduce surgical comorbidities including lower limb lymphoedema. To date, sentinel node removal has not replaced full nodal dissection in routine practice in the United Kingdom, and is pending further evidence on safety and efficacy.

Endometrial Cancer

The majority of women with endometrial cancer will be cured by a total hysterectomy and bilateral salpingo-oophorectomy. A meta-analysis reported lower complication rates and similar recurrence rates and survival after laparoscopic surgery. In addition, long-term survival data from a large randomised-controlled trial suggests that laparoscopic surgery is not inferior to open surgery. Many women with endometrial cancer are obese and are therefore most likely to benefit from the laparoscopic approach to surgery with smaller wounds, lower infection rates and early mobilisation. The main limiting step is the ability of the woman to tolerate an anaesthetic, especially the head down position and its resulting effect on respiratory function. Women with some degree of uterovaginal prolapse are candidates for a laparoscopically assisted vaginal hysterectomy, combined with removal of the ovaries, or

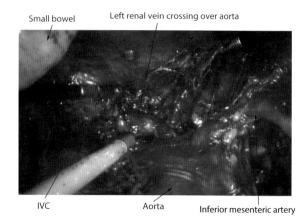

Figure 9.2 Transperitoneal para-aortic node dissection: view from suprapubic port looking cephalad

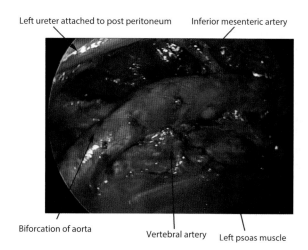

Figure 9.3 Retroperitoneal para-aortic node dissection viewed from left lateral side of patient

occasionally a vaginal hysterectomy alone. Many obese women will have minimal prolapse and limited vaginal access. These women are frequently suitable for a TLH using a gastight vaginal tube or uterine manipulator. While the role of lymphadenectomy is questioned by certain studies, laparoscopic pelvic with/without para-aortic lymph node dissection is considered in addition to hysterectomy, to guide ongoing management in high-risk endometrial cancers (Figures 9.2 and 9.3).

Ovarian Cancer

Laparoscopy is frequently used in the management of adnexal masses by gynaecologists. A number of benign gynaecological conditions such as endometriosis and fibroids can result in a raised serum CA125. Imaging can aid in differentiating between benign and malignant adnexal masses. A pragmatic approach in young women with complex ovarian masses involves the removal of adnexal masses intact in a sealed bag, combined with pelvic washings and careful inspection of the abdominal cavity. Postoperatively, those women with confirmed malignancy should be offered a full staging procedure if this will affect the treatment or prognosis. The role of laparoscopy in advanced stage ovarian cancer is controversial. Laparoscopy can be used to obtain biopsies if the origin of the tumour is in doubt, although biopsies can usually be obtained by using image-guided procedures. Laparoscopy does have the advantage of assessing the potential feasibility of achieving optimal cytoreduction at subsequent laparotomy, or for determining a cancer's response to chemotherapy. However, in advanced disease, laparoscopy also has the potential to cause significant harm, including bowel injury and port-site metastases.

Summary

Minimally invasive surgical techniques in gynaecological oncology have evolved greatly since the introduction of laparoscopy. The advantages of laparoscopy over laparotomy, in the appropriately selected cancer patient, have proven benefits to the patient both intra- and postoperatively, with similar outcomes. Laparoscopic surgery in women with gynaecological cancer requires advanced training with detailed knowledge of anatomy including the retro-peritoneum and the pelvic side wall. With the correct training, MAS surgery has been shown to replicate the radicality of open surgery with reduced morbidity and increased quality of life. New developments such as robotic laparoscopic surgery and the use of small, single-site incisions are being used, but require further scrutiny before becoming part of routine practice. The advent of robotic-assisted surgery may offer the bridge between improved patient perioperative outcomes and surgeon ergonomics.

Further Reading

Mencaglia L, Minelli L, Wattiez A. *Manual of Gynecological Laparoscopic Surgery*. 2nd edition. Tuttlingen, Germany: Endo Press; 2012.

NICE. Laparoscopic radical hysterectomy for early stage cervical cancer. *Interventional Procedures Guidance [IPG338]*. London, England: National Institute of Health Care and Excellence; 2010.

Laparoscopic hysterectomy (including laparoscopic total hysterectomy and laparoscopically assisted vaginal hysterectomy) for endometrial cancer. *Interventional Procedures Guideline [IPG356]*. London, England: National Institute of Health Care and Excellence; 2010.

RCOG. Preventing entry-related gynaecological laparoscopic injuries. *Green-top Guideline No 49*. London: Royal College of Obstetricians and Gynaecologists; 2008.

Endometrial cancer in obese women. *Scientific Impact Paper No. 32*. London: Royal College of Obstetricians and Gynaecologists; 2012.

Chapter 10

Ovarian, Fallopian Tube and Primary Peritoneal Cancer (including Borderline)

Hilary Turnbull and Timothy Duncan

Introduction

Ovarian cancer is the sixth commonest cancer affecting women, with over 7,000 new cases diagnosed in the United Kingdom each year. The lifetime risk of developing ovarian cancer is approximately 2%.

Despite the availability of newer chemotherapeutic agents and more advanced surgical techniques, mortality rates have changed very little. The number of deaths from ovarian cancer is greater than all other gynaecological cancers combined. Ovarian cancer usually presents at an advanced stage, due to a relative lack of specific signs and symptoms at the early stages, coupled with a lack of reliable screening tools. Currently, statistics show that UK survival rates are significantly worse, with 30–40% 5-year survival rates, compared to other developed countries including Canada, Australia, Norway and Sweden (Figure 10.1).

The majority of ovarian cancers arise from epithelial cells, with the remainder originating from other ovarian cell types (i.e. sex cord–stromal tumours, germ cell tumours). High-grade serous epithelial ovarian carcinoma (HGEOC), fallopian tube and peritoneal carcinomas are currently considered to be a single entity due to their similar pathogenesis and clinical characteristics. For the remainder of this chapter, epithelial ovarian cancer (EOC) will refer to this group of malignancies.

Aetiology and Risk Factors

Epidemiological data shows that the risk of ovarian cancer increases with greater numbers of ovulation cycles. Conversely, pregnancies and use of oral contraceptives are associated with a lower risk of ovarian cancer. The following theories explain the association between ovarian cancer and number of ovulation cycles:

1. **The incessant ovulation theory** – Ovulation results in follicular rupture which induces minor trauma, inflammation and subsequent repair to the surface epithelium. Repeated ovulations

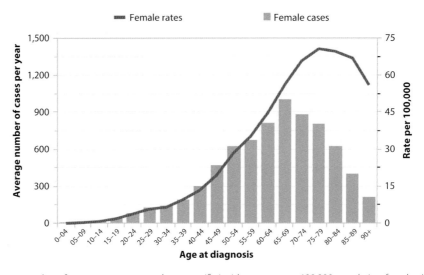

Figure 10.1 Average number of new cases per year and age-specific incidence rates per 100,000 population, females, UK

Cancer Research UK, www.cancerresearchuk.org/health-professional/cancer-statistics/statistics-by-cancer-type/ovarian-cancer/incidence#heading-One. Accessed January 2017

Table 10.1 Factors affecting risk of ovarian cancer

Risk factors	Protective factors
• Increasing age (incidence peaks at ≥60 years)	• History of using the combined oral contraceptive pill
• Early menarche	• Pregnancy
• Late menopause	• Breast-feeding
• Nulliparity	• Salpingectomy
• Subfertility	• Sterilisation
• Genetic pre-disposition	
• Use of hormone replacement therapy	
• Smoking	
• Endometriosis	
• Diabetes	

Table 10.2 Risk of ovarian and breast cancer in BRCA mutation carriers

	Breast cancer risk	Ovarian cancer risk
BRCA1	50–65%	30–45%
BRCA2	45%	11–17%

over a lifetime may increase the likelihood of genetic alterations and subsequent malignant transformation.

2. **Exposure to gonadotropins:** Persistent stimulation of the ovaries by gonadotropins results in an increase in proliferation, and mitotic activity of the surface epithelium. This may increase the risk of malignant transformation.

Most ovarian cancers are sporadic. The most important risk factors are increasing age and a positive family history of ovarian or breast cancer. Factors associated with a reduced lifetime incidence of ovulation, such as multiparty and breast-feeding, are protective. The combined oral contraceptive pill reduces ovarian cancer risk by 10% after 1 year and 50% after 5 years of use. Salpingectomy is protective, in keeping with the theory that the primary site of ovarian cancer is the fimbrial end of the fallopian tube (Table 10.1).

Genetic Pre-disposition to Ovarian Cancer

Familial ovarian cancer accounts for up to 10% of cases of EOC. The lifetime risk for a woman with a history of one affected first-degree relative is 5%, increasing to 7% with two affected relatives. The RCOG recommends that where family history is significant, referral to the Regional Cancer Genetics service should be considered. NICE recommends that every patient with a current or past histological diagnosis of high-grade serous carcinoma or G3 endometrioid ovarian carcinoma should be offered BRCA counselling and testing.

BRCA Mutations 1 and 2

Hereditary ovarian cancer is commonly associated with the breast–ovarian cancer familial syndrome and the autosomal dominant *BRCA1* and *BRCA2* genes (tumour suppressor genes on chromosome 17q and 13q, respectively). Features suggestive of associated gene mutations include early onset ovarian cancer (<50 years), personal history of breast cancer, family history of breast or ovarian cancer and Ashkenazi Jewish ancestry (5–10 times more likely to carry BRCA). Risk of cancer by age 70 is given in Table 10.2.

Despite the younger age at presentation of BRCA carriers, their long-term survival is comparable to non-carriers due to a higher sensitivity to platinum-based chemotherapy and newer biological agents. Their stage at presentation is similar to non-carriers. BRCA carriers should be advised of the symptoms of ovarian cancer and should also be advised to report them to their doctor.

Screening for BRCA carriers – Currently there is no effective screening tool available that has been shown to reliably detect ovarian cancer at an early stage, even in these high-risk women.

• Regular surveillance with serum CA125 levels and ultrasound scanning may be offered for these high-risk women, but limited benefit has been shown to date. Women electing for this approach must be informed that currently there is no evidence that this will be beneficial.

• The UK Familial Cancer Screening Study (UK FOCSS) results reported that annual ultrasonography and CA125 monitoring was too infrequent to identify ovarian cancers at an early stage. Phase 2 of the trial, investigating a more frequent surveillance protocol, is ongoing.

Risk-reducing surgery (RRS) – BRCA carriers should be informed of the option of RRS with bilateral salpingo-oophorectomy (BSO). This has been shown to reduce the risk of ovarian and fallopian tube cancer risk by approximately 90%, and breast cancer by 50%, if performed at around the age of 40. Generally BRCA1 carriers have earlier-onset cancers; hence RRS is advised at approximately 40 years. BRCA2 carriers develop cancers at peri- or post-menopausal age; hence RRS is recommended closer to the age of menopause.

Disadvantages of surgery include premature menopause (osteoporosis, cardiovascular risks) and the psychological impact. RRS does *not* reduce the risk of primary peritoneal cancer in BRCA carriers. Hormone replacement therapy can be given to those without a personal history of breast cancer.

Hereditary Nonpolyposis Colon Cancer Syndrome

EOC is seen in approximately 12% of women with hereditary nonpolyposis colon cancer (HNPCC; Lynch syndrome), in addition to their increased risk of endometrial, colorectal and gastric cancers. HNPCC syndrome results from mutations in DNA mismatch repair genes. RRS for this syndrome includes hysterectomy with BSO.

Screening for Ovarian Cancer in the General Population

The aim of screening programmes is to identify patients with pre-invasive or early stage disease, when treatment can be curative, or can significantly improve outcomes. It is important for any screening test to be specific in case of ovarian cancer, because a positive screening result requires surgical intervention, and therefore has the potential to cause harm if the test is falsely positive. The UK Collaborative Trial of Ovarian Cancer Screening (UKCTOCS) was a very large study that investigated an ovarian cancer screening protocol using a multi-modality approach including CA125, ultrasonography and clinical assessment. Compared to no screening, multi-modal screening detected more cancers at an early stage; however, there was no reduction in mortality. Only one in four women who required surgery was found to have cancer. Therefore the trial concluded that at present there is insufficient evidence to recommend screening for ovarian cancer in the general population. The trial is continuing and will report on the longer follow-up results for women involved in this trial.

Pathology

Primary ovarian tumours can originate from a range of different cell types:

- **Surface epithelium of the ovary** – Serous (70–80%), endometrioid (10%), clear cell (10%), mucinous (3%), transitional cell

- **Germ cells** – Teratoma, dysgerminoma, yolk sac, mixed germ cell, monodermal
- **Sex-cord/stroma** – Granulosa, sertoli cell, thecoma, fibroma.

Serous ovarian carcinomas (SOC) are divided into low-grade (type 1/LGSOC) and high-grade (type 2/HGSOC) originate from the same fallopian tube precursor cells, but differ fundamentally in their behaviour. HGSOC are 20 times more common than LGSOC and account for the majority of deaths from ovarian cancer. LGSOC are slow growing, but may still present at an advanced stage. Contrary to HGSOC subtype, the lower grade tumours are relatively insensitive to platinum-based chemotherapies. Frequently they coexist with non-invasive borderline tumours, having progressed into malignancy.

Mucinous tumours are typically unilateral and large tumours, and are associated with mucin production. They predominantly originate from the appendix, with true ovarian-origin tumours being rare. Appendicectomy is recommended in conjunction with removal of the ovaries if the appendix appears grossly abnormal. A tumour of true appendiceal-origin can be associated with pseudomyxoma peritonei.

Clear cell tumours tend to occur in younger women, with approximately half arising in endometriosis. The tumours are especially aggressive, and typically less responsive to chemotherapy.

Endometrioid tumours also arise from endometriosis and around one third will be bilateral tumours.

Metastases from EOC spread by direct extension (transcoelomic), exfoliation into the peritoneal fluid and lymphatic invasion.

The ovary is a relatively common site of metastatic spread from other primary sites, especially in premenopausal women. Krukenberg tumours are associated with mucinous cancers, and usually arise from the stomach but can also arise from the breast, colon or gallbladder.

Serous Tubal Intraepithelial Carcinoma Lesions and the Fallopian Tube Hypothesis

Currently there is compelling clinical, pathological and molecular evidence to support the hypothesis that the fallopian tube is the site of origin of HGSOC. The precursor lesions to HGSOC are known as serous tubal intraepithelial carcinoma (STIC) lesions. These abnormalities were originally identified in the fimbrial ends of fallopian tubes that had been removed from asymptomatic BRCA carriers with RRS. STIC lesions are characterised by the presence of p53 mutations and high levels of chromosomal instability in affected cells. This pattern is identical to that found in HGSOC.

There are two differing proposed pathways for how STIC lesions result in ovarian carcinoma:

1. Incorporation of Müllerian epithelium from the tube into the ovary with endosalpingiosis, cortical inclusions or endometriosis. This could result in benign, borderline or malignant LGSOC, endometrioid or clear cell tumours, but rarely HGSOC.

2. Malignant transformation of the distal tubal mucosa and the development of STIC. These lesions could exfoliate onto the ovary surface or the peritoneum and result in HGSOC without invasive disease on the tube itself.

TIPS

The RCOG Scientific Paper 44 (2014) recommends 'women who are not at high risk for BRCA mutation and have completed their families should be carefully considered for prophylactic removal of fallopian tubes with conservation of ovaries at the time of gynaecological or other intra-peritoneal surgery'.

If STIC lesions are found incidentally post-operatively, with no associated malignancy, there is no recommendation for further surgical staging or investigation.

Assessment and Diagnosis

Clinical Presentation

The majority of patients who present with symptoms of ovarian cancer already have advanced disease. Ovarian cancer is renowned as the 'silent killer'. Typical symptoms include progressive feelings of:

- Abdominal distension
- Bloating and indigestion
- Bowel symptoms, new onset 'irritable bowel syndrome'
- Urinary symptoms such as frequency and urgency
- Early satiety, weight loss, reduced appetite

Many patients will present in the acute setting with:

- Abdominal/pelvic pain
- Bowel obstruction
- Pleural effusion
- Pulmonary emboli
- Abdominal distension (ascites).

Less common presenting symptoms include vaginal bleeding or discharge and rectal bleeding. Patients may rarely present with symptoms arising from para-neoplastic syndromes. This may include hypercalcaemia, dermatomyositis, nephrotic syndrome and polyneuritis. Occasionally cervical cytology may report atypical glandular cells, which are then identified to be originating from an ovarian carcinoma.

NICE Guidance 122 recommends investigation with the tumour marker Cancer Antigen 125 (CA125) if a patient reports symptoms of persistent distension, bloating, early satiety, loss of appetite, pelvic pain or urinary urgency, especially if she is above 50 years. If the serum CA125 is greater than 35 IU/ml, pelvic USS is recommended, and referral to secondary care if the findings suggest ovarian cysts/cancer. Patients should be referred via the NHS rapid access 2-week-wait pathway, but due to the vagueness of symptoms, they are often seen by other specialties before referral to gynaecology.

RCOG Greentop Guideline 34 recommends:

- A thorough history
    - Risk factors and symptoms suggestive of ovarian cancer
    - Family history of ovarian, bowel or breast cancer
- A full physical examination
    - Body-mass index
    - Abdominal examination (to identify a pelvic/abdominal/omental mass or ascites)
    - Vaginal examination (to identify a pelvic mass or pouch of Douglas involvement).

Investigations

Appropriate investigations usually comprise of:

- Tumour markers
- Ultrasonography
- CT scan if malignancy is suggested by tumour markers or ultrasound scan.

Tumour Markers

CA125 is an antigenic determinant on a high molecular weight glycoprotein expressed by EOC and other tissues of Müllerian origin. A raised level (>35 U/ml) is seen in approximately 80% of EOC. However, it is only raised in 50% of stage-1 cancers, and not consistently raised with less common EOCs (mucinous, clear cell, mixed Müllerian). Raised levels are also found with

Table 10.3 IOTA group ultrasound classification system for ovarian lesions

Benign	Malignant
Unilocular	Irregular solid
Solid components <7 mm	Ascites
Acoustic shadowing	≥4 papillary structures
Smooth multilocular <10 cm	Irregular multilocular solid >10 cm
No blood flow on colour Doppler	Prominent blood flow on colour Doppler

Table 10.4 Formula for calculating RMI score. RMI = $U \times M \times CA125$

Ultrasound scoring (U): solid area, multilocular cyst, bilateral cysts, ascites or distant metastases

	0 = no characteristics
	1 = 1 characteristic
	3 = 2–5 characteristics

Menopausal status (M)

	1 = pre-menopausal
	3 = post-menopausal

CA125

many benign conditions (e.g. menstruation, fibroids, endometriosis), peritoneal inflammation (e.g. pelvic inflammatory disease, ovarian torsion/haemorrhage, peritonitis, pancreatitis) and pregnancy. Therefore, when used in isolation, it only has a pooled sensitivity and specificity of 78% for differentiating benign from malignant masses.

- CA125 is the only tumour marker used for primary evaluation to facilitate Risk of Malignancy Index (RMI) calculation (see below).
- CA125 should not be used in isolation to determine if a cyst is malignant.
- A normal CA125 does not exclude ovarian cancer.
- There is not enough evidence to support other tumour marker use in post-menopausal women.
- Tumour markers including β-hCG, α-FP and LDH should be used when investigating women under the age of 40 years, due to greater risk of germ cell and stromal ovarian tumours in younger women.

Ultrasonography

USS is the investigation of choice to assess adnexal masses and identify suspicious characteristics. Transvaginal USS (TVUS) is the preferred route, but transabdominal scans should be used to supplement images when the cyst is large and to identify associated abdominal disease.

The **International Ovarian Tumor Analysis (IOTA)** group has developed a USS classification system to help differentiate benign and malignant features when an adnexal mass is identified (Table 10.3).

Risk of Malignancy Index

In the United Kingdom, the most widely used tool to evaluate the likelihood of malignancy in an adnexal mass is the RMI I score. This combines the ultrasound

Table 10.5 Example of a protocol for triaging women using the RMI

Risk	RMI	Women (%)	Risk of cancer (%)
Low	<25	40	<3
Moderate	25–250	30	20
High	>250	30	75

features, CA125 level and menopausal status to help predict the risk of ovarian cancer, and consequently provide guidance on subsequent management (Table 10.4).

An example of a protocol for triaging women using the Risk of Malignancy Index is shown in Table 10.5.

- High-risk patients (RMI ≥ 250) should be referred to a gynaecological oncology centre MDT for further management.
- Low/intermediate risk patients (RMI 0–250) should be managed according to their symptoms and ultrasound findings.
- If cancer is diagnosed at laparoscopy, biopsies should be taken (either BSO or peritoneal/omental biopsies) and cytoreductive surgery (CRS) should be undertaken in a cancer centre.

Computed Tomography

A computed tomography (CT) of the abdomen and pelvis is recommended if the CA125 and ultrasound scan are suggestive of malignancy. This is to identify the presence of metastatic disease. A CT of the chest can also be used to identify disease affecting the chest.

MRI and PET/CT are not used routinely in the initial assessment of women presenting with suspected ovarian cancer. MRI may be helpful in the minority of cases where there is still diagnostic uncertainty on USS of an adnexal mass (Figure 10.2).

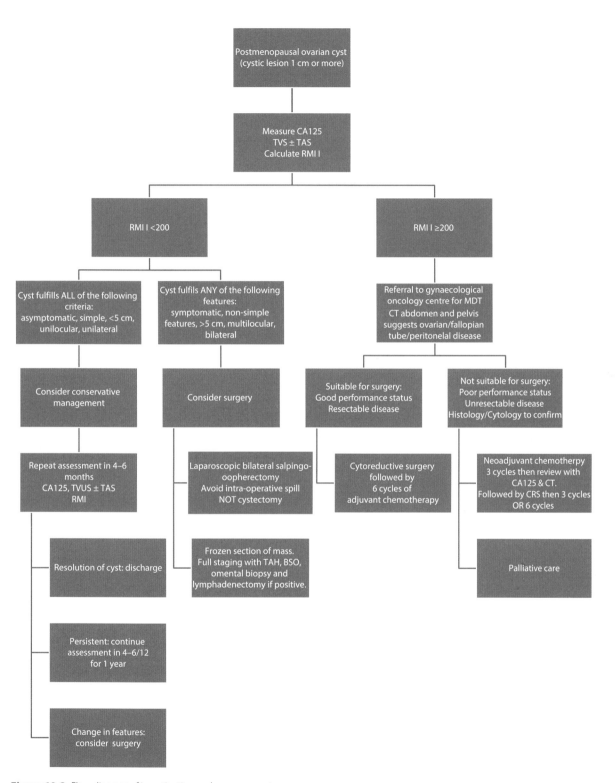

Figure 10.2 Flow diagram of investigation and management

Treatment – Staging and Surgery

The management of patients with EOC begins with accurate diagnosis and staging. A combination of surgery (aiming for optimal cytoreduction of metastatic disease) and platinum-based chemotherapy is used for all but low grade, early stage disease. A small minority of patients may be too unwell for treatment, and best supportive care may be appropriate (Figure 10.3).

Ovarian cancer is staged using the Federation of Gynaecology and Obstetrics (FIGO) system. This was updated in 2014 to encompass ovarian, fallopian tube and peritoneal carcinomas (see Appendix).

Radiological and Histological Staging

CT imaging can indicate the extent of disease in the chest, abdomen and pelvis, prior to surgical staging. If the patient is considered unsuitable for CRS (due to co-morbidities or the location of disease), or if chemotherapy is planned first, then image-guided biopsies or peritoneal/pleural cytology should be collected to

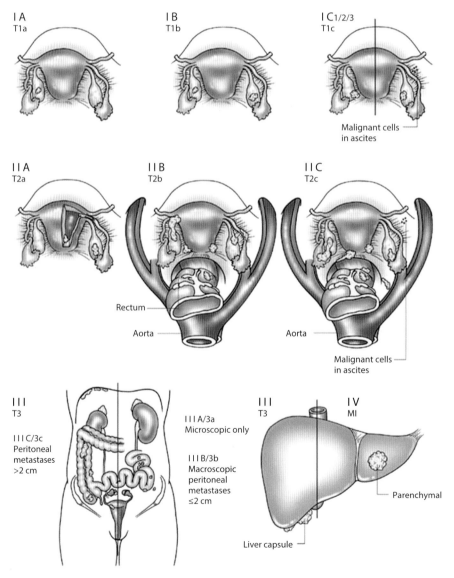

Figure 10.3 Diagrammatic representation of staging for ovarian cancer

confirm diagnosis prior administering chemotherapy. Occasionally an image-guided biopsy may not be technically possible, and laparoscopic biopsies should be considered. Only in exceptional cases, and in agreement with the MDT, should chemotherapy be given based on cytological diagnosis alone. Efforts must be made to attain histology, or consider upfront surgery if appropriate.

Staging and Surgery for Suspected Early Stage Disease (Stage 1)

The aim of staging surgery is to establish the diagnosis, identify any microscopic metastatic spread, and to remove any visible tumour. The standard approach is via midline laparotomy, thus exposing the entire abdomen. Comprehensive surgical staging includes:

- Peritoneal washings
- Total hysterectomy and BSO
- Omentectomy
- Retroperitoneal lymphadenectomy (pelvic and para-aortic)
- Multiple peritoneal biopsies
- Upper abdominal assessment
- Removal of all suspicious looking areas.

Care must be taken to avoid intra-operative cyst rupture, as this will automatically 'upstage' IA/IB disease to IC1, with the latter requiring post-operative adjuvant chemotherapy. In selected cases a laparoscopic approach may be offered, with the aim of reducing morbidity. Although the laparoscopic approach is technically feasible, and there are potential advantages, there is insufficient evidence at present to support this in routine practice. Alternative approaches include laparoscopic BSO with frozen section analysis. If malignancy is confirmed, then full-staging procedures can follow-on immediately avoiding the morbidity of repeated operations. This requires expertise and collaboration with the pathology department.

Stage 1A/B disease with grade 1 or 2 histology does not require adjuvant chemotherapy. If surgical staging is insufficient, the patient may be under-staged, and would be advised to receive adjuvant chemotherapy or a further staging procedure. All cases with high-grade or clear cell histology will be advised to receive adjuvant chemotherapy irrespective of their surgical stage.

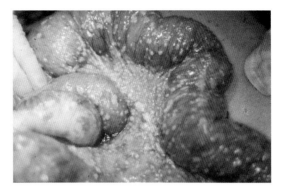

Figure 10.4 Widespread miliary deposits in a case of advanced ovarian cancer

Staging and Surgery for Advanced Disease

The aim of surgery for advanced disease is complete cytoreduction, meaning removal of all visible disease. Surgery may be planned as initial treatment (primary debulking surgery), or after a course of three cycles of neoadjuvant chemotherapy (interval surgical procedure), provided the diagnosis has been confirmed by biopsy. The aim of both approaches is the removal of all visible disease, known as complete cytoreduction (Figure 10.4).

> **TIP**
> Cytoreduction and debulking are terms used interchangeably to describe the surgical removal of tumour deposits.

CRS for Advanced Disease

Complete surgical cytoreduction for EOC results in increased survival. Therefore the aim of surgery should be to remove all macroscopically visible disease. Each 10% increase in patients achieving complete cytoreduction is associated with a 2.3 months increase in mean overall survival. Surgery is typically performed through a large, midline laparotomy incision, often extending to the xiphisternum. At the end of a cytoreductive procedure, it is essential for the surgeon to accurately record the outcome of debulking. The following terms are widely used:

- **Complete cytoreduction** – no visible disease
- **Optimal cytoreduction** – ≤1 cm in maximum tumour diameter remaining

- **Suboptimal cytoreduction** – >1 cm tumour nodules remaining.

Surgical procedures that may be required to achieve complete cytoreduction include:

- BSO
- Total abdominal hysterectomy (TAH)
- Supra-colic omentectomy
- Bowel resection
  - Rectosigmoid resection with anastomosis or colostomy
  - Total colectomy with ileostomy[1]
  - Small bowel resection with anastomosis[1]
  - Radical oophorectomy (en-bloc retroperitoneal resection of pelvic peritoneum, uterus, cervix, tubes, ovaries, rectosigmoid)[1]
- Pelvic and para-aortic lymphadenectomy (of enlarged nodes only)
- Peritonectomy[1]
  - Diaphragmatic and Morison's pouch (following mobilisation of the liver)
  - Pelvic – including bladder peritoneum, sigmoid, pouch of Douglas, etc.
- Splenectomy[1]
- Cholecystectomy[1]
- Partial gastrectomy[1]
- Excision of disease from porta-hepatis[1]
- Liver resection[1]

Primary surgery may be the preferred approach if complete resection is judged to be achievable. However, feasibility of CRS must be carefully considered on an individual case-by-case basis according to disease resectability and the fitness of the patient to withstand such surgery. Some disease is not readily amenable to surgical resection, such as bulky disease at the porta-hepatis, extensive small bowel disease and parenchymal liver involvement. Additionally some patients are unable to tolerate such extensive surgery due to age, medical co-morbidities and nutritional status. Despite the potential survival benefit associated with primary CRS, surgical morbidity can be extensive, with significant risks of complications. When complications do arise, the extended recovery period can cause delay in commencing chemotherapy, which may offset the benefits gained from their surgery.

Unfortunately, at present there is no reliable preoperative tool to determine the likelihood of surgical resectability. Sometimes during primary laparotomy, optimal cytoreduction is found to be unachievable. In this scenario biopsies should be taken and the procedure abandoned (open and close laparotomy). This decision relates to evidence that leaving even a single area of disease >1 cm carries the same prognosis as leaving multiple sites of disease. Therefore surgical morbidity must be minimised, and patients should be considered for chemotherapy.

Patients who receive neoadjuvant chemotherapy followed by CRS have a significantly lower risk of perioperative complications and mortality.

Treatment – Chemotherapy

The standard management for the majority of patients with ovarian cancer is a CRS approach combined with chemotherapy. There are two principle treatment approaches:

- Primary CRS – debulking first, followed by six cycles of chemotherapy
- Interval CRS – biopsy to confirm disease, three cycles of neoadjuvant chemotherapy, followed by surgery and then another three cycles of chemotherapy.

Long-term prognosis may be better in carefully selected women who receive successful primary surgery with post-operative chemotherapy compared to those undergoing upfront chemotherapy with interval CRS. However, the perioperative morbidity and mortality is significantly lower in those having upfront chemotherapy followed by surgery.

'Neoadjuvant' (upfront) chemotherapy is used before surgery for patients unsuitable for primary surgery, due to either radiologically detected unresectable disease or poor performance status with associated perioperative morbidity and mortality risk. 'Adjuvant' chemotherapy is used following CRS and is ideally commenced within 4 weeks of surgery.

First-line chemotherapy is *carboplatin* (a platinum compound alkylating agent). Cisplatin, an alternative platinum agent, is equally efficacious but has a worse toxicity profile. Paclitaxel (a taxane derivative) is used in combination therapy. Normally both drugs are given intravenously, every 3 weeks for six cycles. However,

---

[1] These procedures are often referred to as 'ultra-radical'.

dosing can vary according to higher risk histology, adjuvant or neoadjuvant courses and stage.

Chemotherapy for Early Stage Disease

The risk of relapse in patients with low-risk disease (comprehensively staged 1A/B with grade 1–2 tumours) is minimal. Therefore, patients are not routinely given adjuvant chemotherapy and receive follow-up for approximately 5 years with a combination of observation, serum CA125 and imaging. Stage 1C, grade 3, or clear cell tumours have a higher relapse rate and poorer prognosis, so adjuvant chemotherapy is recommended. These patients have 40–80% 5-year disease-free survival rates, compared to >90% for low-risk disease. Most commonly six cycles of carboplatin monotherapy are used, avoiding the toxicity of taxane agents. Clear cell tumours are insensitive to platinum-based chemotherapy, so other agents are sometimes used including temsirolimus with carboplatin and paclitaxel. Research continues to search for the most efficacious combination.

Chemotherapy for Advanced-Stage Disease

Most women with stage 3–4 EOC are incurable, even with complete surgical cytoreduction. Most will receive a total of six cycles of combination therapy carboplatin and paclitaxel. In patients who receive neoadjuvant chemotherapy, their response to treatment is assessed after three cycles with repeat measures of CA125 levels and CT imaging. If patients are medically fit for surgery, and imaging suggests a response, CRS is performed, followed by a further three cycles of chemotherapy.

Attempts to introduce targeted molecular agents have had limited success. The addition of bevacizumab (a monoclonal antibody to vascular endothelial growth factor) has been investigated and has shown some benefits, but has significant side-effects. It cannot be used between 28 days before or after surgery. At present it is predominantly used in selected patients for maintenance therapy with some benefit. PARP inhibitors are showing promise for use in patients with BRCA mutations, and in those with recurrent disease.

Hyperthermic Intra-peritoneal Chemotherapy

As advanced ovarian cancer is often limited to the peritoneal cavity, direct intra-peritoneal chemotherapy has the potential to increase drug delivery directly to the tumour. Hyperthermic intra-peritoneal chemotherapy (HIPEC) delivered intraoperatively following CRS showed promising results. It is associated with high morbidity. Currently, HIPEC is not routinely used in clinical practice, and is generally reserved for selected patients in specialist centres, in the context of clinical trials.

Recurrent Disease

The overall likelihood of relapse for all stages of EOC is 62%; however, this is >85% for those who are diagnosed at stage 3–4. Recurrence rates also depend on the disease distribution at the time of diagnosis, the success of surgical cytoreduction, and the response to chemotherapy. Median survival time after recurrence is 2 years. Recurrence can be diagnosed either when the patient is investigated after becoming symptomatic or prior to symptoms when surveillance detects rising CA125 markers or disease on CT imaging.

Chemotherapy for Recurrent Disease

Recurrent disease is usually treated with further chemotherapy. Because cure is not possible in recurrent disease, the primary goal of therapy must be the management of symptoms, and prolonging good quality of life. This can be problematic for patients who have had their recurrence detected on surveillance prior to developing symptoms. Evidence suggests that these patients have a worse quality of life if chemotherapy is administered prior to symptoms, with no increase in survival benefit. It has therefore been advocated that routine surveillance with CA125 is unhelpful for follow-up in asymptomatic patients.

The length of platinum-free interval (i.e. the relapse-free interval after completion of chemotherapy) is a predictor of the likelihood of subsequent response to chemotherapy. Recurrent disease is classified as follows:

- Platinum-sensitive – Platinum-free interval is greater than 6 months. There is a high chance of the disease responding to further platinum-based chemotherapy.
- Platinum-resistant – Platinum-free interval <6 months.
- Platinum refractory – Disease progression when taking platinum.

Platinum-sensitive patients can be considered for further platinum agents with the addition of other drugs such as paclitaxel, topotecan, liposomal doxorubicin, gemcitabine and etoposide. Platinum-resistant patients are often treated with a combination of paclitaxel, doxorubicin and bevacizumab.The issue of how many treatment regimens to use in patients with advanced ovarian cancer is an area of controversy. With low response rates with subsequent chemotherapies, patients need to decide whether to continue chemotherapy or receive only best supportive care.

Surgery for Recurrent Disease

The role of surgery in patients with recurrent disease is debated and appropriate patient selection is vital. Imaging with CT and PET/CT is used to identify the exact site of disease, with any distant recurrence sites. MDT discussion must take place to decide if complete cytoreduction is achievable, and if this is the correct approach for the individual patient. Ideal candidates for secondary surgery include those with disease-free interval longer than 12 months, a solitary tumour, cytoreductable distribution and absent or low volume ascites. Surgery is rarely indicated for patients who have platinum resistant or refractory disease. The preliminary reports from the DESKTOP III trial suggest selected patients may benefit from surgery at the time of their first relapse, provided that complete cytoreduction is achieved. The full trial results are pending and will guide future management of relapsed disease.

Consolidation and Maintenance Therapy

To improve survival, maintenance therapy, novel cytotoxic agents and biologic agents are current areas of research. Hormonal therapies can be used for patients with BRCA mutations. Olaparib, a poly-ADP ribose polymerase (PARP) inhibitor, is recommended for use in platinum-sensitive EOC patients as maintenance treatment for patients with either a germ line or somatic BRCA mutation. Tamoxifen can be used with some benefit when there is a CA125 increase but no radiological evidence of recurrent disease, but this is not a true maintenance therapy. Oestrogen receptor status of the primary tumour can be used to guide hormonal therapy but it is unclear what the receptor status of the recurrent tumour is as it is unusual to take biopsies of the tumour at recurrence. The Scottish SIGN Guidance suggests hormonal therapy, tamoxifen or an aromatase inhibitor can be used for platinum-resistant patients when the original tumour expressed the oestrogen receptor.

Fertility-Sparing Procedures

A minority of younger patients will present with ovarian cancer and wish to retain their fertility. Any decision to carry out conservative surgery requires expert counselling, to ensure that the patient understands, and is willing to accept, the risks and uncertainties of incomplete staging or treatment. The risk of disease in the contra-lateral ovary has been reported as 2.5% but prognostic data are unclear. Fertility preservation may be a realistic option for patients with:

- Borderline tumours (see *BOT* section)
- Non-EOCs
- Early stage 1A EOCs

  Fertility-sparing surgery includes:
- Unilateral salpingo-oopherectomy
- Conservation of the uterus, contra-lateral tube and ovary
- Full surgical staging including peritoneal washings, omental biopsy, unilateral pelvic and full para-aortic lymphadenectomy, peritoneal biopsies
- Biopsy of the remaining ovary is indicated only if it appears abnormal.

Palliative Care

Support from palliative care professionals and gynaecological clinical nurse specialists is essential for delivery of holistic care. Early involvement can be beneficial for patients far in advance of the end-of-life phase.

Bowel obstruction is the commonest end-of-life complication, and may result in hospital admissions with pain, colic, nausea, vomiting, anorexia and dehydration. Bowel obstruction may result from a range of underlying causes including intraluminal, intramural and extramural obstruction, motility disorders from nerve infiltration and constipation. Early investigation with CT may be helpful in selected patients in order to identify the small minority of relatively fit patients with single site obstruction who may benefit from surgery. There appears to be no value for parenteral nutrition for these women in their terminal phase.

Conservative measures are normally used first to reduce the frequency and severity of vomiting.

Therapeutic interventions may include:

- Limiting oral intake
- Antiemetics
- Antisecretory agents such as hyoscine bromide or octreotide

- Analgesics
- Corticosteroids
- Mouth care preparations for comfort
- Fluids for hydration (subcutaneous, or intravenous if appropriate).

Medications are often administered via a subcutaneous continuous infusion (syringe driver). Nasogastric tubes are usually an ineffective way of controlling vomiting caused by malignant bowel obstruction. However, they may provide significant symptomatic relief for patients experiencing faeculant vomiting, gastric outflow obstruction and persistent vomiting when drugs have failed. Laxatives can be helpful for patients in partial obstruction or with constipation.

If conservative measures are unsuccessful, the decision for surgery must take into account available further chemotherapy, overall health, extent of disease, suitable length of unaffected bowel for de-functioning stoma and patient choice. Surgical intervention may not prolong life but it has the potential to significantly improve quality of life and end-of-life experience. Such decisions should take place in a multidisciplinary setting and on discussion with the patient.

Borderline Ovarian Tumours

Borderline ovarian tumours (BOTs) are also known as tumours of low-malignant potential. The neoplasms are a heterogeneous group of tumours comprising atypical epithelium without stromal invasion. These tumours can be associated with peritoneal spread.

> **TIPS**
> Borderline ovarian tumours are different from low-grade ovarian carcinomas. Their clinical behaviour is distinct.

These account for approximately 15% of all primary ovarian neoplasms. They tend to affect younger women, which make issues related to fertility of particular importance in the management of these tumours.

The majority of these tumours are slow growing, with the overall 10-year survival rate over 90%. The majority will present with stage-I disease, confined to the ovary, but the prognosis still remains good for patients with more advanced disease.

BOTs are staged by the same FIGO classification system as ovarian, fallopian tube and primary peritoneal carcinomas.

Pathological Features

BOT tumours occur in the same range of sub-types as those in epithelial ovarian carcinomas. The majority will be serous or mucinous tumours. Endometrioid, clear cell and transitional cell sub-types do occur, but are extremely rare.

Microscopically these tumours comprise of atypical epithelial proliferation, in the absence of destructive stromal invasion. If there are associated peritoneal implants, then it is essential for the pathologist to examine these closely for evidence of invasion. Typically these deposits are not invasive, and are therefore classified as 'non-invasive peritoneal implants', although they may have a macroscopic resembling metastatic carcinoma. Evidence of invasion in either the ovarian tumour, or in peritoneal deposits, would qualify the tumour to be classified as a low-grade carcinoma.

Serous borderline tumours account for 65% of all BOT. They are slow growing and generally confined to the ovary, but approximately 20% of cases have non-invasive peritoneal implants. Around half will be bilateral. Age at presentation is commonly 35–40 years old.

Mucinous borderline tumours are nearly always confined to the ovary at presentation, unlike the serous sub-type. Those that are associated with pseudomyxoma peritonei are usually apendiceal in origin, rather than true ovarian tumours.

Clinical Presentation and Diagnosis

BOTs typically present with the same features as any other adnexal mass, such as abdominal pain, distension, dyparaeunia or urinary frequency. Asymptomatic patients may be diagnosed incidentally with imaging. Ultrasonography does not easily distinguish a BOT from a benign tumour. However, they are often unilateral, solid or with fluid components and papillary projections. Tumour markers are unreliable. CA125 may be normal or elevated. Definitive diagnosis is only possible with post-operative histology.

> **TIP**
> The diagnostic approach for borderline ovarian tumours is identical to that for ovarian cancer.

Surgical Management

Borderline tumours usually present as an adnexal mass with features suspicious for malignancy, and therefore surgery is recommended. The goal of surgery is to remove the affected ovary and tube, confirm the histology, and proceed to the most appropriate surgical procedure.

The choice between full-staging or ovarian conserving surgery can be challenging, and should be discussed and agreed with the patient prior to surgery. Due to the relative rarity of these tumours, there is often limited data to guide management.

For pre-menopausal women who wish to preserve fertility and ovarian function, the contra-lateral adnexa should be preserved. This should be carried out in combination with additional staging procedures that include pelvic washings, omental and peritoneal biopsies. If there are any peritoneal implants present, these should be removed and sent for histology. There is a 7–30% risk of recurrence following unilateral salpingo-oopherectomy alone. Some centres consider/recommend removal of the remaining ovary and tube after completion of the patient's family. For women with bilateral ovarian involvement the decision can be even more challenging. Ovarian cystectomy remains an option, but there is limited data to help guide management for these patients, as borderline tumours are relatively rare. Patients should be informed of these uncertainties, and advised that there may be a higher risk of recurrence, which could include malignancy. Consultation with a fertility expert may be helpful. These women may elect to proceed to completion surgery when they no longer desire fertility.

In post- or peri-menopausal women, surgical treatment should include BSO, and consideration of a full-staging procedure including TAH, peritoneal washings, omentectomy and peritoneal biopsies. Lymphadenectomy is not usually carried out in borderline tumours, as lymph node involvement is uncommon, and survival is excellent even if the lymph nodes are involved. If advanced disease is identified, then CRS of all peritoneal implants is carried out.

Frozen section – This can be a useful tool in the intra-operative management of women with suspected BOTs, especially if fertility preservation is desirable. Performing frozen section on the ovarian tissue can help direct the intra-operative decision regarding the most appropriate procedure, and avoid return for further surgery if a carcinoma is identified. Pathological expertise must be available, and clinicians and patients must be aware that this approach is not 100% accurate.

TIPS

Women who wish to preserve ovarian tissue for a suspected borderline adnexal mass must be counselled of the potential risks for malignancy. Pre-operative discussions must include options regarding conservative surgery versus complete staging. If frozen section is planned, patients must agree on the surgical decisions that will be made with the different possible results.

Adjuvant Treatment

Adjuvant treatment is rarely indicated for women with BOTs.

Follow-Up

Routine follow-up is not currently practised in the United Kingdom because recurrence risk is low, and often occurs late. Cases should be managed on an individual basis. Those patients who have had conservative therapy, or who have risk factors for recurrent disease may be considered for individualised follow-up plans.

Risk factors for recurrence include:

- Advanced disease (II, II or IV) at presentation
- Invasive implants
- Incomplete or conservative surgery
- Increasing age
- Higher grade histology features.

Relapse – If relapse occurs, it is usually treated with further CRS. Relapse may be with invasive carcinoma.

Conclusion

Symptoms of ovarian cancer are often nonspecific and usually occur after the disease has spread. The presence of a pelvic mass in a post-menopausal woman is the most important sign of ovarian cancer. CA125 and USS are used to triage for a possible EOC in the primary assessment of a pelvic mass. Management of EOC should be at a cancer centre, directed by the multidisciplinary team who can offer accurate diagnosis, staging, and surgical expertise together with platinum/taxane combination chemotherapy. CA125 measurement is used to assess response to treatment and for detection of early recurrence. By developing our understanding of the biology of ovarian cancer and its response to treatment, new treatment strategies are being investigated.

Further Reading

Berek J, Crum C, Friedlander M. 2015. Cancer of the ovary, fallopian tube, and peritoneum. FIGO Cancer Report. *International Journal of Gynecology and Obstetrics* 131; 111–22.

NICE. 2011. Ovarian cancer: recognition and initial management. *NICE Clinical Guideline [CG122]*. London: National Institute for Health and Clinical Excellence.

RCOG. 2014. High-grade serous carcinomas. The distal fallopian tube as the origin of non-uterine pelvic.

Scientific Impact Paper No. 44. London: Royal College of Obstetricians and Gynaecologists.

2016. The management of ovarian cysts in postmenopausal women. *RCOG Greentop Guideline 34*. London: Royal College of Obstetricians and Gynaecologists.

SIGN. 2013. Management of epithelial ovarian cancer. *SIGN Guideline 135*. Scotland: Scottish Intercollegiate Guidelines Network.

Endometrial Cancer

Cathrine Holland

Epidemiology

Endometrial cancer is more common in industrialised, developed Western societies where it is the most common gynaecological cancer. The incidence of endometrial cancer rose by 43% between 1993 and 2009, which is believed to be linked to the increasing rates of obesity. Approximately 75% of women diagnosed with endometrial cancer are post-menopausal with the incidence rising steeply over the age of 50, with the median age at presentation being 61 years. However, approximately 20–5% of women are premenopausal at diagnosis, with up to 5% of them below the age of 40.

Aetiology

At least three quarters of endometrial cancers are endometrioid endometrial adenocarcinomas. Atypical endometrial hyperplasia is a precursor lesion for endometrioid-type tumours and is frequently seen in the uterine specimens removed as a treatment for endometrial cancer. The underpinning link between the risk factors for atypical hyperplasia and endometrioid endometrial cancer (EEC) is the effect of unopposed oestrogen on the endometrium.

Endometrial hyperplasia
- Precursor lesion for endometrioid-type tumours.
- The risk of malignant progression is the highest for atypical hyperplasia (8–28% from 4 to 19 years after diagnosis).
- The long-term risk of malignant progression from hyperplasia without atypia is low (only 3%).

Although cigarette smoking is associated with a lower risk of developing EEC, smoking concurrently with exogenous oestrogen use multiplies the risk of developing endometrial cancer.

Risk factors for EEC
- Obesity
- Prolonged anovulation
- Early menarche
- Late menopause
- Use of unopposed oestrogen replacement therapy
- Polycystic ovarian syndrome
- Nulliparity
- Infertility
- Diabetes
- Hypertension
- Tamoxifen use
- Oestrogen-secreting granulosa cell tumour of ovary
- Genetic predisposition, e.g. Lynch syndrome (see Genetic Associations)

The risk factors for non-endometrioid cancers are less well established. Although these tumours frequently arise in non-obese, multiparous women, recent epidemiological evidence suggests that the risk factors for both endometrioid and non-EECs may overlap.

Genetic Associations

Lynch Syndrome

Lynch syndrome (previously known as hereditary nonpolyposis colorectal cancer syndrome) is caused by germline mutations in mismatch repair (MMR) genes (*MSH2*, *MLH1*, *MSH6*, and *PMS2*). The germline mutation is passed on via autosomal dominant inheritance. Lynch syndrome is associated with an increased risk of early onset of endometrial and colorectal cancers. The lifetime risk of developing endometrial cancer with Lynch syndrome is 40–60%, compared to 3% in the general population. There is also an increased risk of ovarian cancer (10–12% compared to 1.4% in the general population). Other associated cancers are small bowel,

Box 11.1 Amsterdam II guidelines for a clinical diagnosis of Lynch syndrome

At least three relatives with a Lynch-associated cancer (endometrium, colorectal, small bowel, ureter, renal pelvis) and:
- One should be a first-degree relative to the other two.
- At least two successive generations should be affected.
- At least one should be diagnosed before age 50.
- Familial adenomatous polyposis should be excluded.
- Tumours should be verified by pathological examination.

Box 11.2 Revised Bethesda guidelines for identification of patients for whom MSI testing is warranted

Tumours from individuals should be tested for MSI in the following situations:
- Individuals in families that satisfy the Amsterdam II criteria
- Colorectal cancer or endometrial cancer diagnosed in a patient below the age of 50
- Individuals of any age with two Lynch-associated cancers (including synchronous, metachronous colorectal or other Lynch-associated cancers)
- Colorectal cancer with the MSI-high[a] histology diagnosed in a patient below the age of 60
- Colorectal cancer diagnosed in one or more first-degree relatives with HNPCC-related tumour, with one of the cancers being diagnosed below the age of 50
- Colorectal cancer diagnosed in two or more first- or second-degree relatives with HNPCC-related tumours, regardless of age

[a]Presence of tumour infiltrating lymphocytes, Crohn's-like lymphocytic reaction, mucinous/signet-ring differentiation or medullary growth pattern.

hepato-pancreatico-biliary, brain, ureteric and renal pelvis cancers. Endometrial cancers with Lynch syndrome are often well to moderately differentiated and early stage at presentation. MMR mutations occur in 9% of women with endometrial cancer diagnosed below the age of 50. Women of any age with endometrial cancer having two or more first-degree relatives with endometrial cancer have approximately 9% chance of MMR abnormality.

Criteria have been developed to aid clinicians in identifying women with possible Lynch syndrome, and select out those that warrant testing for microsatellite instability (MSI) on their tumours (Boxes 11.1 and 11.2). Those at risk should be referred for genetic counselling and testing. Identification of affected families is important as affected individuals may benefit from screening for colorectal cancer or risk-reducing surgery (see *Prevention*).

TIP

Any woman presenting with an endometrial cancer below the age of 50 and any woman with synchronous endometrial and ovarian cancer should be referred for genetic counselling and testing for MMR abnormalities should be performed on their tumours.

Cowden Syndrome

Cowden syndrome is caused by a germline mutation in the tumour suppressor gene, PTEN. The germline mutation is passed on via autosomal dominant inheritance. Cowden syndrome is characterised by multiple hamartomas (benign tumours) and macrocephaly. Women with Cowden syndrome have an increased risk of other tumours, including endometrial, breast, thyroid, colorectal, renal cell carcinoma and melanoma. The lifetime risk for developing endometrial cancer is up to 30%. Tumours arising in this group are typically low-grade endometrioid endometrial adenocarcinomas.

Diagnosis

'Red flags' symptoms of endometrial cancer
- The most common presenting symptom for endometrial cancer is post-menopausal bleeding. At least 90% of women present with this symptom.
- Unexplained post-menopausal vaginal discharge (may indicate a pyometra secondary to endometrial pathology).
- Persistent intermenstrual bleeding in women over the age of 40.
- Failure of treatment for heavy or problematic menstrual bleeding in women above the age of 45.

TIPS

The presence of abnormal non-cervical glandular cells on a routine cervical smear is strongly associated with an underlying endometrial abnormality (atypical hyperplasia or cancer). A woman with this cervical cytology result should be referred for urgent hysteroscopy and endometrial sampling under the 2-week rule for suspected cancers (not colposcopy).

Referral Guidelines and Diagnostic Testing

According to current NICE guidance, women with post-menopausal bleeding (unexplained vaginal bleeding more than 12 months after menstruation has stopped because of the menopause) over the age of 55

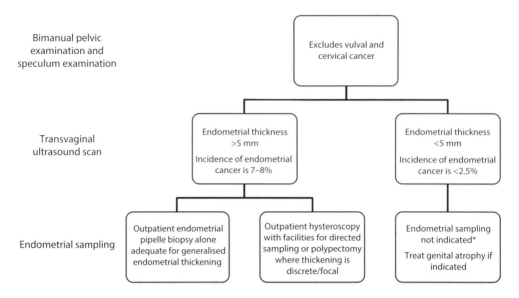

Bimanual pelvic examination and speculum examination

Transvaginal ultrasound scan

Endometrial sampling

Excludes vulval and cervical cancer

Endometrial thickness >5 mm

Incidence of endometrial cancer is 7–8%

Endometrial thickness <5 mm

Incidence of endometrial cancer is <2.5%

Outpatient endometrial pipelle biopsy alone adequate for generalised endometrial thickening

Outpatient hysteroscopy with facilities for directed sampling or polypectomy where thickening is discrete/focal

Endometrial sampling not indicated*

Treat genital atrophy if indicated

Figure 11.1 Algorithm for the assessment of post-menopausal bleeding. *Women re-presenting with further post-menopausal bleeding, despite previous normal pelvic examination and transvaginal ultrasound scan, should be re-referred directly for out-patient hysteroscopy

should be referred to a gynaecologist using a suspected cancer pathway referral (HSC205/2-week wait pathway) for assessment within 2 weeks. Consideration should also be given to women with post-menopausal bleeding below the age of 55. It is also important to consider the possibility of endometrial pathology in pre-menopausal women with new onset of chaotic menses particularly in the presence of known risk factors (see *Risk factors*). Women on tamoxifen after a diagnosis of breast cancer have an increased risk of developing endometrial cancer and should therefore be referred using a suspected cancer pathway if they experience any abnormal bleeding.

Physical examination, including direct visualisation of the cervix with a Cusco bivalve speculum, is required to exclude obvious vulval or cervical pathology as a cause of bleeding.

Trans-vaginal ultrasound scan is the initial diagnostic tool to assess endometrial thickness and contour and to exclude ovarian pathology (Figure 11.1).

While endometrial thickening has a poor positive predictive value for endometrial pathology (hyperplasia or cancer), the negative predictive value of a thin endometrium is high (98%).

Many studies have sought to determine the endometrial thickness that should be used as a cut-off value for directing further investigations. Most gynaecological services use 4 mm as the cut-off value for trans-vaginal ultrasound scan.

The post-test probabilities for endometrial pathology after a negative (normal) ultrasound result are only 1.2% and 2.3% when normal values for double-layer endometrial thickness of 4 mm and 5 mm are used, respectively. Where the endometrium is thickened, outpatient aspiration endometrial biopsy is required. Diagnostic hysteroscopy is useful if 'blind' outpatient endometrial sampling fails or is non-diagnostic. It is usually carried out as an outpatient procedure (Figure 11.2).

TIPS

Tamoxifen use can cause benign changes beneath the endometrium that manifest as endometrial thickening on transvaginal ultrasound scan. As a result, ultrasound is less useful for assessment of abnormal bleeding in this group and women on tamoxifen with abnormal bleeding should be directly investigated with hysteroscopy and endometrial biopsy.

Pathology

Primary endometrial cancers arise from the epithelial elements within the endometrium comprising of the cells forming the endometrial glandular structures. Tumours can rarely occur in the connective tissue (mesenchymal) elements within the endometrium. These are endometrial stromal sarcomas and account for only 0.2% of all endometrial cancers.

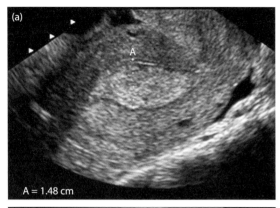

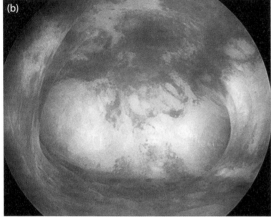

Figure 11.2 Outpatient hysteroscopy: (a) transvaginal ultrasound scan showing thickened endometrium (A) and (b) normal endometrial appearance at hysteroscopy

Classification of Endometrial Cancers

The World Health Organisation (WHO) classification of endometrial tumours is based on architectural features and cellular morphology.

Endometrioid tumours are further classified according to the degree of architectural and nuclear abnormality (grade), with grade 1 tumours most closely resembling the normal endometrial glandular epithelium, and grade 3 tumours showing a much greater degree of architectural and nuclear abnormality (Table 11.1).

Additional tests such as oestrogen receptor (ER) and progesterone receptor (PR) expression are sometimes used to aid diagnosis.

All non-endometrioid tumours are classified as high-grade tumours.

Carcinosarcoma accounts for <5% of all endometrial cancers and is an aggressive tumour composed of epithelial and mesenchymal elements. Although not currently included within the WHO classification of

Table 11.1 WHO classification of endometrial cancers

Primary	Secondary
Endometrioid carcinoma (75–80%) – several variants exist – secretory variant, villoglandular variant, ciliated cell variant, with squamous differentiation	Metastases to endometrium – usually by direct extension from primary cervix or fallopian cancer; rarely from breast, colon, stomach, melanoma
Mucinous adenocarcinoma	
Serous carcinoma (5–10%)	
Clear cell carcinoma (1–5%)	
Adenosquamous carcinoma	
Undifferentiated carcinoma	
Mixed endometrial carcinoma	

epithelial endometrial tumours, evidence from molecular studies suggests that this is an epithelial rather than a mesenchymal (sarcomatous) tumour. The prognosis is significantly worse than that for other types of endometrial cancer.

Although the traditional WHO classification of endometrial cancer is based on morphological appearances, the concept of Type 1 and 2 cancers has been used to differentiate between tumours with differing clinical behaviour, expression of hormone receptors in addition to morphological appearances.

- **Type 1 tumours** generally comprise grade 1 or grade 2 endometrioid tumours and occur in pre-, peri- or younger post-menopausal women. They often arise on a background of the precursor lesion atypical hyperplasia and are usually early stage at diagnosis.
- **Type 2 tumours** include grade 3 endometrioid tumours, undifferentiated tumours and non-endometrioid variants, which are all considered to be high grade. These usually occur in older post-menopausal women, are not associated with atypical hyperplasia and are more frequently of higher stage at presentation. Type 2 tumours have a poorer prognosis overall than Type 1 tumours.

More recent genomic studies suggest the future possibility of a classification system based on genetic signature and herald the potential for future personalised medicine, with treatments targeted against specific molecular anomalies.

Clinical Behaviour of Endometrial Cancers

Endometrial cancer can grow and spread beyond the endometrium by numerous different methods as follows:

Direct extension: First into the myometrium and then through the uterine serosa. Tumours arising in

115

the lower or isthmic portion of the uterus may extend into the cervical stroma and finally to the paracervical and parametrial tissues and structures of the pelvic side wall.

- **Trans-tubal spread** – To fallopian tubes, ovaries and peritoneal cavity.
- **Lymphatic spread** – The pelvic lymph nodes (obturator and iliac nodes) are most commonly affected. Fundal tumours may spread directly to para-aortic nodes. Para-aortic node metastasis is uncommon (<2%) when the pelvic nodes are free of disease. Tumour grade is correlated with the risk of lymph node metastasis. High-grade tumours are associated with an increased risk of lymph node metastasis.
- **Haematogenous spread** – Vaginal metastases can occur as separate lesions from the primary tumour and occur via haematogenous (and possibly lymphatic) spread. The lungs are the most common site for distant haematogenous spread.

> **TIP**
> Serous and clear cell cancers have a tendency to metastasize early, even when the primary tumour is small, including intra-peritoneal spread.

Staging for endometrial cancers – Two staging systems are in use worldwide, the International Federation of Obstetrics and Gynaecology (FIGO) system and the American Joint Committee on Cancer (AJCC) Tumour, Node, Metastasis (TNM) system. These two systems are very similar. Most gynaecologists use the FIGO system to treat women with cancer, but the TNM system is also in widespread use internationally (Figure 11.3).

Prevention

There are a number of modifiable risk factors for endometrial cancer. Women attending consultation at fertility or other gynaecological services with polycystic ovarian syndrome (PCOS), anovulation and other menstrual problems should be advised about the impact of obesity on endometrial cancer risk. Women that are anovulatory with less than four menses per year are at increased risk, and should be treated with a hormonal regime that will provide regular menstruation,

withdrawal bleeds and/or protection for the endometrium, e.g. levonorgestrel intra-uterine system (LNG-IUS).

Risk-Reducing Surgery for Women with Genetic Predisposition

There is proven benefit for risk-reducing surgery in women with Lynch syndrome. Total hysterectomy and bilateral salpingo-oophorectomy (BSO) should be offered to the affected women once they have completed their family. Laparoscopic surgery should be performed unless contraindicated. Women below the age of 45 having risk-reducing surgery are at significant risk of the effects of menopause, and hormone replacement therapy (HRT) should be recommended for them at least until the age of 50. Data regarding the efficacy of risk-reducing surgery for women with Cowden syndrome is lacking.

Screening
Population Screening

There have been no large population-based studies of screening for endometrial cancer. Only published series reporting significant numbers of undiagnosed endometrial abnormalities, including cancer, in asymptomatic women attending for bariatric surgery, are available. However, currently there is insufficient evidence from large, randomised-controlled trials to support the introduction of routine screening in asymptomatic women with obesity.

Women on tamoxifen do not require routine screening but should be referred for assessment if they experience abnormal vaginal bleeding.

Screening for Women with Genetic Predisposition

Most women that develop endometrial cancer on a background of Lynch syndrome present with early stage disease and typically have low-grade tumours with a good overall prognosis. Therefore it is not known whether detection of the tumour via annual screening with trans-vaginal ultrasound, hysteroscopy and endometrial biopsy offers any survival advantage. To date, the efficacy of screening for endometrial cancer in asymptomatic women with genetic predisposition (e.g. Lynch syndrome) remains unproven.

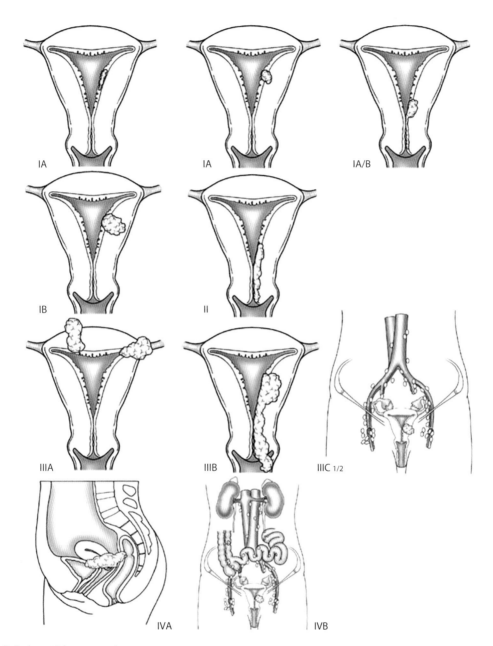

Figure 11.3 Endometrial cancer staging

Management of Pre-malignant Endometrial Disease (Atypical Hyperplasia)

WHO has classified endometrial hyperplasia into two groups based on the presence or absence of cytological atypia, i.e. hyperplasia without atypia and atypical hyperplasia. It is a histological diagnosis and cannot be diagnosed by imaging.

Endometrial hyperplasia without atypia has a low risk of progression to endometrial cancer (<5% over 20 years) and most cases regress spontaneously over time.

Contributing factors such as polycystic ovarian syndrome or unopposed oestrogen use should

117

be addressed as part of management. Women with BMI > 30 kg/m^2 should be advised to lose weight.

Progesterone is used as treatment for those women with hyperplasia without atypia, who have symptoms of abnormal uterine bleeding or where there is failure to regress spontaneously.

Women with atypical hyperplasia should be advised to undergo total hysterectomy, as the risk of an associated underlying malignancy is high (up to 43%). Post-menopausal and peri-menopausal women should also have their ovaries and fallopian tubes removed. The removal of ovaries in pre-menopausal women should be individualised. HRT may be used after total hysterectomy in the absence of endometrial cancer. Laparoscopic hysterectomy is preferable.

Endometrial ablation is contraindicated because post-operative intra-uterine adhesions prevent ongoing endometrial surveillance with histological sampling and complete and permanent endometrial destruction cannot be guaranteed.

Women who prefer to retain fertility should be counselled about the risk of concomitant endometrial cancer and the risk of progression to endometrial cancer. The evidence for the efficacy of fertility-sparing treatment is weak and is based mainly on small observational studies.

Although reported rates for disease regression in small observational studies is high (approximately 85%), the risk of relapse following fertility-sparing treatment is substantial (26%). This treatment is associated with a live birth rate of approximately 26%.

Before embarking on fertility-sparing treatment for atypical hyperplasia, imaging should be performed to exclude both coexisting ovarian malignancy and tumour invasion of the myometrium. A trans-vaginal ultrasound scan is used to assess the ovaries and a magnetic resonance imaging (MRI) scan of the pelvis is used to assess for any myometrial invasion.

The first-line treatment for women desiring fertility-preserving treatment is the LNG-IUS because systemic side effects are less when compared with oral progestogens and also a higher concentration of progesterone is achieved at the endometrium.

Continuous oral progestogens should be used for women who decline the LNG-IUS. Suitable regimens are medroxyprogesterone 10–20 mg/day or norethisterone 10–15 mg/day.

Where disease regression is confirmed histologically on a minimum of two consecutive endometrial biopsies, long-term follow-up with further endometrial biopsies every 6–12 months is recommended until hysterectomy is performed.

The length of follow-up in most studies is short and the true risk of long-term relapse is uncertain. Therefore, once fertility is no longer required, total hysterectomy should be offered (Figure 11.4).

Management of Endometrial Cancer

Once a histological diagnosis of endometrial cancer has been made, the next steps in management are aimed at excluding distant metastases (which may alter the plan for surgical treatment) and preparing the patient for surgery, as this is the preferred treatment in the great majority of cases.

Clinical History and Examination

A comprehensive history should be taken, to include co-morbidities, history of previous abdominal or vaginal surgery and family history of cancer.

Physical examination should include inspection of the cervix (which may detect gross involvement of the cervix) and a bimanual pelvic examination to determine the size of the uterus. The latter is relevant because a grossly enlarged uterus may be a contraindication to laparoscopic surgery for endometrial cancer. Delivery of a disrupted uterus makes histopathological interpretation more difficult, resulting in an adverse effect on post-surgical decision making with regard to post-operative radiotherapy or chemotherapy. There is also a theoretical risk of disseminating tumour intra-abdominally.

Basic pre-operative investigations include:

- Full blood count
- Serum urea and electrolytes
- Serum liver function tests
- Electrocardiogram.

Because of the risk factors associated with the development of endometrial cancer, some women will require more extensive pre-operative preparation and assessment due to other factors such as diabetes, obesity and hypertension.

Pre-operative Imaging

Imaging is used to exclude distant metastases which may indicate the need for non-surgical treatment is some cases. It is also used to assign a 'provisional stage' which aids decisions about the correct setting for

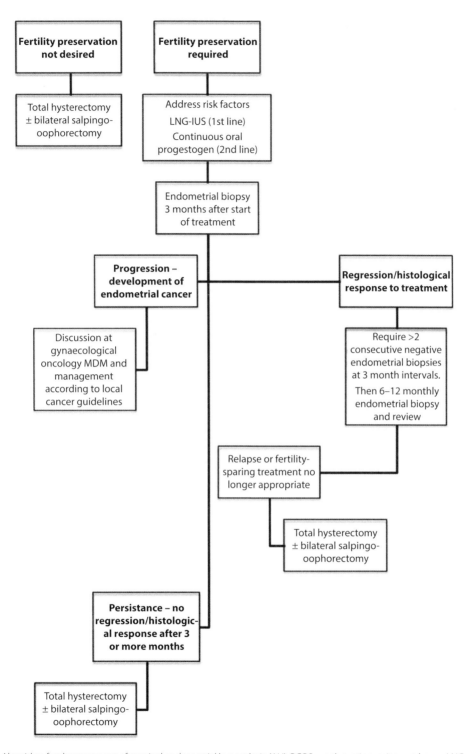

Figure 11.4 Algorithm for the treatment of atypical endometrial hyperplasia (AH). PCOS = polycystic ovarian syndrome; LNG-IUS = levonorgestrel containing intra-uterine system; MDM = multi-disciplinary meeting (adapted from RCOG Green-top Guideline No. 67. Management of endometrial hyperplasia)

surgery (local hospital or cancer centre) and the extent of surgery.

It should be noted that staging for endometrial cancer is surgical, i.e. final disease stage depends upon the histopathology of the surgical specimens. Therefore, the pre-operative findings are only a guide and a tumour may be up- or down-staged following surgery and receipt of pathology results.

Ultrasound – Although ultrasound is an important tool in the investigation of post-menopausal bleeding, it has limited, if any, role in the further management of endometrial cancer.

Plain X-ray or computerised-tomography (CT) scan – A plain chest X-ray is required for all women prior to surgery in order to detect pulmonary metastases. CT scan of the thorax is preferred for high-grade (behaviourally more aggressive) tumours.

MRI scan – MRI is the main imaging modality for further evaluation of proven endometrial cancer pre-operatively, although its use is not universal. MRI is mainly used to assess myometrial invasion pre-operatively. This information, together with tumour grade, determines whether the woman requires surgery in a tertiary level cancer centre by a sub-specialist gynaecological oncologist, or whether the surgery can be performed at secondary care cancer unit. MRI of the pelvis is more accurate than clinical examination, ultrasound scan or CT scan and correctly correlates with post-operative histology in 85–95% of cases. MRI is superior to CT scan for imaging the cervix and surrounding soft tissues. If cervical extension of tumour is seen, there is a need for an extended or radical hysterectomy to effect full tumour clearance, although other factors such as obesity and patient fitness may preclude this (Figure 11.5).

Pelvic lymph nodes are also imaged by MRI scan, and where nodes are significantly enlarged or morphologically abnormal, removal of lymph nodes is indicated. MRI scan has the advantage that it does not involve the use of ionising radiation but it may not be possible for women with claustrophobia.

CT scan – Indications for CT scan in the management of endometrial cancer are to identify enlarged extra-pelvic lymph nodes and distant metastases in women with initial MRI findings or clinical features suggestive of advanced disease. CT is also routinely indicated in the pre-operative assessment for intra-abdominal spread and distant metastases in women with high grade and non-endometrioid type

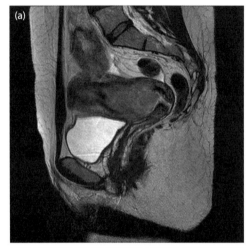

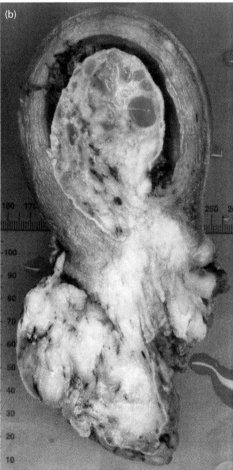

Figure 11.5 MRI scan for pre-treatment evaluation of endometrial cancer: (a) saggital view shows tumour invading and expanding the cervical stroma and (b) hysterectomy specimen shows a large endometrial tumour replacing the cervix and prolapsing into the vagina

endometrial cancers. CT is also used in the management of recurrent disease, to document sites of extrapelvic metastasis and plan appropriate management.

Surgery for Endometrial Cancer

In almost all cases, surgery is the initial treatment for endometrial cancer. Total hysterectomy and BSO are standard components of the surgery. Peritoneal cytology is no longer necessary for staging purposes.

For low grade (G1 and G2 endometrioid cancers) with <50% myometrial invasion on MRI scan (provisional stage IA tumours), total hysterectomy and BSO is sufficient as the risk of lymph node metastases is low (<5%). For high grade or more deeply invasive tumours, the risk of lymph node involvement is higher. Lymphadenectomy provides helpful prognostic information, but evidence from randomised-controlled trials shows that there is no reduction in death or recurrence of cancer when systematic lymphadenectomy is performed, i.e. there is no evidence of therapeutic benefit. In addition, women having lymphadenectomy experience more complications from surgery. However, lymphadenectomy can be used to help identify those women who may benefit from adjuvant pelvic radiotherapy in selected cases. Consequently, there is variable practice regarding pelvic lymphadenectomy in women with high grade, or locally advanced endometrial cancer. Enlarged or morphologically abnormal lymph nodes on pre-operative imaging should be removed where possible.

Omental biopsy/infracolic omentectomy is indicated for women with serous endometrial cancers as these have a predilection for intra-peritoneal spread. Laparoscopic hysterectomy is associated with similar overall survival and disease-free survival when compared to open hysterectomy for women with presumed early stage (stage I) endometrial cancer.

Laparoscopic surgery is associated with reduced operative morbidity and reduced hospital stay compared to open hysterectomy and should be offered in the absence of contraindications. Radical (extended) hysterectomy and BSO with pelvic lymphadenectomy alone, with subsequent adequate tumour-free margins and negative nodes, may be curative in women with suspected stage II disease. Radical hysterectomy is more morbid than 'simple' extra-fascial hysterectomy and some women with endometrial cancer will not be suitable for radical surgery due to co-morbidity, including significant obesity.

Advanced endometrial cancer – Women with more advanced endometrial cancer (stages III and IV) are a diverse group and, within these two stage groups, prognosis varies considerably. Examination under anaesthetic may be indicated for women with locally advanced disease, to determine operability. Surgery, followed by chemotherapy, radiotherapy or both, remains the standard initial treatment approach for women with advanced disease, although the role of aggressive debulking of all tumour deposits with widespread metastases is uncertain. Good palliation of bleeding and pelvic symptoms can be achieved with hysterectomy, even if distant metastases are present, but the correct treatment should be determined after multi-disciplinary discussion taking into account the woman's symptoms, pre-operative histology and imaging and physical condition.

Recurrence – Radiotherapy is usually the first choice in this situation. Cure is possible for isolated vaginal vault recurrence. Occasionally surgery may be appropriate for women with recurrent endometrial cancer, if the disease is confined to the vaginal vault and if the woman has previously received radiotherapy to the pelvis. Surgery is rarely used for other instances of recurrence. There may be a role for surgery if there is a limited area of recurrent disease when there has been a long disease-free interval and the patient has a good performance status. This is an uncommon situation.

Complications of Surgery

Complications of surgery can occur intra-operatively, in the early or late post-operative phase. To minimise the risks:

- A urinary catheter should be placed intra-operatively.
- Peri-operative antibiotics should be administered.
- Prophylactic measures against venous thrombo-embolism (VTE) should be used peri-operatively and for 28 days post-operatively in accordance with NICE guidance.

Intra-operative complications include:

- Primary haemorrhage
- Bladder injury, 0.05–0.66%
- Bowel injury, <0.5%
- Ureteric injury, 0.02–0.4%
- Neurological damage.

The ureter is at the risk of damage as it passes behind the ovarian blood vessels and beneath the uterine vessels. Damage at the pelvic brim can be simply avoided by dividing the round ligament and then extending the peritoneal incision to open the broad ligament in a cephalad direction. The ureter is then easily identified retro-peritoneally as it crosses the bifurcation of the common iliac vessels. The ovarian vessels can then be isolated and cut with the ureter in full view. Risk of ureteric damage near the cervix is minimised by opening the utero-vesical peritoneum and reflecting the bladder caudally down the cervix in the midline with sharp dissection. This moves the bladder inferiorly taking the ureter with it and allows clamping/sealing of the uterine vessels close to the uterus at the cervico-isthmic junction.

Early post-operative complications include:
- Pulmonary complications, e.g. hospital acquired pneumonia, basal atelectasis
- Venous thromboembolism
- Pelvic haematoma
- Wound infection
- Urinary tract infection
- Urinary retention – bladder dysfunction is more common after radical hysterectomy due to disruption of autonomic nerve supply
- Paralytic ileus.

TIPS
Unrecognised intra-operative bowel injury may not be apparent in the immediate post-operative period. This complication should be considered in women treated laparoscopically that appear slow to recover, particularly if they are not making good post-operative progress by day 2 or 3. Typical symptoms are peritonitis, severe abdominal pain, fever and abdominal distension. Prompt recourse to CT scan of the abdomen and pelvis is advised to rule out bowel injury under these circumstances.

Late post-operative complications include:
- Lymphoedema – following pelvic lymphadenectomy (5–38%).
- Pelvic lymphocysts/lymphocoele – following pelvic lymphadenectomy.
- Vesico-vaginal fistula – especially following radical hysterectomy.
- Ureteric fistula – more common following radical hysterectomy and often secondary to ureteric ischaemia; increased risk with post-operative (adjuvant) radiotherapy.

- Incisional hernia – more common following midline abdominal incision.
- Port-site hernia – risk with laparoscopic port sites >7 mm in diameter. These should be closed intra-operatively. Herniation of bowel may lead to ischaemia, bowel obstruction or peritonitis.

The Role of Radiotherapy

Radiotherapy is a directed or regional treatment which may be used in the following ways for treatment of endometrial cancer:

Adjuvant (after initial or primary treatment such as surgery) – to increase the chance of cure or reduce local relapse in the vagina as this is the most common site of recurrence. This is the most common indication in endometrial cancer.

Palliative – for the relief of symptoms such as bleeding from recurrent pelvic disease or to provide pain relief for a bony metastasis.

Salvage – given with the aim of cure for isolated vaginal vault recurrence. The cure rate is 70–80%.

Radical or curative radiotherapy – seldom used but may be indicated as the primary treatment where a woman has such severe co-morbidity that surgery cannot be considered. Cure rates of approximately 65% have been reported but the risk of recurrence is high (20%).

Radiotherapy can be delivered as external beam radiotherapy (EBRT) (also known as teletherapy). X-rays are generated by a linear accelerator machine (linac) and focused into a treatment beam at a distance from the area to be treated. Radiotherapy can also be delivered as brachytherapy whereby the radioactive source is placed into or adjacent to the area that requires treatment. When brachytherapy is given after hysterectomy for endometrial cancer, the radioactive source is placed at the vaginal vault inside a vaginal applicator.

Efficacy of Radiotherapy

The efficacy of radiotherapy has been well established in large, randomised-controlled trials.

Adjuvant radiotherapy after surgery is effective at reducing local recurrence of cancer in the pelvis but does not increase survival in women at low or intermediate risk of recurrence. Vaginal brachytherapy is as effective as EBRT in reducing vaginal recurrence and

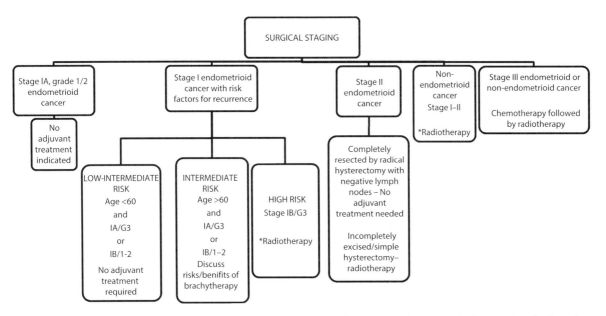

Figure 11.6 Use of adjuvant (post-operative) radiotherapy and chemotherapy for endometrial cancer. *Radiotherapy is beneficial in reducing the risk of loco-regional relapse. The use of adjuvant chemotherapy in addition to radiotherapy for women at high risk of recurrence has not yet been fully defined in randomised controlled trials. The PORTEC3 trial (awaiting analysis of results) examined the benefits of adjuvant chemotherapy in addition to pelvic radiotherapy for women at high risk of distant recurrence. While the data is not yet mature, many cancer centres consider the use of adjuvant chemotherapy in women with indicators for increased risk of distant recurrence, e.g. high grade/non-endometrioid histology with myometrial invasion

has fewer side effects. There may be a survival advantage when adjuvant EBRT is given to women at high risk of recurrence (outer half myometrial invasion and grade 3 disease). This has not been absolutely confirmed by meta-analyses, because in the trials assessed, not all women included were truly at high risk of recurrence.

The routine use of EBRT is not advocated in stage I endometrial cancer as there is a risk of lasting side effects and no conclusive evidence of a survival benefit (Figure 11.6).

Side Effects and Complications of Radiotherapy

Acute side effects following radiotherapy affect approximately a quarter to a third of all women. Common acute side effects are fatigue, bowel symptoms (frequent bowel motions, diarrhoea) and urinary symptoms (frequency and cystitis). Symptoms range from mild (can be managed with simple measures) to severe (requiring modification or cessation of treatment). Most acute side effects resolve or reduce within 6–8 weeks.

Stenosis of the vagina is a common side effect in women treated with pelvic radiotherapy and most

often develops in the first year after treatment. Women are trained in the regular use of vaginal dilators. In addition to assisting women in maintaining sexual function, it is important that the vagina must be accessible for follow-up examination because approximately 50% of recurrences occur at this site.

The risk of severe late toxicity, requiring surgery, is approximately 3%. These complications include fistula formation involving bowel and bladder and are more common following EBRT compared with brachytherapy.

Role of Chemotherapy

Chemotherapy is used for the following indications:

Adjuvant treatment for advanced disease (stage III and IV) – Clinical trials show a modest improvement in survival.

Adjuvant treatment for early stage disease – Chemotherapy may be used following surgery for high-grade tumours where the risk of distant relapse is significantly increased, e.g. carcinosarcoma, serous carcinoma. Many centres use chemotherapy in this setting although the evidence base for this approach is currently not strong. Results from a large, randomised-controlled trial (PORTEC3), addressing the role of chemotherapy and radiotherapy compared to radiotherapy alone, are awaited. There has generally been an increased use of adjuvant chemotherapy for both high-risk stage I disease and stage II disease, pending the outcome of this trial.

Palliative treatment for recurrent disease – Particularly extra-pelvic recurrence or where there is no scope for further radiotherapy.

Neo-adjuvant (prior to surgery) chemotherapy – Occasionally used as initial treatment for advanced disease where the primary (uterine) tumour is thought to be inoperable due to direct extension into surrounding structures. Surgery may be possible subsequently if the response to chemotherapy is good.

The most common chemotherapy agents in use for endometrial cancer given intra-venously are as follows:

- Platinum-based, e.g. carboplatin
- Taxanes, e.g. paclitaxel
- Anthracyclines, e.g. doxorubicin.

A combination of carboplatin and paclitaxel is the most common regimen and is typically given as four treatments (cycles), at three-weekly intervals.

Hormonal (Endocrine) Therapy

There is no indication for the use of hormonal agents as an adjuvant (post-surgery) treatment. Adjuvant progestogen treatment does not reduce recurrence or improve survival. The main role of hormonal therapy is in the palliative treatment of women with recurrent or advanced disease where chemotherapy is considered too toxic. Hormonal therapy is often used for the treatment of pulmonary metastases as it is generally well tolerated. There is an initial response rate of 10–25%. Low-grade tumours are more likely to respond as they more frequently express hormone receptors. Assessment of hormone receptor status on the diagnostic tumour sample is useful in determining the likely benefit from progestogen therapy for advanced or recurrent disease.

Recommended drug regimens are as follows:

- Medroxyprogesterone acetate (MPA) 200–400 mg daily in divided doses, or
- Megestrol acetate 40–320 mg daily in divided doses.

Median overall survival is 10 months. Down-regulation of PRs within the tumour may occur after a period of treatment, leading to reduced effect.

> **TIPS**
> High-dose progestogens are thrombogenic. Many women with endometrial cancer have significant risk factors for VTE, and therefore they must be prescribed with caution. Previous VTE is a contraindication to hormonal therapy.

Gonadotropin-releasing hormone analogues (GnRHa) and aromatase inhibitors are used less often but may be helpful in progesterone refractory disease.

Fertility-Sparing Treatment

A number of young women with anovulation secondary to PCOS are diagnosed with endometrial cancer in the fertility clinic. These women present a management dilemma as many will be reluctant to consider hysterectomy under these circumstances. There has been increased use of progestogen treatment (e.g. LNG-IUS or high-dose MPA) for the treatment of young women with established endometrial cancer that wish to retain their fertility. While response rate across all studies combined is 75%, recurrence rates are high (23%). The evidence base is weak and studies have been small.

It is only appropriate to consider fertility-sparing treatment where there is no evidence of myometrial invasion on MRI scan and for low-grade endometrioid tumours. However, MRI scan is not 100% accurate for staging. There is no consensus about the appropriate treatment regimen or duration of treatment.

> **TIP**
> Hysterectomy remains the standard treatment for endometrial cancer and women need to be fully counselled about the risks of embarking on fertility-sparing treatment.

A realistic assessment of the chance of achieving a live birth with assisted conception is important in counselling women properly. Close collaboration between the gynaecological cancer team and the fertility team is essential in the management of these women.

Prognosis

It is often said that endometrial cancer has a better prognosis than other gynaecological cancers. This is

Table 11.2 Five-year survival following a diagnosis of endometrial cancer

	Endometrioid (%)	Serous/clear cell (%)
Stage I	85–90	60
Stage II	70	50
Stage III	40–50	20
Stage IV	15–20	5–10

simplistic and somewhat inaccurate, and is based on the assumptions that post-menopausal bleeding is a well-recognised sign of possible cancer and that there is usually prompt assessment and diagnosis at an early stage.

Women with early stage, low-grade disease do have an excellent prognosis but women with advanced or high-grade disease may have 5-year survival rates that are similar to those for advanced ovarian cancer (Table 11.2).

Prognosis is related to the following factors:

- Depth of myometrial invasion
- Overall stage
- Grade of tumour and histological sub-type
- Age.

Further Reading

Frost JA, Webster KE, Bryant A, Morrison J. Lymphadenectomy for the management of endometrial cancer. *Cochrane Database of Systematic Reviews* 2015, Issue 9, Art. No.: CD007585. DOI:10.1002/14651858. CD007585.pub3.

Galaal K, Al Moundhri M, Bryant A, Lopes AD, Lawrie TA. Adjuvant chemotherapy for advanced endometrial cancer. *Cochrane Database of Systematic Reviews* 2012, Issue 5, Art. No.: CD010681. DOI:10.1002/14651858. CD010681.pub2.

Galaal K, Bryant A, Fisher AD et al. Laparoscopy versus laparotomy for the management of early stage endometrial cancer. *Cochrane Database of Systematic Reviews* 2012, Issue 9, Art. No.: CD006655. DOI:10.1002/14651858. CD006655.pub2.

Kong A, Johnson N, Kitchener HC, Lawrie TA. Adjuvant radiotherapy for stage I endometrial cancer. *Cochrane Database of Systematic Reviews* 2012, Issue 4, Art. No.: CD003916. DOI:10.1002/14651858. CD003916.pub4.

Royal College of Obstetricians and Gynaecologists/ British Society for Gynaecological Endoscopy. *Green-Top Guideline No. 67. Management of Endometrial Hyperplasia*. London: RCOG, 2016.

Chapter 12

Cervical and Vaginal Cancer

Claire Louise Newton and Tim Mould

Introduction

There are significant similarities between the patho-physiology of cervical and vaginal cancers as the majority are squamous cell carcinomas caused by persistent infection with high-risk human papillomavirus (HPV). The introduction of the HPV vaccination programme aims to reduce the number of cancers caused by HPV including cervical, vagina, vulva, penile, anal and laryngeal cancers.

Both cervical and vaginal cancers are treated by a multidisciplinary team (MDT) that includes gynaecological oncologists, medical oncologists, clinical oncologists, pathologists, radiologists and clinical nurse specialists. Both tumours are staged clinically by an examination under anaesthesia. Although lymph-node involvement is of paramount importance in determining appropriate treatment approaches, and outcome, it does not form part of the International Federation of Gynecology and Obstetrics (FIGO) staging system.

Human Papilloma Virus

HPV is a DNA virus and is the most common sexually transmitted infection globally. The virus is ubiquitous, and consequently most individuals get infected at some stage of their lives. However, the vast majority of infections resolve spontaneously without ever developing symptoms, as HPV is eliminated by their immune system. Individuals with HIV infection or other immune deficiency states (such as transplant recipient on immunosuppression, drug usage) and smoking act as cofactors that prevent the elimination of HPV by the immune system. Persistent HPV infection with high-risk oncogenic subtypes causes precancerous lesions such as cervical intraepithelial neoplasia (CIN), vulval intraepithelial neoplasia (VIN), anal intraepithelial neoplasia (AIN) and vaginal intraepithelial neoplasia (VaIN). These lesions may either progress into invasive cancer or can regress spontaneously

if HPV is subsequently eliminated. The longer an oncogenic HPV subtype is present and the greater the viral load, the higher the chance of developing a precancerous lesion.

HPV is detected in 99% of cervical tumours and 75% of vaginal tumours. HPV subtypes 16 and 18 account for 70% of all cervical tumours. Other oncogenic subtypes of HPV include 31, 33, 35, 39, 45, 51, 52, 53, 56, 58, 59, 66, 68, 73 and 82.

Cervical cancer is more common than other HPV-derived cancers (vagina, vulva, penile, anal and laryngeal) due to the presence of the transformation zone on the cervix. The transformation zone is the area of exposed columnar tissue present on the surface of the cervix that undergoes the process of squamous metaplasia, and transforms into squamous tissue. This area is particularly susceptible to the effects of oncogenic HPV infection.

HPV is typically spread by sustained skin-to-skin contact with vaginal and anal intercourse being the most common route of spread. Condoms do not prevent the spread of HPV infection, although they do reduce the risk. HPV infects the epithelial tissue through micro-abrasions or other trauma that expose the basement membrane. The viral genome is then transported to the cellular nucleus by unknown mechanisms.

The HPV genome comprises open reading frames (E1, 2, 4, 5, 6, 7 and L1, 2), where E denotes proteins that are expressed early in the HPV life cycle, and L denotes proteins expressed later. The two main oncoproteins of high-risk HPV types are E6 and E7. E6 inactivates the tumour suppressor protein p53, which has an important function in protecting the cell from DNA damage by preventing cell growth, promoting cell death and upregulating p21 to block the cell cycle. The oncogenic protein E7 competes with and binds to the retinoblastoma protein which frees E2F, a transcription factor which is involved in pushing the cell cycle forward. Therefore the actions of E6 and E7 cause unregulated cell growth, division and survival that can lead to cancer.

HPV Vaccination

The aim of HPV vaccination is to prevent infection with HPV and thus reduce the risk of developing HPV-associated cancers such as cervical, vagina, vulva, penile, anal, and laryngeal cancers. In the United Kingdom, it is estimated that vaccinating girls against HPV could save up to 400 lives per year.

The currently available vaccines are as follows:

- Cervarix – a bivalent vaccine active against HPV 16 and 18
- Gardasil – a quadrivalent vaccine active against HPV 6, 11, plus 16 and 18
- Gardasil 9 – a nonavalent vaccine against 6, 11 plus 16, 18, 31, 33, 45, 52 and 58.

HPV subtypes 6 and 11 are not oncogenic, and therefore do not cause malignancy. However, they are the major cause of genital warts, which are a significant burden on sexual health clinics, and the individual. Therefore some of the vaccines have been developed to include protection against these viruses.

The current UK vaccination programme uses Gardasil and advises vaccination of all girls between the age 12 and 13 as part of the national childhood vaccination programme. The vaccine is administered as a series of two injections given at 6–24 months interval. The vaccine is given before the onset of sexually activity, and therefore prior to exposure of HPV. At present girls until the age of 18 can receive the HPV vaccine on the NHS. However, those above the age of 14 are given a series of three injections because the immune response to the vaccinations may not be as effective in older girls.

In Australia, where the quadrivalent vaccine has been used to vaccinate young girls since 2007, there has been a 90% reduction in genital warts in heterosexual men and women below the age of 21 years. This is because of the herd immunity that vaccinating girls creates. Men who have sex with men (MSM) will get less benefit from this effect.

TIPS

It is still crucial that women are advised to attend for cervical screening, even if they have been vaccinated, because not all cervical cancers are caused by HPV 16 and 18. Vaccination should reduce the risk of cancer by 70%.

Cervical Cancer

Cervical cancer is the second most common cancer affecting women worldwide. In developed countries, the prevalence of cervical cancer is low due to screening programmes. In the United Kingdom, approximately 2,800 women are diagnosed with, and 1,000 women die from, cervical cancer each year. The national screening programme is estimated to save up to 5,000 lives per year.

Pathology of Cervical Cancer

The most common types of cervical cancer are as follows:

- Squamous cell carcinoma (approximately 70%)
- Adenocarcinoma (approximately 25%).

Rarer pathological subtypes include small cell and large cell neuroendocrine tumours, sarcoma, lymphoma and melanoma.

Squamous cell carcinomas arise from precursor CIN lesions affecting the cervical squamous cells, and adenocarcinomas arise from precursor cervical glandular intraepithelial neoplasia (CGIN) affecting the glandular cells.

The histological features are associated with higher risk of metastatic disease and poorer prognosis include:

- Tumour grade
- Tumour size
- Depth of invasion
- Presence of lymphovascular space invasion
- Status of lymph nodes.

Clinical Presentation and Diagnosis

Diagnosis of cervical cancer is made by history, examination and biopsy. Early stage cancers can be detected before symptoms arise, as abnormal cytology, colposcopy and biopsy are included in the National Screening Programme.

Clinical History

Symptoms associated with cervical cancer are common and non-specific. Similar symptoms are associated with *Chlamydia trachomatis* infection and therefore it is important to test for this infection particularly in young women where it is highly prevalent.

Signs and symptoms suggestive of cervical cancer are as follows:

- Post-coital bleeding (PCB) – the most common symptom

- Intermenstrual bleeding (IMB)
- Postmenopausal bleeding (PMB)
- Vaginal discharge (usually blood stained)
- Pelvic pain
- Suspicious cervix on examination.

In later stages of cervical cancer, women can experience signs and symptoms as a result of extensive pelvic and systemic disease. These symptoms include:

- Loin pain from hydronephrosis secondary to ureteric obstruction from lateral spread of the tumour
- Sciatica as the cancer compresses nerve roots
- Swollen, painful leg secondary to deep vein thrombosis.

PCB is a common symptom, with the prevalence in the community estimated between 0.7% and 9%. The majority of women with PCB do not have cervical cancer. However, PCB is the most common presenting symptom of cervical cancer. Therefore, cervical cancer should be considered in all women with these symptoms. The NHS Cervical Screening Programme advises referral to a gynaecologist if a woman presents with PCB and is over 40 years old, or if their cervix looks abnormal. NHS suspected cancer guidelines suggest that PCB for more than 4 weeks in women above 35 years should be immediately referred within 2 weeks, and for all other cases of repeated unexplained PCB referral should be early within 4–6 weeks.

Post-menopausal bleeding can also herald an endometrial cancer. Women require an ultrasound, to measure the endometrial thickness, and an endometrial biopsy if the endometrial thickness is ≥4 mm.

Examination Findings

Examination of the cervix with a speculum is mandatory for any patient presenting with symptoms suggestive of cervical cancer. Colposcopy is required for those referred with abnormal cervical cytology.

In early stage cancer, inspection of the cervix may not reveal any abnormalities. Colposcopy features suggestive of microinvasive disease include large areas of high-grade disease, often extending into the endocervical canal, together with irregular surfaces, necrosis and atypical blood vessels. The surface epithelium may be fragile, with contact bleeding.

As the disease progresses, the cervix becomes abnormal in appearance and the tumour may be visible as an irregular mass, ulcer or erosion (see Figure 12.1).

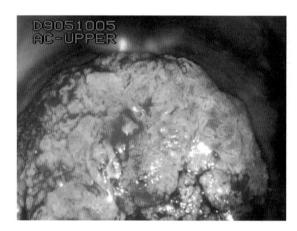

Figure 12.1 Cervical cancer

Bimanual examination may reveal a bulky, irregular pelvic mass.

The diagnosis is confirmed by tissue biopsies. Microinvasive and smaller lesions may be suitable for excision biopsy by large loop excision of the transformation zone (LLETZ).

Investigations

Once the diagnosis has been established, baseline blood tests should be ordered, including full blood count, urea and electrolytes and others as clinically indicated.

Imaging studies are then carried out to assist with clinical staging. All patients, with the exception of stage IA1 disease, should have an MRI of the pelvis to help define the extent of local spread within the cervix, parametrium and pelvis. Computerised tomography (CT) of the chest and abdomen may be indicated to evaluate for signs of distant spread including abnormally enlarged lymph nodes. A newer technique called diffusion-weighted imaging (DWI) is a form of MR-based imaging that assesses the water diffusion properties of tissue. Generally, densely cellular tissues or those with cellular swelling exhibit lower diffusion coefficients, and this difference has helped to differentiate between normal tissue and cancer. This can be especially helpful to determine if lymph nodes are involved with disease, or if there is any residual tumour or recurrence following treatment (Figure 12.2).

Imaging of lymph nodes – Criteria for probable lymph-node involvement on CT and MRI are based on their size and morphology. A lymph node is judged to be suspicious when its shape is spherical (rather than

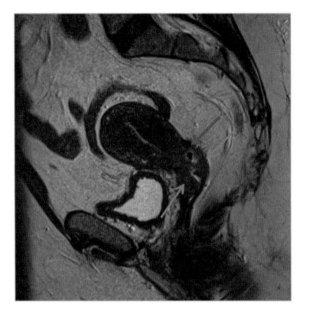
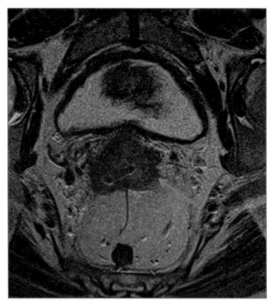

Figure 12.2 Picture of MRI cervix. Sagittal T2W images shows abnormal intermediate T2W signal intensity tumour in the anterior and posterior lips of the cervix (blue arrows). Small focus of low T2W signal intensity is in keeping with a biopsy artefact (red arrows). Axial oblique T2W image shows loss of the normal low T2W signal intensity stroma on the left compatible with parametrial invasion (blue arrow)

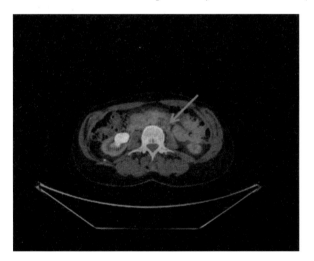
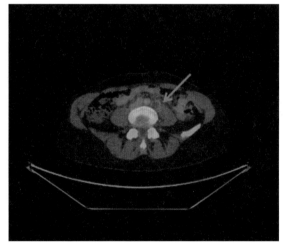

Figure 12.3 Picture of PET/CT of nodal disease. Images from FDG-PET CT show an FDG avid lymph node in the left paraaortic region (left hand image) and a cluster of FDG avid nodes in the left common iliac station (image on the right)

ovoid) and its shortest measured diameter is >10 mm. More recently, positron emission tomography/computed tomography (PET/CT) imaging has been utilised to help define the extent of both local and distal with high sensitivity and specificity. PET/CT is especially useful in detecting lymph-node involvement and is more sensitive than CT or MRI alone, especially in assessing the para-aortic nodes (see Figure 12.3).

Examination under Anaesthetic and Clinical Staging

Unlike the other gynaecological malignancies, the FIGO staging system for both cervical and vaginal cancers is clinical, rather than surgical, and does not include information obtained from CT or MRI studies. Therefore, this staging system does not take into account lymph-node status, even though it is well

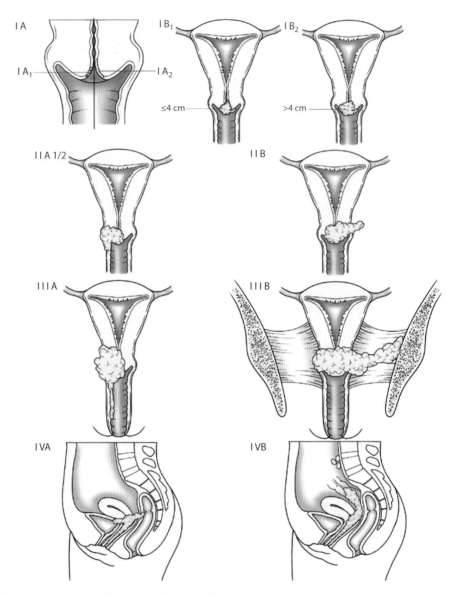

Figure 12.4 Diagrammatic representation of staging for cervical cancer

established that lymph-node status does affect prognosis and survival. The rationale for the clinical staging approach is because the majority of cervical cancer cases occur in developing countries with poor resources. Clinical staging therefore allows direct comparisons of data between different countries. The FIGO staging system is based on clinical examination performed under anaesthetic. During this examination, the tumour is assessed for size, involvement of the vagina and/or parametrium, the pelvic side walls,

and direct spread to the bladder and/or rectum. Chest radiography, intravenous pyelography, cystoscopy and proctoscopy (if apparent bladder or rectal involvement) are permitted.

Spread of cervical cancer is usually direct to parametrium (which may cause ureteric obstruction), bladder and bowel. It can also spread via the lymphatics to pelvic and para-aortic lymph nodes. Spread via the blood to the lungs and liver occurs late (Figure 12.4).

Management of Cervical Cancer

Every patient with a diagnosis of cervical cancer should be discussed through the MDT at a cancer centre. Management depends on the stage of disease and may also be influenced by the fertility wishes of the patient. In general, combined treatment with radical surgery followed by post-operative chemoradiation results in increased morbidity than either treatment alone, but with no survival advantage. If parametrial or lymph node spread is suspected on pre-treatment imaging and assessment then chemoradiation is usually recommended as the primary treatment modality, and surgery is not undertaken.

Treatment by Stage

Stage IA1 – Cone biopsy, or LLETZ if the margins are clear of disease, or simple hysterectomy for women who have completed their family. The risk of lymph-node involvement is only 0.4% and therefore lymphadenectomy is unnecessary.

Stage IA2 – This can be treated by simple hysterectomy for women who have completed their family and a pelvic node dissection. For women who have not completed their family, a cone biopsy or a simple trachelectomy can be offered. The risk of parametrial involvement in this group is only 0.6%. The risk of lymph-node involvement becomes clinically significant at 5%, and therefore bilateral pelvic lymphadenectomy is recommended. No further treatment is required if there is no residual tumour and negative lymph nodes. Women with positive nodes will require external beam radiotherapy.

Stage IB1 – This group of tumours includes a wide variation of tumour volumes ranging from microscopic to tumours up to 4 cm. There is a significant risk of lymph-node involvement in these tumours (approximately 15%), and therefore bilateral pelvic lymphadenectomy should be undertaken in all cases.

- Tumours <1 cm diameter are only just bigger than 1A2 and can be treated in a similar way.
- Tumours between 1 and 2 cm may be treated with either radical hysterectomy or (where fertility is desired) radical trachelectomy (resection of the cervix and parametrium, with uterine preservation). Bilateral pelvic lymphadenectomy should be carried out. Tumours >2 cm are usually treated with radical hysterectomy and bilateral pelvic lymphadenectomy. A radical trachelectomy is not usually advised as the recurrence rates are higher.

Adjuvant treatment after surgery – Women are advised to have adjuvant chemoradiotherapy following surgery if they are found to have either positive pelvic lymph nodes, or tumour at the surgical resection margins. Women with tumours >4 cm, LVSI and close vaginal surgical resection margins (<5 mm), have worse progression-free and overall survival and should be considered for adjuvant chemoradiation.

Stage IB2 to stage IIIB – Standard treatment for these tumours is with radical chemoradiotherapy.

Stage IV – These patients require a highly individualised approach, according to the pattern of spread. Spread to bladder or rectum may be treated with defunctioning stoma and chemoradiation if the patient is fit, or palliative radiation to the pelvis if not. In rare cases, localised disease may have extended to bladder or rectum without reaching the pelvic side wall, and without distant spread. Radical surgery to remove the cancer with likely adjuvant chemoradiotherapy can be considered, provided distant spread has been excluded on specialist imaging. Exenterative surgical approaches are covered later in this chapter. In cases where distant spread has occurred, primary chemotherapy would be recommended followed by palliative radiation to the pelvis. If the response to primary chemotherapy is good, chemoradiotherapy to the pelvis may be considered.

Surgical Management of Cervical Cancer

Cone Biopsy

Cone biopsy can be performed by cold knife, laser, or electrocautery needle under local or general anaesthesia. The difference between cone biopsy and LLETZ is primarily the size and the depth of excision, which would usually be considerably deeper with a cone biopsy.

Complications include primary haemorrhage, which is unusual, or secondary haemorrhage, which occurs as a significant bleed in 3%. Pre-term delivery is increased following a cone biopsy and is directly related to the depth of the cone biopsy.

Radical Trachelectomy

Radical trachelectomy is performed in patients who want to retain their fertility and have stage IB1 tumours <2 cm in size. A radical trachelectomy can be carried out through a vaginal, abdominal or laparoscopic approach, or with the assistance of the surgical robot. The procedure involves removal of the cervix, parametrium and a cuff of vagina (usually 1–2 cm). To reduce the risk of future pre-term delivery, a permanent, non-absorbable cervical cerclage suture is placed at the uterine isthmus, where the uterus joins the endocervix. The vaginal edge is then sutured to the uterine isthmus taking care to maintain the patency of the isthmus. Uterine isthmic stenosis can cause haematometra.

Other complications include primary haemorrhage, ureteric, bladder and bowel damage.

Although more than 70% of pregnancies are carried to ≥37 weeks, late miscarriages and pre-term deliveries are common complications of subsequent pregnancies and women must be advised of this prior to their surgery. First trimester miscarriage rates are not increased. Women will require delivery by lower segment caesarean section.

The rates of recurrence following trachelectomy are comparable to radical hysterectomy providing the cervical cancer measures <2 cm and there is no lymphovascular space invasion.

Radical Hysterectomy

Radical hysterectomy can be carried out abdominally, laparoscopically or robotically. The uterus, cervix, parametrium and cuff of vagina are removed. Different levels of radicality describe the amount of parametrium removed, which is in turn determined by the size of the tumour. Ovarian transposition may also be carried out, to lift the ovaries out of the pelvis, in case future radiation treatment is required, and thus avoiding damage to them.

Complications include primary haemorrhage, ureteric, bladder and bowel damage.

Bladder dysfunction with voiding difficulties and bladder hypotonia can occur due to damage to the hypogastric nerves that lie within the uterosacral ligaments and parametria. A catheter is usually placed for a minimum of 48 hours following the procedure, and bladder emptying is checked on removal of the catheter.

Ovarian conservation – Ovaries will be conserved in all women undergoing fertility-sparing surgery. Premenopausal women who have completed their families may still benefit from ovarian preservation. Squamous cell carcinoma is not hormone-dependent, and ovarian metastases are rare; therefore ovarian conservation is usually recommended. Although adenocarcinomas of the cervix are not thought to be hormone dependent, they may be more likely to metastasize to the ovaries; therefore the decision to conserve ovaries is individualised.

Pelvic Lymph Node Dissection

Pelvic lymph-node dissection can be approached abdominally, laparoscopically or robotically. The pelvic lymph-node groups that should be removed include the obturator nodes and the common, internal, and external iliac nodes. Presacral nodes are included by many centres.

Complications of node dissection include primary haemorrhage and damage to the obturator or genitofemoral nerves. A significant late chronic complication is lymphoedema of the mons pubis, groin and leg. This occurs in 10% of women and is severe in 1%.

Sentinel lymph-node mapping in cervical cancer – The sentinel lymph node is defined as the first lymph node to receive lymphatic drainage from the tumour. If this node is clear of tumour (negative), then the remaining lymph nodes are deemed to be clear and do not need removal. If this is the case, then the risk of lymphoedema can be significantly reduced. Sentinel node mapping is now standard practice in breast cancer, and becoming standard in vulval cancer.

The application and validity of sentinel lymph-node biopsy is not yet established in routine clinical practice and usually practised in the context of clinical trials. As the cervix is a midline structure its lymphatic drainage is more complicated. The histopathological analysis of the sentinel lymph node requires ultrasection and immunohistochemistry in addition to the routine H&E staining which gives higher detection rates. The results of published trials for sentinel node mapping in cervical cancer are promising, and it is likely that this approach may soon become standard practice.

Non-surgical Management

Primary Chemoradiotherapy

Chemoradiotherapy has been shown to be superior to radiation for cervical cancer, and is now the standard of care for women with cervical cancer.

Radiation is given as a combination of external beam radiotherapy (EBRT) and vaginal brachytherapy (BT). EBRT is usually administered on weekdays for 5 weeks. Each daily session lasts 30 minutes. The dose of radiation delivered to the pelvis by EBRT is approximately 45 Gy. In the sixth week, BT is administered to the target site by insertion of applicators into the cervical canal, placed while under anaesthesia. Once the position of the applicator is checked by further imaging, it can then be attached to an implant that contains radiation. The implant is left in the applicator for a few minutes, and can be repeated over several days. This is known as high dose-rate BT. BT boosts the local radiation dose to the cervix to 90 Gy. Chemotherapy is given simultaneously with radiotherapy, and usually includes cisplatin administered once a week for 6 weeks during the course of radiotherapy.

Wherever possible it is important that there are no interruptions to the radiotherapy treatment regime. Treatment that takes 8 weeks or more is associated with worse tumour control and survival. The haemoglobin should be checked and maintained above 100 g/l.

Pelvic radiotherapy will result in loss of fertility. The ovaries are very sensitive to radiation and lose their function permanently after the first few fractions of treatment. The uterus is also permanently damaged by the level of radiotherapy required for cervical cancer treatment, and cannot maintain a pregnancy. Chemotherapy agents can also affect gonadal function; however, cisplatin (the agent commonly used in chemoradiotherapy) spares ovarian function.

Ovarian transposition – It is a laparoscopic procedure that is carried out to reposition the ovaries from the pelvis up to the paracolic gutters within the abdominal cavity. The aim is to minimise the effects of radiotherapy (if needed) on them, while still maintaining their blood supply. This procedure results in ovarian function preservation in approximately 20–50% of patients. The potential consequences of the procedure include ovarian metastases (approximately 1% usually in adenocarcinomas) and symptomatic ovarian cysts in a minority of women.

During chemoradiotherapy other pelvic organs receive a significant dose of radiation which results in acute and late toxicities. Acute radiation proctitis with symptoms of diarrhoea, rectal bleeding, urgency and tenesmus is frequently experienced during radiotherapy. Late toxicities occur 3 months and beyond following radiotherapy and arise as a result of small vessel damage with endothelial damage, inflammation, ischaemia and necrosis. Symptoms of late radiation effects to the bladder include urinary frequency, urgency, dysuria and detrusor instability, haematuria, ulceration and fistulation. Frequency of bowel opening, rectal bleeding and fistulation are late bowel effects.

Neoadjuvant Chemotherapy

Neoadjuvant chemotherapy is sometimes given before chemoradiation or radical surgery in locally advanced cervical cancer, but this is not a standard approach. It is currently given in highly individualised cases, after discussion and agreement by the MDT.

Adjuvant Treatment

Adjuvant treatment is usually given after surgery if there are positive lymph nodes or positive surgical margins. Adjuvant treatment is usually given as a combination of radiation and cisplatin. Radiation consists of EBRT and vaginal BT but the BT is to the vaginal vault using a different shaped applicator rather than a cervical insertion, as the cervix has been removed at surgery.

Vaginal Cancer

Carcinomas of the vagina are rare and account for only 1% of all gynaecological malignancies. Around 260 women are diagnosed with a primary vaginal carcinoma each year in the United Kingdom. Consequently there is limited data to guide on management, as most published studies contain small numbers and are not randomised. Vaginal metastases are more common than primary vaginal carcinoma. Care must be taken in making the correct diagnosis of a primary vaginal cancer, and in excluding the possibility of metastatic disease from an underlying cervical tumour.

Pathology

This is based on the type of cell from which the cancer arises:

- Squamous cell carcinomas (85%)
- Adenocarcinomas (10%) – including clear-cell adenocarcinomas associated with diethylstilbestrol (DES) exposure *in utero*.

Melanomas, sarcomas, and vaginal germ-cell tumours (e.g. endodermal sinus tumour, teratoma <1%) are rare.

Risk factors for Vaginal Cancer

- Increasing age – mostly occurs in patients over the age of 60 years
- VAIN
- Exposure to DES *in utero*
- Prior hysterectomy for CIN
- Risks for HPV infection including smoking, HIV and immune suppressing drugs.

Between 1940 and 1971 DES was given to pregnant women hoping that it would reduce miscarriages. In 1971 it was shown that DES caused a 40-fold increase in vaginal and cervical clear-cell adenocarcinoma in women exposed to this drug while *in utero,* and it was subsequently withdrawn from use. DES exposure *in utero* also increases the risk of other abnormalities such as vaginal adenosis (columnar cells present in the vagina), larger cervical transformation zone, uterine fibroids, cervical incompetence and T-shaped uterus which contribute to the increase of infertility and adverse pregnancy outcomes in these women. DES exposure *in utero* is also thought to increase the risk of breast cancer. The NHS Cervical Screening Programme advises that women exposed to DES *in utero* should undergo an initial colposcopic assessment of the cervix and vagina. If this is normal then they can be managed with routine cervical screening. If they show any abnormalities then they will require annual assessments in a specialist setting, and managed on a case-by-case basis.

Clinical Presentation and Diagnosis

Like cervical cancer, diagnosis of vaginal cancer is made by history, examination and biopsy.

Clinical History

Early vaginal cancer may not cause any symptoms but as the cancer progresses the following symptoms can be experienced:

- PCB
- Intermenstrual bleeding
- Post-menopausal bleeding
- Abnormal vaginal discharge
- Dyspareunia
- Pelvic pain
- Dysuria
- Vaginal lump
- Tenesmus/PR bleeding/constipation particularly for lesions developing on the posterior wall of the vagina.

Examination Findings

Similar to cervical cancer, examination with a speculum is mandatory. An examination including colposcopy, vaginoscopy and vulvoscopy with biopsies of suspicious areas of the vagina should be performed. Cervical cytology should be taken if due, even if the cervix appears normal. If the cervix looks macroscopically abnormal biopsies should be taken even with a history of normal cervical cytology.

Investigations

Once vaginal cancer is diagnosed, an examination under anaesthetic is performed to assess the spread of the disease. Cystoscopy and/or sigmoidoscopy may be performed if bladder and/or bowel involvement are suspected. Staging is clinical, similar to cervical cancer.

A CT chest/abdomen/pelvis is also performed to assess spread and to evaluate for potential lymph-node involvement (even though lymph-node status is not part of FIGO staging). As with all gynaecological cancers, a lymph node is judged suspicious when shape is spherical and the shortest diameter is greater than 10 mm. An MRI pelvis is performed to assess spread particularly into adjacent structures such as the bladder and bowel.

Staging for Vaginal Cancer

Squamous cell carcinomas of the vagina initially spread locally but can spread to distant organs such as the lungs and liver. Adenocarcinomas of the vagina frequently spread to the lung, pelvic and supraclavicular lymph nodes (Figure 12.5).

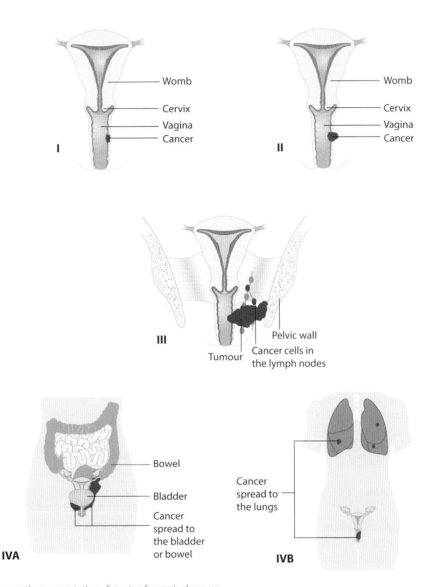

Figure 12.5 Diagrammatic representation of staging for vaginal cancer

Management of Vaginal Cancer

Surgical Management

Chemoradiation is usually the preferred mode of treatment for vaginal cancer, due to the close proximity of the vagina to critical pelvic and perineal structures. Chemoradiotherapy is highly effective and avoids surgical morbidity. However for small tumours located in the upper one-third of the vagina with no muscular mucosa involvement, a wide local excision may be appropriate. Patients with bulky tumours (>5 cm) or inferior involvement may require a total vaginectomy.

Neoadjuvant chemotherapy followed by radical surgery is another alternative, although less widely adopted.

Radiotherapy and Chemotherapy

Radiotherapy with or without chemotherapy is the treatment of choice for primary vaginal cancer. Chemotherapy regimens vary, and agents such as cisplatin or 5-flurouracil have been used. Chemotherapy is often used with radiotherapy by extrapolating cervical cancer data in which concurrent chemoradiotherapy is superior to radiotherapy alone; however, no randomised trial has been undertaken in vaginal cancer due to its

135

rarity. In 2014 the National Cancer Database of the USA reported on 8,000 patients with vaginal cancer, and demonstrated the superiority of concurrent chemoradiotherapy. Radiotherapy consists of interstitial and intracavity radiotherapy up to 75 Gy in stage I disease and with additional EBRT for women with more advanced disease.

Lymphatic involvement is relatively common in vaginal cancer with node involvement in 6–14% of patients in stage I, and 26–32% in patients with stage II disease. Therefore the relevant lymph nodes need to be included in the radiotherapy field. The vagina is usually divided into thirds, reflecting the lymphatic drainage and its embryological origins. The upper third drains into the external iliac and para-aortic lymph-node chains, the middle third into the common and internal iliac lymph-node chains and the lower third drains into the superficial inguinal, femoral and perirectal lymph-node chains. However these patterns are highly variable.

Complications of Treatment

Radiation-induced bladder, vaginal and rectal toxicity is common, and is proportional to the extent of invasion, tumour size and FIGO stage. Complication rates have been reported at 8–14% for stage I–II and between 23% and 40% for stage III/IV disease. Late complications of radiotherapy include vesicovaginal and rectovaginal fistulas which are best visualised with MRI imaging.

Prognosis of Vaginal Cancer

Prognostic factors for vaginal cancer include stage, tumours >5 cm, type (malignant melanomas of the vagina carry an increase in mortality), advanced age and lymph-node involvement. Grade, HPV status and location of the lesion have conflicting evidence with regard to prognostic factors.

> **TIP**
> The mainstay of vaginal cancer treatment is chemoradiotherapy which is highly effective and prevents surgical morbidity.

Prognosis and Recurrence of Cervical and Vaginal Cancer

The 5-year survival rates for cervical cancer depend on the stage:

- Stage IA – 93%
- Stage IB – 80%
- Stage IIA – 63%

- Stage IIB – 56%
- Stage IIIA – 35%
- Stage IV – 16%.

If recurrences occur, around half do so within 2 years, and the majority (50–60%) present with disease outside the pelvis which is no longer curable. Therefore management approaches are usually palliative.

The 5-year survival rates for vaginal cancer also depend on stage: 84% (stage I), 75% (stage II) and 57% (stage III/IV). Approximately 68% of patients with stage I–II and 86% of patients with stage III–IV vaginal cancer have a locoregional recurrence. The vast majority of vaginal cancer recurrences occur in the first few years – 80% by 2 years and 90% by 5 years.

Exenterative Surgery

Patients who relapse with localised pelvic disease after chemoradiotherapy cannot receive any more radiotherapy. Pelvic exenteration is the only potentially curative approach for these patients, provided that there is no evidence of disease outside the pelvis. Exenterative surgery involves removing the uterus and cervix (if not already done so) along with the bladder (anterior exenteration), rectosigmoid colon (posterior exenteration) or both bladder and bowel (total exenteration). Pre-operative imaging is essential to exclude distant metastases. If no distant disease is seen on routine imaging, then PET/CT should also be carried out to exclude distant metastases prior to consideration of an exenteration. Exenterative surgery is not appropriate in patients with metastatic disease.

The 5-year survival rate following exenterative surgery is estimated to be between 30% and 60%. The prognosis is better for patients with a disease-free interval of more than 6 months, tumour size <3 cm and no pelvic side wall fixation.

Palliative Treatment

Stage IV disease is incurable, and therefore management is palliative with the primary objective of symptom control and quality of life. Symptoms that may need control include pain, diarrhoea, constipation, shortness of breath, dysuria, and offensive odours and discharge. Palliative chemotherapy may be considered, although the response rates are worse in patients who have already received chemotherapy. Several regimens are used in the palliative setting including cisplatin-paclitaxel, cisplatin – topotecan, or cisplatin monotherapy. Response rates are 20–30% and survival is usually only around 7 months.

Follow-Up

There is a lack of evidence for any follow-up regimes for patients following treatment for cervical or vaginal cancer. Currently there is no national guidance, and most cancer centres have their own regional protocols. At the clinic appointment a history is taken with respect to vaginal bleeding, weight loss, abdominal pain and change in bowel habit or urination. An abdominal and pelvic examination is undertaken including a speculum examination to look for signs of recurrence. As 90% of recurrences occur within 5 years, the majority of patients are discharged after 5 years.

TIPS

The use of vault cytology to detect recurrences may be inappropriate. There is no published evidence of benefit, and samples can be difficult to interpret after radiotherapy and may even give false reassurance. Cervical cytology testing is a screening test for cervical precancer, and there is no convincing argument for its use in follow-up of cancer. However, liquid-based cytology from isthmic and vaginal vault area may be recommended in the follow-up of trachelectomy patients, but is highly individualised.

Further Reading

Colombo N, Carinelli S, Colombo A et al. On behalf of the ESMO guidelines working group. Cervical cancer: ESMO clinical practice guidelines for diagnosis, treatment and follow-up. *Annals of Oncology* (2012) 23(supplement 7), 27–32.

Donato V, Bellati F, Fischetti M et al. Vaginal cancer. Critical reviews in oncology. *Haematology* (2012) 81, 286–95.

Management of cervical cancer, *SIGN Guideline* (Scottish Intercollegiate Guidelines Network) (January 2008).

Rajaram S, Maheshwari A, Srivatava A. Staging for vaginal cancer. Best practice and research. *Clinical Obstetrics and Gynaecology* (2015) 29, 822–32.

Wu Y, Li Z, Wu H, Yu J. Sentinel lymph node biopsy in cervical cancer: a meta-analysis. *Molecular and Clinical Oncology* (2013) 1, 1025–30.

Vulval Cancer

Chapter 13

Carmen Gan and Ketan Gajjar

Introduction

Vulval cancer is predominantly a disease of older population. In 2014, there were 1289 new cases of vulval cancer in the United Kingdom, accounting for <1% of all cancers. The lifetime risk of developing vulval cancer is 1 in 275 women and age-standardised (AS) rate is 2.5 per 100,000 of female population. Although vulval cancer is rare, it is anticipated that the incidence will rise alongside the increasingly ageing population in the United Kingdom. More than half of all vulval cancers diagnosed in 2014 were in women aged 70 years and above. The incidence of vulval cancer is also rising in the younger population. A retrospective population study in the United Kingdom has identified an upward trend of new cases diagnosed in the 20–69 year age group over the last 20 years.

Survival is dependent on several factors including pathological staging and histological subtype. In the United Kingdom, the mortality due to vulval cancer remained stable over the last 10 years, and overall 5- and 10-year AS survivals for vulval cancer are 63.6% and 52.6%, respectively.

Anatomical Considerations

A good knowledge of the anatomy of vulva is essential to understand the patterns of spread in vulval cancer, and is the basis of the pathological staging using the International Federation of Gynecology and Obstetrics (FIGO) classification (see Appendix) (Figure 13.1).

Arteries – The arterial supply of the vulva is derived from the internal pudendal artery (branch of internal iliac artery) and superficial and deep external pudendal artery (both are branches of femoral artery). As the internal pudendal artery enters the lesser sciatic foramen within the Alcock's canal, it divides into inferior rectal, perineal and bulbar branches, where the latter will go on to supply the crus and glans of the vulva through deep arteries of clitoris and dorsal clitoral artery, respectively.

Veins – Venous drainage is mainly through the internal pudendal vein and deep dorsal vein of clitoris, with additional drainage by the external pudendal vein.

Lymphatic drainage – The lymphatic drainage of the vulva follows the external pudendal blood vessels to the inguinal lymph nodes (superficial and deep), the external iliac nodes and then the common iliac and para-aortic nodes. Midline structures have a higher tendency to drain into lymph nodes bilaterally. There are usually 3–5 deep inguinal lymph nodes. Cloquet's node is the most superior node of the deep inguinal lymph nodes, which is also the most inferior of the external iliac nodes (Figure 13.2).

Nerve supply – The sensory nerve supply of vulva is derived from ilioinguinal nerve (L1), genitofemoral nerve (L1–2) anteriorly and pudendal nerves (S2–4) posteriorly.

Role of Screening

Currently there is no effective screening strategy beneficial in the diagnosis of vulval carcinoma. Women at a higher risk of developing vulval cancer, such as those with complicated lichen sclerosus (LS) [a form of non-neoplastic epithelial disorder (NNED)], Paget's disease of the vulva and vulval intraepithelial neoplasia (VIN), should have long-term follow-up at the vulva clinic or by the gynaecology team experienced in dealing with vulval conditions. Vulvoscopy with acetic acid (synonymous with colposcopy) are useful adjuncts to aid follow-up.

Aetiology

The cause of vulval carcinoma remains poorly understood. Risk factors include:

- Smoking
- Human papilloma virus (HPV) infection
- VIN
- Lichen sclerosus
- Immunosuppression
- Northern European ancestry.

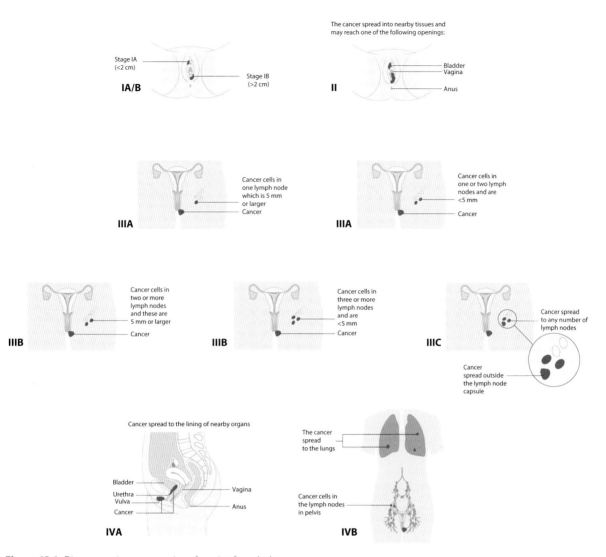

Figure 13.1 Diagrammatic representation of staging for vulval cancer

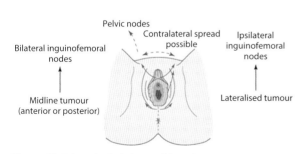

Figure 13.2 Lymphatic drainage of the vulva

Source: Vulval illustration courtesy of *The Sourcebook of Medical Illustration, Parthenon*, 1991

Pathology

The most common sub-type of vulval cancer is squamous cell carcinoma (SCC), but rarer sub-types exist.

Squamous Cell Carcinoma

About 90% of vulval carcinoma is squamous cell-type in origin. This can be further divided into two sub-types based on aetiology:

1. **HPV-related disease** which is more common in younger women owing to HPV infections. These lesions tend to be warty in appearance and are

139

Table 13.1 Comparison of clinicopathological features between two VINs

	Usual-type VIN (classic, undifferentiated, bowenoid, basaloid and warty)	Differentiated (simplex)-type VIN
Prevalence	More common	Less common
Age	Younger females	Older females
Distribution	Often multifocal	Usually unifocal
Association with multifocal lower genital tract neoplasia	Yes, frequently	Rarely
HPV associated	Yes	No
Association with vulval dystrophy	Rare	Common
Risk of progression to squamous carcinoma	Low risk of progression to HPV-related squamous carcinoma (approximately 9–16% untreated; 3% treated)	High risk of progression to non-HPV-related squamous carcinoma
Immunohistochemistry	p16 positive; p53 'wild-type'	Some cases diffusely p53 positive or totally negative; p16 negative; MIB1 largely confined to basal layers
Molecular	HPV E6 inactivation of p53; HPV E7 inactivation of retinoblastoma tumour suppressor gene	TP53 mutation in some cases

typically multifocal and multicentric. There may be associated cervical intraepithelial neoplasia (CIN)/vaginal intraepithelial neoplasia (VaIN) and therefore thorough assessment of the genital tract is necessary. This is commonly associated with HPV 16, but other viral sub-types such as HPV 18 and 33 have been isolated.

2. **Differentiated or keratinising lesions** are unrelated to HPV and associated with vulval epithelial dystrophies such as LS. Patients with LS have a 4% risk of developing invasive vulval cancer. Histological evidence of LS is seen in up to 60% cases of vulval cancer. This subtype is more commonly found in older women.

Vulval intra-epithelial neoplasia - It is a premalignant lesion of the vulva, homologous with CIN. Usual-type VIN (uVIN) is classically associated with HPV, whereas differentiated-type VIN (dVIN) is associated with the vulval epithelial dystrophies. dVIN is rare and accounts for less than 10% of all VINs. Table 13.1 summarises the difference between these two premalignant conditions.

Verrucous carcinoma – It is a variant of well-differentiated SCC of vulva. It runs a slightly more indolent course, rarely metastasizes but can be locally destructive. It adopts a cauliflower-like exophytic appearance. Lymph node metastasis is rare but may result in an inflammatory reaction of the regional lymph nodes.

Management involves wide local excision with adequate margins without lymphadenectomy.

Malignant melanoma – Although rare, this is the second most common histological subtype of vulval cancer. It accounts for <10% of all vulval malignancies and is more common in Caucasian women. Although the cellular origin is melanocytes, approximately one quarter of these lesions will not be pigmented. Vulval melanoma, similarly to its cutaneous counterparts, is staged using the Breslow criteria (Table 13.2).

Prognosis worsens with increasing depth of invasion. Other poor prognostic indicators are ulcerative lesions and high mitotic count. Primary treatment is surgical, and includes a wide local excision of primary lesion with or without groin lymphadenectomy or sentinel lymph node (SLN) biopsy. The cases should be managed in collaboration with the specialist melanoma multidisciplinary team (MDT).

Basal cell carcinoma (BCC) – It is a variant of vulval SCC and accounts for approximately 2% of all vulval carcinoma. The lesion typically presents with pruritus or a lump. These tumours are locally invasive and usually without lymph node involvement. It has a typical 'rodent' ulcer appearance and carries an excellent prognosis. Surgical excision with adequate margins without need for lymphadenectomy is the usual course of management. The BCC must be distinguished from basaloid type SCC which is more aggressive and should be treated as an SCC.

Table 13.2 Breslow classification of tumour stage in melanoma based on depth of invasion

Stage	Depth
Stage I	≤0.75 mm
Stage II	0.76–1.50 mm
Stage III	1.51–2.25 mm
Stage IV	2.26–3.0 mm
Stage V	>3.0 mm

Paget's disease of the vulva – Extramammary Paget's disease (EPD) represents 1–2% of all vulval cancers and typically affects Caucasian women in their 60–70s. These are eczematous, weepy, erythematous plaques with typical white scaling and are frequently associated with an underlying vulval adenocarcinoma (4–8%) or adenocarcinoma elsewhere (<15%). Multiple diagnostic biopsies may be necessary to ascertain the extent of the lesion since tumour cells can be seen within the epidermis from skin that appears to be unremarkable on clinical examination, and also to assess for an invasive adenocarcinoma. Paget's disease of the vulva can be classified as primary Paget's disease of the vulva (majority of cases) or secondary involvement of overlying skin by the underlying adenocarcinoma (25% of cases). Associated adenocarcinomas may be located in the adjacent skin, adnexa, Bartholin's gland, cervix, vagina, colon, rectum or lower urinary tract. Surgical excision of invasive Paget's disease with adequate margins is the mainstay of treatment but recurrences are common. It is essential to perform a full assessment to identify any associated malignancies.

Bartholin's gland cancer – It is a rare type of vulval cancer, although it accounts for the majority of vulval adenocarcinomas. Most common histological subtypes are squamous and adenocarcinoma. It usually affects women above the age of 50; therefore persistent Bartholin's abscess or cysts in women of older age groups should be excised. These tumours are usually deep-seated and approximately 20% of women will present with lymph node metastasis. Treatment is similar to SCC of vulva.

Sarcoma – These are rare cancers affecting the vulva and carry poor prognosis. They include leiomyosarcoma and rhabdomyosarcoma. Leiomyosarcomas are most common and often present as an enlarging, painful mass, usually on the labia majora. Treatment is wide local excision, and adjuvant radiotherapy may be beneficial.

Clinical Presentation

Typical symptoms and signs of vulval cancer include:

- Vulval lump or growth
- Bleeding or discharge
- Ulceration
- Vulval pain and itching.

The vulval lump may be a flat plaque, condylomatous, or ulcerated with raised, rolled or everted edges. The carcinoma is frequently present on the labium majus and is often solitary. There may be surrounding field change associated with underlying VIN or dermatoses. Younger patient with HPV-related malignancy are more likely to have multifocal disease.

The most commonly associated symptom is vulval pruritus and soreness leading to repeated treatments for candidiasis or inflammatory skin conditions. However, vulval cancer can be relatively asymptomatic in early stage disease and is occasionally an incidental finding at the time of gynaecological examination for other indications. This is especially so in older patients. Despite the high incidence of symptomatic lesions, delay in diagnosis and referral (typically of four to six months) is common in this group of women with vulval SCC. Many women will delay presentation due to embarrassment, and primary care physicians may delay an examination for similar reasons or because of the practical limitations of examination in the available settings.

> **TIPS**
> Clinicians should have a high index of suspicion for vulval cancer. A thorough inspection of the entire vulva should be carried out for women with symptoms of pain, bleeding, itching or soreness.

Women with an unexplained vulval lump, ulceration or bleeding seen in primary care should be referred for specialist assessment via the suspected cancer pathway (within 2 weeks). Patients with confirmed vulval cancer should be managed within a specialist gynaecological oncology centre with their specialist MDT.

Diagnosis and Investigations

Women presenting with symptoms suggestive of vulval cancer warrant a thorough clinical examination, including the vulva and perianal regions. The clinical examination findings must be clearly documented and should include:

- Characteristics of the lesion – site, dimensions
- Distance from, or involvement of, midline structures (urethra, clitoris, vagina, anus)
- Appearance of surrounding skin
- Presence and characteristics of palpable groin nodes.

Cervical cytology, if due, should be performed at the same time.

Diagnostic Biopsy

Incisional biopsy is paramount and should include a representative sample of the lesion together with an area of normal epithelium adjacent to abnormality. This can be carried out in an office setting with the use of local anaesthesia and punch biopsy forceps. Tissue measuring 3–4 mm is usually adequate to obtain histological diagnosis provided there is no sampling error. Multiple 'mapping' biopsies are often necessary for multifocal disease (Figures 13.3 and 13.4).

Excisional biopsy of a suspicious lesion must be avoided as this may preclude adequate surgical margins and patient's suitability for SLN identification procedure.

Examination under anaesthesia – Selected patients such as the elderly or those with symptomatic large lesions may benefit from an examination under anaesthesia due to discomfort leading to limited assessment of extent of the lesion.

Assessment of Groin Nodes

Clinical palpation for groin node status carries low sensitivity (35–57.1%) and specificity (61.5–94.3%), unless the patient presents at an advanced stage with large, fixed nodes.

Imaging and biopsy of lymph nodes – Either ultrasound or magnetic resonance imaging (MRI) should be used to evaluate the groin lymph nodes. Ultrasound assessment carries a sensitivity of 45–100% and specificity of 58–96%. MRI was shown to carry better pooled sensitivity and specificity of groin node assessment at

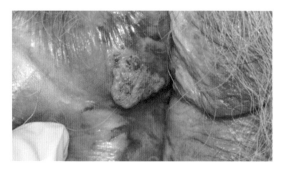

Figure 13.3 Squamous cell carcinoma of right labia

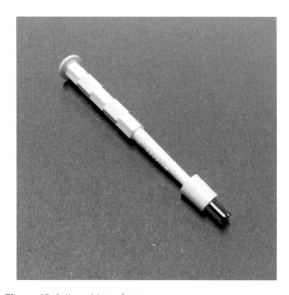

Figure 13.4 Keyes biopsy forceps

86% (95% CI 0.57–0.98) and 87% (95% CI 0.74–0.95), respectively. Suspicious nodes (at palpation or imaging) should be further analysed by fine-needle aspiration (FNA) or core biopsy when this would alter primary treatment.

Imaging for Distal Disease

Further staging with CT scan of chest, abdomen and pelvis is recommended where there is a clinical suspicion of or proven (nodal) metastatic disease and/or advanced stage disease.

Staging and Spread

Staging of vulval cancer is based on FIGO revised classification from 2009 (see Appendix). The depth of invasion is defined as the measurement of the tumour from the epithelial–stromal junction of the adjacent most superficial dermal papilla to the deepest point of invasion.

Vulval carcinoma can spread through:

- Direct extension to adjacent structures including the vagina, anus and urethra
- Embolisation through the lymphatics – which can occur even in early disease
- Haematogenous spread to distant organs – occurs late, and rarely.

Management of Vulval Cancer

Vulval cancer is typically managed surgically, with additional radiotherapy and chemotherapy in selected cases. Management of patients with vulval cancer should be managed through the specialist MDT and individualised according to stage, histological subtype, comorbidities and patients' preferences. Involvement of the specialist nurses is helpful for both patient education and to provide much needed psychological support.

Principles of Surgical Management

Primary surgical treatment of the vulval lesion – Surgery has become increasingly conservative and individualised. The aim of surgical treatment must be for radical excision with the aim of achieving adequate, tumour-free resection margins of at least 8 mm (after fixation). Tissue shrinks after fixation; therefore this requires a fresh surgical margin of approximately 15 mm. Achieving an adequate surgical margin will reduce the risk of local recurrence within the vulva.

Treatment of the groin nodes – The greatest single factor associated with mortality from vulval cancer is groin node involvement. Appropriate groin node treatment is therefore essential. The groin nodes should be treated in all but the earliest stage disease (stage IA where the risk of groin node metastases is negligible).

Early Stage Cancer (Stages I and II)

Surgery in early stage disease (stages I and II) should always be with curative intent. Lesions <2 cm in diameter with <1 mm depth of invasion (FIGO stage IA) carry lymph node metastatic risk of <1%. Therefore wide local excision with adequate surgical margins without the need for lymphadenectomy can be safely undertaken.

Dissection of the superficial and deep groin nodes should be performed in all but stage IA tumours. The triple incision technique can be employed for patients with more extensive disease requiring wide local excision and inguino-femoral lymphadenectomy. Bilateral groin lymphadenectomy must be undertaken if lesion is close to the midline owing to extensive crossover of lymphatic channels from the vulva. Ipsilateral groin node dissection is permissible provided the tumour is lateralised. This is defined as tumours that are located at least 2 cm away from midline structures (urethra/clitoris/anus/perineal body) or excision margin is not within 1 cm of these structures. Lateralised tumours are less likely to drain to contralateral groin nodes and this negates the need for bilateral groin lymphadenectomy. However, contralateral groin lymphadenectomy will need to be subsequently performed if ipsilateral nodes are found to be positive.

> **TIP**
> Excision of abnormal skin (such as LS or VIN) should be considered alongside radical local excision of the tumour, to minimise the risk of further tumours arising.

SLN excision – It may be appropriate in selected early stage cases. Groin lymph node dissection carries an approximately 30% risk of lymphoedema and similar risk of wound infection. The sentinel node is the first lymph node to which cancer cells are most likely to spread from primary tumour. Removing SLN and evaluating it for the presence of tumour may eliminate the need for full groin node dissection in node-negative patients, and therefore reduce adverse effects and potentially improve their quality of life.

Eligibility criteria for SLN biopsy are as follows:

- Primary SCC of vulva
- Cancer measuring a maximum diameter of <4 cm
- Unifocal tumour
- No clinical or radiological evidence of lymph node metastasis
- No known safety issues for the use of the tracer (blue dye or technetium-99).

If SLN cannot be identified, or is found to contain metastatic disease, a full groin node dissection should be carried out. Those with negative sentinel nodes do not require any further treatment, but will require close surveillance.

143

Locally Advanced Vulval Cancer

Management of locally advanced vulval cancer is challenging by virtue of its spread to surrounding structures such as the urethra, anus and involvement of groin nodes. Treatment requires careful planning including input from colorectal and plastic surgeons if surgical treatment is desired. Examination under anaesthesia is usually necessary for pre-procedural planning. The size and location of the tumour will dictate the appropriate surgical approach. If surgery is undertaken with curative intent, adequate margins of at least 15 mm will be necessary. Reconstructive surgical techniques may be required to enable primary surgical closure.

Radical local excision to achieve clear surgical margins may result in damage to the sphincters leading to urinary or faecal incontinence. In these cases, decisions are complex and require careful consideration. Radical excision with exenterative procedures may be required, with inevitable significant physical and psychological morbidity afterwards. Preoperative radiation therapy and/or chemotherapy may be used as an alternative approach to reduce the need for stoma, but this is not without risk. Post-radiation skin changes pose a significant risk to wound healing for reconstructive procedures involving plastic surgeons following radical surgery. Early recourse to involve palliative care team should be initiated for patients who are not suitable for, or have chosen not to embark on, radical procedures. Symptoms may be managed with adequate analgesia, topical treatment for discharge and odours, indwelling catheter for urinary obstruction and assistance in managing bowel function.

Reconstructive surgical options – These are required whenever wide local excision is achieved at the expense of cosmesis and function. Closure of the vulval wound must be achieved without tension, otherwise wound breakdown inevitably follows. This can lead to secondary healing with disfigurement and further loss of function. Disfigurement following vulval cancer surgery may affect sexual function and can have a major impact on the patient's psychology. Reconstructive techniques have been developed to improve the cosmetic outcome and to an extent, the function following radical vulval surgery. Techniques vary according to size and depth of defect as well as the quality of surrounding tissues. Options include skin grafts, and local or distant tissue flaps. Flaps can be performed as a secondary procedure. Complications from plastic procedures could occur at the donor or recipient site and include wound dehiscence, hernias and flap necrosis.

Patients and relatives will need upfront information and realistic expectations about recovery and prognosis from any radical treatment.

Management of clinically suspicious groin nodes – Treatment should be surgical wherever possible, even in the case of fixed or ulcerated nodes. Postoperative radiation is likely to be necessary. Women with advanced vulval cancer who are not fit for surgery can have their nodes treated with primary radiotherapy, after pathological assessment with FNA.

Complications of Surgery

While newer and more conservative approaches to surgical treatment have improved morbidity, there are still significant problems that result from treatment. Perioperative complications include:

- Wound breakdown
- Wound infection
- Deep vein thrombosis and pulmonary embolism
- Pressure sores.

Other morbidities may become apparent at a later stage; therefore follow-up is essential for assessing longer term problems, in addition to checking for recurrence. Chronic problems that may arise include:

- Introital stenosis
- Incontinence (urinary and faecal)
- Rectocoele
- Lymphocoele (Figure 13.5)
- Lymphoedema (Figure 13.6)
- Hernia
- Psychosexual problems.

Every effort should be taken to minimise morbidity associated with surgery. Adequate pre-operative counselling and support is essential to ensure the patient is fully informed of the potential consequences of the treatment.

Radiotherapy for Vulval Cancer

SCCs of the vulva are known to be radiosensitive tumours. It is most commonly used in the adjuvant setting, but occasionally it may be utilised in a primary setting. Vulval skin tolerates radiation poorly and is

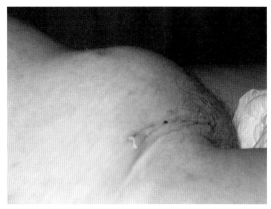

Figure 13.5 Right lymphocoele following lymphadenectomy on the same side

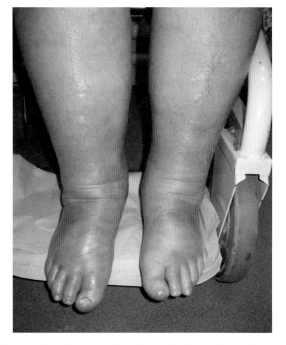

Figure 13.6 Chronic lymphoedema of both lower limbs which is often debilitating and difficult to manage

susceptible to both dry and wet desquamation. Vulval cancers are generally treated by surgery in the first instance for these reasons.

Adjuvant Radiotherapy

Indications for adjuvant radiotherapy include:

- Positive surgical margins at the vulval excision site
- Positive groin nodes (two or more micrometastases, replacement of node, extracapsular spread).

> **TIP**
> There is no evidence to routinely recommend adjuvant radio-therapy to women with close surgical margins, despite the higher risk of recurrence.

Primary Radiotherapy

This can be used in the management of advanced tumours or in patients with comorbidities unsuitable for surgical intervention. External beam radiotherapy is given to irradiate inguinal and lower pelvic nodes followed by brachytherapy usually with the dose of 45–50 Gy. Primary radiotherapy can also be used in highly selected cases to allow for sphincter-preserving surgery.

Chemotherapy

There is limited data to guide on the role of chemotherapy for vulval cancer. It has been used in the neo-adjuvant setting to reduce the extent of surgery, and in the adjuvant setting after surgery, either alone or in combination with radiotherapy. It has also been used in recurrent and metastatic disease. Responses are variable, and toxicity may be a problem in the elderly with co-morbidities.

The European Society of Gynaecological Oncology (ESGO) has recently made the following recommendations regarding chemoradiation:

- Definitive chemoradiation (with radiation dose escalation) is the treatment of choice in patients with unresectable disease.
- In advanced stage disease neoadjuvant chemoradiation should be considered to avoid exenterative surgery.
- Radiosensitising chemotherapy, preferably with weekly cisplatin, is recommended.

Recurrent Disease

Most vulval recurrence occurs within 2 years of primary treatment, predominantly within the vulva. The risk is increased for women with positive groin nodes at primary surgery, involved or close surgical margins, VIN in adjacent tumour tissue, higher tumour grade and lymphovascular space invasion. Survival following recurrence is poor, and treatment can be challenging.

Management will depend on various factors including the site and extent of recurrence, and previous treatments. Surgery with curative intent can be performed if the recurrence is localised to the vulva. Radiotherapy should be considered if surgery would impair sphincter function or require exenterative procedures. Excision may be the only option if the area has already received maximum dose of radiation in the past. The palliative care team should be involved if symptom control is difficult.

Groin recurrences are difficult to manage and have a poorer prognosis. Radiotherapy should be given to women who have not previously been treated with this. There are limited options for women who have previously received irradiation. Palliation, which may include surgery, should be offered.

Chemotherapy may be considered in selected cases, but data is lacking, and many patients may not be fit enough to tolerate this treatment.

> **TIPS**
> Survival following recurrence is poor, and symptoms are difficult to palliate. Therefore all attempts to prevent recurrence must be made at the time of primary treatment.

Conclusion

Vulval cancer is a rare disease but the incidence is rising secondary to HPV infection. Presenting symptoms should prompt clinicians to perform a careful vulval and pelvic examination and instigate appropriate referral. There has been a trend to adopt more conservative and patient-centred surgical approaches with wide local excision and individualised management of groin nodes. Techniques such as SLN sampling are becoming a standard of care for tumours <4 cm. Surgery is the mainstay of treatment, including management of the groin nodes, with radiotherapy mostly utilised in the adjuvant setting. Management of recurrences can be difficult and are associated with poor outcomes. Every effort must be made to prevent recurrence at the time of initial treatment. A highly individualised approach is required in the management of vulval cancer.

Further Reading

Ayhan A, Reed N, Gultekin M, Dursun P, editors. *Section V: Diseases of vulva. In: Textbook of Gynaecological Oncology.* 3rd ed. Ankara, Turkey: GUNES Publishing, 2016; pp. 897–944.

Grootenhuis NC, van der Zee AGJ, van Doorn HC et al. Sentinel nodes in vulvar cancer: Long-term follow-up of the GROningen INternational Study on Sentinel nodes in Vulvar cancer (GROINSS-V) I. *Gynecol Oncol* 2016; 140: 8–14.

Lu SM, Yashar CM. The vulva. In: Levine DA, Dizon DS, Yashar CM et al., editors. *Handbook for Principles and Practice of Gynecologic Oncology.* 2nd ed. Philadelphia: Wolters Kluwer, 2015; pp. 72–95.

Royal College of Obstetricians and Gynaecologists. *Guidelines for the Diagnosis and Management of Vulval Carcinoma,* May 2014. London: RCOG.

Selman TJ, Luesley DM, Acheson N et al. A systematic review of the accuracy of diagnostic tests for inguinal lymph node status in vulvar cancer. *Gynecol Oncol* 2005; 99: 206–14.

Chapter 14

Uterine Sarcomas

Helen Bolton and Mahmood Shafi

Background

Uterine sarcomas are uncommon gynaecological cancers. They are a small but important group of tumours because their management may require a different approach compared to some of the more common cancers of the female genital tract. Due to small numbers, there is limited evidence to guide treatments. From the patient's perspective having a rarer type of cancer may feel more challenging to cope with for several reasons, for example, they may feel more isolated; it might take longer to make a diagnosis; and it can be more difficult for them to find information about their type of tumour.

Sarcomas can occur anywhere within the female genital tract, but the most common site is the uterus. These tumours account for <1% of all gynaecological cancers. They usually behave aggressively and are associated with a poor prognosis.

Terminology and Pathology

The accurate histological assessment of uncommon gynaecological tumours requires expert review by specialist pathologists at cancer centres. A correct pathological diagnosis is essential for planning appropriate management.

The terminology of uncommon cancers can be confusing, as their nomenclature has evolved with improvements in understanding of the pathology. All cancers are classified by both the primary location of tumour (primary site) and the cell type from which the cancer originates (histological type). *Carcinomas* are malignant cells that arise from *epithelial* cells and account for the majority of gynaecological cancers. In contrast, *sarcomas* are malignant cells that arise from *mesenchymal tissues* such as smooth muscle, connective tissue, fibrous tissue, fat and endothelial cells. In addition to identifying the underlying cell type of the tumour, it is also important to grade the tumour, usually as low (G1, well differentiated) or high (G3, poorly

differentiated). Grading is generally based on the degree of cellular abnormality, the presence of necrosis and the rate of cellular proliferation (the mitotic index, measured by the number of mitotic figures identified within a given magnification field). Tumour grading helps to predict how the tumour is likely to behave and respond to treatment.

Carcinosarcoma is a term used to describe a tumour that contains a mixture of both malignant epithelial and mesenchymal cell types. These were previously referred to as malignant mixed Mullerian tumours (MMMTs). However, with advances in molecular diagnostic techniques, it is now apparent that these tumours arise from malignant epithelial cells that have undergone metaplasia (the transformation of one cell type to another) to form a tumour that contains mixed cellular elements. These tumours are now classified as carcinomas (rather than sarcomas) as they arise from a monoclonal neoplastic epithelial cell. Further details on carcinosarcoma are discussed in Chapter 11.

> **TIP**
> Endometrial carcinosarcomas are considered to be a high-risk variant of endometrial adenocarcinoma, rather than sarcomas, and share similar risk factors.

Uterine Sarcomas

Gynaecological sarcomas most commonly originate within the uterus. Uterine sarcomas usually originate from the smooth muscle of the uterine wall (leiomyosarcomas), but they can also arise within the stromal tissue of the endometrium (endometrial stromal tumours).

Epidemiology and Risk Factors

Uterine sarcomas are rare and therefore identification of clear risk factors is difficult due to lack of large studies. Increasing age is a significant risk factor for uterine sarcomas, with the average age at diagnosis being 60 years. Therefore most women will present after the menopause, but young age and pre-menopausal status does not exclude the diagnosis of sarcoma. Long-term use of tamoxifen is a risk factor for sarcoma, although the absolute risk remains small. Black race is also a risk factor for uterine leiomyosarcoma (but not other sarcomas) with an approximately two-fold higher incidence than women of white race.

Uterine Smooth Muscle Tumours

Leiomyosarcomas are the most common malignant smooth muscle tumour of the uterus. They may arise *de novo*, or from pre-existing fibroids. These are high-grade tumours, and typically aggressive with early spread to lymph nodes and blood-borne metastases to the lung, liver and bones. Pre-operative diagnosis can be difficult, as benign tumours (fibroids) are so common. Although pre-operative imaging with CT or MRI can raise suspicions, many of these tumours are still detected post-operatively by the histopathologists.

> **TIPS**
> Benign leiomyomas (fibroids) are the most common pelvic neoplasm in women. Clinically they can be difficult to distinguish from uterine sarcomas, and consequently many are diagnosed post-operatively by the histopathologists.

Smooth muscle tumours of uncertain malignant potential (STUMP) are uterine tumours that cannot be reliably diagnosed as benign or malignant despite expert pathological review. The clinical behaviour of these lesions is difficult to predict, which can pose challenges to management, especially in pre-menopausal women who want to retain their fertility.

Endometrial Stromal Tumours

Tumours arising from the stromal layer of the endometrium account for <10% of uterine sarcomas, and approximately 1% of all uterine malignancies. The World Health Organisation (WHO) classifies endometrial stromal neoplasms into the following three groups:

- **Endometrial stromal nodules (ESN)** – These comprise a well-defined, non-invasive nodule, usually within the myometrium. These are usually benign; however, definitive diagnosis requires complete excision of the nodule (usually hysterectomy) as invasive features cannot reliably be excluded by imaging or biopsy alone.
- **Endometrial stromal sarcomas (ESS)** – These are low-grade sarcomas with metastatic potential. The majority are ER/PR positive, and have an indolent course with recurrences that often present many years later. Overall the prognosis is good. These patients should undergo total hysterectomy with oophorectomy, together with resection of any extra-uterine disease where possible. Metastatic or recurrent disease may respond well to cytoreductive surgery and adjuvant treatment with progestins or aromatase inhibitors. Conversely, patients with a history of ESS should not receive oestrogens or tamoxifen.
- **Undifferentiated endometrial stromal sarcoma (UES)** – These are high-grade aggressive tumours that are usually ER/PR negative, with a poor overall prognosis, regardless of stage.

Staging of Uterine Sarcomas

The staging for uterine sarcomas was re-classified in 2009 by International Federation of Gynecology and Obstetrics (FIGO) and is found in Appendix.

Clinical Presentation, Staging and Pre-operative Assessment

Clinical Presentation

Common symptoms and signs of uterine sarcoma
- Abnormal uterine bleeding
- Abdominal pain or distension
- Pelvic mass
- Rapidly enlarging uterus.

Uterine sarcomas typically present with symptoms of abnormal vaginal bleeding and/or symptoms from an enlarging uterus such as pelvic pressure, distension pain or a pelvic mass. Some women may present without symptoms, with a co-incidental finding of a pelvic mass identified on pelvic examination or at the time of imaging. Some cases will be discovered only after surgery, usually as an unexpected finding after a hysterectomy or myomectomy for presumed benign fibroids.

Consequently women with sarcomas may present through various routes. Pre-menopausal women may present via the menstrual dysfunction or reproductive medicine clinic with a history of abnormal uterine bleeding or presumed fibroids. Post-menopausal women are more likely to present via the rapid access clinic with symptoms of post-menopausal bleeding or a pelvic mass. Pre-operatively it can be difficult to distinguish between benign fibroids and sarcoma, especially in pre-menopausal women. Women may rarely experience symptoms related to metastatic disease.

Pre-operative Assessment

The initial assessment should include a thorough, focused history and physical examination, which will then direct further specialist investigations including imaging. Abdominal and pelvic examination usually reveals an enlarged uterus. Visualisation of the vulva, vagina and cervix should be included to identify any other causes for vaginal bleeding. A more general physical examination should be carried out, including an assessment of fitness for surgery. It is uncommon to identify metastatic disease on physical examination at presentation; however, it is good practice to examine the chest and to evaluate for groin and supraclavicular lymph nodes. Imaging studies are carried out to characterise the uterus, endometrium and adnexae.

First-line imaging is usually by pelvic ultrasound scan, using the vaginal approach, to give clear images of the uterus, endometrium and adnexae. Endometrial biopsy should be undertaken for post-menopausal women if the endometrium is poorly visualised, thickened (4 mm or above) or otherwise appears abnormal. For pre-menopausal women an endometrial biopsy should be taken if she is above 45 years with irregular vaginal bleeding, and must be also considered in younger women with irregular bleeding in the presence of other risk factors for endometrial pathology. A hysteroscopy may be required and sometimes the diagnosis is revealed after the histology of a hysteroscopic trans-cervical resection of fibroid. Although endometrial biopsy does not usually detect sarcoma, it is important to exclude endometrial cancer if present. Occasionally, a sarcoma may prolapse through the cervix and be amenable to direct biopsy.

Further imaging is required if the ultrasound scan reveals myometrial abnormalities or sarcoma is suspected. The definitive imaging modality for suspected sarcoma is MRI assessment (Figure 14.1). This allows a detailed assessment of the pelvic mass, including assessment of localised extension or spread to the parametrium, pelvic peritoneum and lymph nodes. Although MRI is helpful, it cannot reliably differentiate between sarcoma and a benign fibroid undergoing degeneration or other uterine abnormalities.

If sarcoma is suspected then a CT scan of the abdomen and chest should be carried out to evaluate for the presence of metastases. Common sites of metastases are the lung, liver and upper abdomen.

As surgery is usually required for treatment, assessment must also include routine pre-operative tests to evaluate and maximise fitness for surgery. Anaesthetic review should be arranged for patients who are obese, unfit, elderly or with significant co-morbidities.

Multidisciplinary Team Review

Where sarcoma is suspected pre-operatively, it is essential to arrange for the case to be reviewed at the regional centre gynaecological oncology multidisciplinary team (MDT) meeting and subsequently referred to sarcoma MDT. All clinical information including imaging and any available histology must be considered by the team so that an individualised management plan can be recommended. The MDT will continue to have an ongoing role in reviewing the case and re-evaluating management plans as the treatment progresses.

Management of Uterine Sarcomas

Wherever possible, women with suspected uterine sarcomas should be managed in a specialist cancer centre. In some cases the disease would have been diagnosed after surgery for presumed benign fibroids. These cases will require referral to the cancer centre MDT for subsequent management. The approach to management will depend upon whether the disease appears to be confined to the uterus at the time of presentation. Most cases are treated with upfront surgery, followed by consideration of adjuvant treatment.

Surgery for disease confined to the uterus – For disease that appears to be confined to the uterus, a total hysterectomy including bilateral salpingectomy should be carried out. Bulky lymph nodes should be removed if identified on imaging or at surgery, but routine lymphadenectomy is not indicated as lymph node metastases are rare in stage I disease. Most experts would recommend that standard surgical treatment should include bilateral oophorectomy in peri- or post-menopausal women. For younger women who want to avoid premature menopause or retain their ovaries for fertility preservation, it is usually acceptable to retain the ovaries. However, decisions must be individualised. While metastases to the ovaries are rare in sarcoma (unlike in carcinomas), many tumours express oestrogen and/or progesterone receptors, and data is limited regarding the impact of

149

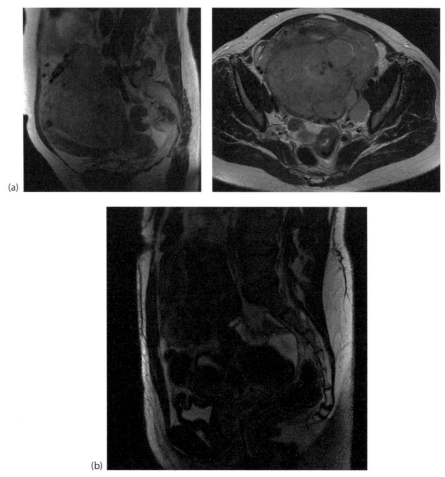

Figure 14.1 (a) **MRI of leiomyosarcoma**. Sagittal and axial T2 weighted images through the uterus. Heterogeneous intermediate signal intensity uterine mass. Lobulated contour, signal intensity and presence of haemorrhage on T1 weighted sequence are suspicious for LMS. The pathological left external iliac node is supportive of this diagnosis and (b) **MRI of benign fibroids**. Sagittal T2 weighted images reveal multiple low signal intensity lesions throughout all locations of the uterus (SM, IM and fundal pedunculated SS). These homogenous, well defined lesions are consistent with fibroids

ovarian conservation on outcomes in uterine sarcoma. Individualised decisions must be made according to the women's preferences after detailed discussion with her about the uncertainties of ovarian preservation on long-term outcomes.

Surgery for disease extending beyond the uterus – For women whose disease has spread beyond the uterus, the role of surgery is less clear and options regarding surgery require a highly individualised approach. Decisions usually depend upon fitness for surgery, and whether or not complete surgical resection is possible. For women with resectable disease a total abdominal hysterectomy with resection of metastatic disease can be carried out, with the aim of total cytoreduction leaving no evidence of the disease. For women with distant metastatic disease, or disease not amenable to complete cytoreduction, then surgery may not be beneficial. Moreover, surgery may delay the start of adjuvant treatment. However, in selected cases, palliative surgery may be appropriate for women who are experiencing significant pelvic symptoms such as pain or bleeding. These symptoms may be relieved by hysterectomy. While the role of extensive cytoreductive surgery is unclear, gynaecological oncology MDT may sometime consider referring a patient to supraregional sarcoma centre for a surgical opinion.

Women diagnosed post-operatively – Women who are unexpectedly diagnosed with leiomyosarcoma after hysterectomy for presumed benign disease should undergo imaging with CT of the chest, abdomen and pelvis with the aim of detecting any residual or metastatic disease. Routine second surgery solely for staging purposes is not indicated. However further surgery may be considered to remove residual ovaries after ovarian preservation or to remove the cervix after subtotal hysterectomy. Where imaging shows evidence of residual disease that is amenable to optimal resection, a further second surgical staging procedure with cytoreduction is indicated.

> **TIP**
> Repeat surgery for staging purposes is not routinely indicated for most women who have been diagnosed with sarcoma post-operatively.

Adjuvant Treatment for Uterine Sarcomas

Although the mainstay treatment for uterine sarcomas is surgery, adjuvant treatment is usually considered on a case-by-case basis. Treatments that may be considered include radiotherapy, chemotherapy and hormonal treatment. Unlike surgical treatment, the benefits of adjuvant treatment in uterine sarcomas are less clear. Gynaecological sarcomas are rare diseases, and therefore robust data on the impact of adjuvant treatment are limited. Patients should be encouraged to consider taking part in suitable clinical trials run by the major gynaecological oncology groups, so that further data becomes available to guide management of these patients.

For patients with early stage disease, confined to the uterus, who have undergone complete surgical resection, there is no clear proven benefit to adjuvant treatment. Surveillance only may be a reasonable option, as chemotherapy and radiotherapy have not yet been proven to improve overall survival. Uterine leiomyosarcomas are aggressive tumours with a high risk of relapse, usually within the first 2 years after diagnosis. In contrast, ESS may relapse many years later, and require prolonged follow-up.

Pelvic radiotherapy – The use of adjuvant radiotherapy has not been proven to improve survival or local recurrences rates, even in early stage disease based on EORTC 55874 study. Radiotherapy is therefore rarely justified for the treatment of uterine sarcomas. The use of combined radiotherapy with chemotherapy is still investigational.

Chemotherapy – Although high-quality evidence is limited, chemotherapy is usually offered to women with advanced disease, and for those with distant metastases. First-line treatments usually include gemcitabine plus docetaxel, or doxorubicin. Additional clinical trials with larger numbers are required to optimise the role of chemotherapy in the treatment of uterine sarcomas.

Hormonal treatment – ESS are usually oestrogen receptor (ER) and/or progesterone receptor (PR) positive; therefore hormone replacement therapy (HRT) and tamoxifen is contraindicated for these patients. Women with advanced or recurrent disease usually respond well to progestins or aromatase inhibitors and these may be helpful in controlling the disease for many years if cytoreductive surgery is not appropriate. Aromatase inhibitors may be more appropriate for women who experience side-effects from progestins. For women with uterine leiomyosarcomas, hormonal therapy can be considered if their tumour is hormone receptor positive, although the benefits are uncertain.

Prognosis

The overall prognosis for most sarcomas is poor, with surgery as the only curative treatment. Even with early stage disease, recurrence is common and usually occurs within the first 2 years. Low-grade ESS and STUMP tend to follow a more favourable disease course.

Summary

- Gynaecological sarcomas are rare malignancies.
- They can be difficult to distinguish pre-operatively from benign fibroids.
- All sarcomas must be managed in specialist cancer centres and reviewed at the MDT.
- Many sarcomas are diagnosed post-operatively following surgery for presumed benign fibroids.
- Surgery is the mainstay of treatment for early stage disease.
- The role of surgery is less clear in advanced disease but may be considered if complete removal of disease is achievable, or to palliate symptoms in advanced disease.
- Adjuvant chemotherapy has a role in advanced disease, but the role of radiotherapy is less certain.
- Further good quality clinical trials are needed to assist in the management of these rare tumours.

- Prognosis tends to be poor, even in early stage disease, except for the low-grade ESS which have a more favourable prognosis.
- Hormonal treatment may be considered in selected cases.

Clinical practice point: fibroids and the role of power morcellation in the surgical management of benign fibroids

Morcellation is a surgical technique that can be employed to enable large specimens to be removed through small incisions (usually laparoscopic) at the time of hysterectomy or myomectomy. In 2014, concerns were raised by the US Food and Drug Administration (FDA) that power morcellation (using rapidly rotating blades) may inadvertently disseminate tumour cells within the abdominal cavity in women with unsuspected malignancies, and thus upstage their disease and worsen their prognosis. This followed a high-profile campaign by a patient, herself a doctor, who was found to have leiomyosarcoma after hysterectomy. Consequently, the FDA issued a warning to discourage the use of power morcellator devices to minimise the risk of inadvertent spread of malignancy. This triggered much debate within the international medical community and there has been a subsequent decline in the use of power morcellation. Consequently, many women with benign disease are undergoing laparotomy, whereas previously they would have benefited from a minimal access approach. In the United Kingdom, the British Society of Gynaecological Endoscopists (BSGE) issued a statement acknowledging these potential risks and advised gynaecologists to be aware of the latest evidence and to avoid the use of power morcellation where malignancy is suspected. Gynaecologists should review each case on individual merit, and if considering offering power morcellation must ensure that their patients are counselled appropriately so that they can make an informed choice about their surgery. In light of these concerns, 'in-bag' morcellation techniques are being developed which may reduce the risks, although safety data is in its infancy.

Further Reading

Hall T, Lee SI, Boruta DM et al. Medical device safety and surgical dissemination of unrecognized uterine malignancy: Morcellation in minimally invasive gynecologic surgery. *Oncologist.* 2015; 20(11): 1274–82.

Prat J. Mbatani. Uterine sarcomas. *Int J Gynaecol Obstet.* 2015; 131(Suppl 2): S105–10.

Non-epithelial Ovarian Tumours and Gestational Trophoblastic Neoplasia

Michael J. Seckl and Christina Fotopoulou

Non-epithelial Ovarian Tumours

Non-epithelial ovarian tumours (NEOTs) are derived from the germ cell and non-epithelial components of the gonads, as opposed to the epithelial ovarian cancers which arise from ovarian epithelium. They represent very rare tumour entities comprising a heterogeneous group of benign or malignant tumours. There are two main groups, namely germ cell tumours and sex cord–stromal tumours (see Table 15.1). Malignant ovarian sex cord–stromal tumours comprise only 1.2% of all primary ovarian malignancies, while malignant germ cell tumours account for only about 5% of all malignant ovarian neoplasms. They usually affect younger women and thus present clinicians and patients with a therapeutic dilemma in regards to fertility-sparing options when the disease is locally advanced or metastatic.

Malignant Germ Cell Tumours

Ovarian germ cell tumours (OGCTs) primarily affect young, premenopausal women until the third decade of life, and represent approximately 70% of all

Table 15.1 Classification of non-epithelial ovarian tumours

Germ cell tumours	Sex cord–stromal tumours
Dysgerminoma	Granulosa-cell tumour
Endodermal sinus tumour (yolk sac tumour)	Fibroma
Embryonal carcinoma	Thecoma
Polyembryoma	Fibrothecoma
Ovarian choriocarcinoma	Sertoli–Leydig cell tumours

Teratoma
  Immature (solid, cystic, both)
  Mature (solid, cystic)
	Sertoli cell

Monodermal
  Struma ovarii
  Carcinoid
	Gynandroblastoma

Mixed forms	

ovarian neoplasms in this age group. However, germ cell tumours may also affect postmenopausal women and should be considered in the differential diagnosis in older women with suspected ovarian tumours. In most instances, no predisposing factors are found. However in rare cases some may arise from fully differentiated mature teratomas, otherwise known as dermoid cysts. Dysgerminomas are more common in phenotypic females who have a Y chromosome, such as those with gonadal dysgenesis or complete androgen insensitivity and rarely in Turner syndrome.

Pathology

OGCTs can be broadly divided into:

- those that differentiate towards embryo-like neoplasms – including teratomas and their subtypes, and dysgerminomas
- those that differentiate towards extraembryonic foetal-derived (placenta-like) cell populations or
- a mixture of both.

They are best thought of as a spectrum of disorders ranging from the pre-malignant dermoid and immature grade I/II OGCT through to the malignant immature grade III malignant germ cell tumours, dysgerminomas (equivalent to male seminomas), non-dysgerminomatous and mixed forms. Since germ cells can differentiate to form all cell types seen in the neonate and adult any combination of pathologies are possible, although some are more common than others. For example, elements of yolk sac tumour, choriocarcinoma and dysgerminoma are more commonly seen than embryonal or rhabdomyosarcoma. The cellular elements present can help to predict clinical behaviour, and determine the production of tumour markers. Very rarely, cancers from a variety of other origins can have histological elements that mimic malignant germ cell tumours, including tumour marker secretion, and this can produce diagnostic dilemmas. In addition, ovarian choriocarcinomas may indeed turn out to be gestational in origin, rather than non-gestational and/ or epithelial in origin.

Clinical Presentation and Diagnostic Pathways

Presentation may be with:

- localised symptoms from the pelvic mass
- coincidental finding on imaging
- systemic symptoms from hypercalcaemia (in dysgerminoma).

Patients typically present with a short history of lower abdominal swelling and pain arising from the pelvis as these tumours frequently may grow rapidly with all the associated symptoms of local pressure such as urinary frequency, change of bowel habits and pain. In addition, hypercalcaemia rarely seen in patients with dysgerminomas may be associated with systemic symptoms. Menstrual irregularity is common. Patients may present as acute admissions and an ultrasound (transabdominal and transvaginal) often reveals or confirms the clinical suspicion of a pelvic mass.

Tumour markers – OGCTs are usually associated with elevated tumour markers:

- **Human chorionic gonadotropin (hCG)** – embryonal cell carcinomas, ovarian choriocarcinomas, mixed germ cell tumours and dysgerminomas (approximately 10%)
- **α-Fetoprotein (AFP)** – yolk sac tumours, embryonal cell tumours, polyembryomas, mixed germ cell tumours and some immature teratomas
- **Lactate dehydrogenase (LDH)** – dysgerminomas.

Patients with choriocarcinoma/trophoblastic tumour elements will usually have an elevated serum hCG and those with yolk sac tumours will produce α-fetoprotein (AFP). Elevation of either or both of the latter two markers is seen in approximately 85% of non-dysgerminomatous forms and hCG but not AFP is raised in about 10% of dysgerminomatous cases. In addition, CA125 and lactate dehydrogenase (LDH) may be non-specifically raised in any histological subtype. It follows that measurement of AFP, hCG and CA125 can help in the diagnostic work-up of patients with a suspected ovarian mass and should be done in any woman under the age of 50 years who is still planning a family.

Investigations – An early assessment of tumour markers including AFP, hCG and CA125 should be requested in addition to other blood tests, an MRI pelvis and a CT chest and abdomen. An MRI head

should be carried out in those with disease above the diaphragm or clinical symptoms of central nervous system (CNS) involvement.

Recommendations for Management

Surgery

Similar to epithelial ovarian cancer, the fundamental goal of surgical treatment for malignant ovarian germ cell tumours (MOGCTs) is complete tumour resection with adequate surgical staging. Peritoneal surgical staging includes cytology, at least infracolic omentectomy, and multiple peritoneal biopsies even when the peritoneum appears macroscopically normal. In contrast to epithelial ovarian tumours, lymph node staging is not required in OGCTs; however, bulky lymph node disease should be resected.

Fertility-sparing surgery – In early stages of the disease a fertility-sparing approach is oncologically safe, and should be discussed and offered to women who wish to retain their fertility. In these cases, the contralateral ovary is spared. It is not necessary to perform a biopsy from the contralateral ovary, provided it appears normal.

For women presenting with advanced disease, neoadjuvant chemotherapy should be considered. This may downstage the disease prior to surgery, and thus minimise the extent or need to carry out ultraradical resection surgery for complete tumour clearance. This approach enables a fertility-sparing approach in selected cases.

> **TIP**
> Fertility-sparing surgery is usually possible in women undergoing treatment for OGCTs.

Systemic Treatment and Follow-Up

Early stage disease – stage IA/B – These patients can be considered for surveillance, irrespective of the underlying pathological subtype or presence of lymphovascular space invasion. Surveillance involves regular clinic visits, tumour marker measurements and imaging. The relapse rate is approximately 20–25% and these relapses are virtually all cured with subsequent chemotherapy. Consequently, surveillance is one strategy to prevent 75–80% of patients being unnecessarily exposed to toxic chemotherapy. However, in those rare patients unable or unwilling to undergo a surveillance programme, adjuvant therapy with two cycles of 5-day BEP (bleomycin, etoposide, cisplatin) chemotherapy can be given for non-dysgerminomatous tumours and it is possible that single-agent carboplatin AUC7 is sufficient for those with dysgerminomatous disease.

The overall survival in patients with stage IA/B disease whether managed with surveillance or with adjuvant therapy is almost 100%.

Stage IC and above disease – These patients are treated with adjuvant chemotherapy. Standard treatment is with three cycles of 5-day BEP. In selected cases of advanced disease, three cycles of neoadjuvant chemotherapy can be given prior to debulking surgery to remove any remaining disease. Histological review of the post-operative pathology will determine if further chemotherapy is required. If there is no active residual tumour, then further chemotherapy is not necessary. Otherwise a further three cycles of chemotherapy should be administered.

Post-treatment surveillance will be organised as shared care between the MOGCT centre and local gynaecological oncology centre.

The overall outcome for patients with stage IV disease remains disappointing with only a 65% 5-year survival rate. Therefore new therapeutic approaches are urgently required. This will likely arise from improved disease understanding achieved through the new centralised malignant germ cell service.

Follow-up – All patients are advised to avoid pregnancy during the first 2 years after treatment. Due to their tendency for late relapse patients with malignant germ cell tumours should receive long-term follow-up. This involves:

- serial monitoring of tumour markers until they normalise
- three monthly pelvic ultrasounds in cases of fertility-sparing surgery.

Relapsed Disease

Surgical debulking should be considered in all patients with potentially resectable disease as retrospective data shows improvement in survival.

In male patients with testicular germ cell tumours who relapse following initial chemotherapy, the salvage rates are relatively high at approximately 60%. In contrast, <10% of women with relapsed malignant germ cell tumours are salvaged despite the use of similar chemotherapy regimens, suggesting different tumour biology. It is therefore essential that relapsed disease is managed in specialised ovarian germ cell centres so that outcomes can be improved. Chemotherapy is usually given, but is rarely curative. Radiotherapy

may provide palliation in selected cases. Experimental treatments are therefore required together with better identification of patients most likely to relapse so that more aggressive therapies can be deployed earlier to prevent relapse.

Sex Cord–Stromal Tumours

Ovarian sex cord–stromal tumours comprise a range of benign and malignant tumours that arise from the supporting tissue of the ovary, including cells that produce hormones. These tumours are rare and account for only 1.2% of all cases of ovarian neoplasms, with granulosa-cell tumours (GCTs) being the most common malignant histological subtype.

Like MOGCT, the average age at diagnosis for sex cord–stromal tumours is considerably younger than the epithelial ovarian cancer. In the SEER database, 12% of the patients were younger than 30 years, while 57% were between 30 and 59 years of age.

Histopathology and Genetics

Morphologically, sex cord–stromal tumours display nonspecific and equivocal features and the histopathological diagnosis may be difficult, leading not uncommonly to misdiagnosis especially in non-expert centres. GCTs are almost always associated with mutations in the *FOXL2* gene, and this mutation may be a potential driver in the pathogenesis of adult-type GCTs.

Mutations in DICER1 are associated with Sertoli–Leydig cell tumours and other non-epithelial ovarian cancers. Germline DICER1 mutations have been shown to be associated with a number of clinical conditions other than ovarian Sertoli–Leydig cell tumours, including pleuropulmonary blastoma, lung cysts, cystic nephroma, thyroid nodular hyperplasia and differentiated carcinomas, and cervical sarcoma botryoides.

Clinical Presentation and Diagnostic Pathways

Patients may present with:

- Symptoms of pelvic and abdominal disease – pain, bloating and distension
- Manifestations of hormonal secretion – sex cord–stromal tumours may secrete oestrogens or androgens and patients may present endocrine-dependent clinical manifestations such as

155

virilisation, abnormal uterine bleeding and endometrial hyperplasia.

Tumour markers – Sex cord–stromal tumours may secrete hormones, inhibin, AFP or specific tumour markers may include hormonal levels, inhibin and anti-Müllerian hormone.

The diagnostic and clinical pathways are otherwise identical to those described for malignant OGCTs.

> **TIP**
> GCTs may be associated with complex atypical hyperplasia or carcinoma of the endometrium in up to 25% of patients.

Management

Surgical management relies on the basic principles as presented above for the MOGCTs but with the recognition that chemotherapy and other systemic therapies are much less successful. Consequently, the initial surgical approach needs to be curative in intent wherever possible. However, in young patients who desire their fertility, a fertility-sparing approach with uterine preservation should be attempted. However, it is essential to evaluate the endometrium to exclude a hormonal-induced endometrial pathology such as complex atypical hyperplasia or even cancer.

Adjuvant treatment – Systemic treatment guidelines have been controversial especially in regards to the value of cytotoxic chemotherapy and targeted agents. Many clinicians now save systemic therapies for inoperable relapses, as they do not appear to achieve sustained cures. Hormonal treatment may be of benefit, such as those agents used in oestrogen-receptor positive breast cancer, including the aromatase inhibitors letrozole or anastrozole. Current studies are also investigating the role of anti-angiogenetic agents such as bevacizumab in recurrent disease.

In terms of cytotoxic agents, historically these tumours were treated with the BEP or PEI (*cisplatin*, etoposide, ifosfamide) regimen analogous to the MOGCTs. However, in recent years these have been replaced by less toxic regimens such as carboplatin and paclitaxel.

Recurrent Disease

At presentation, sex cord–stromal tumours tend to be localised to the pelvis. In contrast, relapsed disease tends to present as diffuse, disseminated disease,

which may be multi-focal. GCTs may recur many years after the initial presentation, and the years between subsequent relapses tend to get progressively shorter. Surgery is the cornerstone of management, with the aim of leaving no residual disease, since no systemic agent has been proven to be especially effective. Some patients may require multiple operations. There is no evidence that post-operative adjuvant treatment offers a survival benefit. Once the disease becomes inoperable, deployment of hormonal or systemic chemotherapy seems reasonable. Emerging data suggests that among the hormonal therapies of leuprolide acetate, tamoxifen, medroxyprogesterone or the aromatase inhibitors, the latter may be the most promising, particularly for the treatment of adult-type GCTs.

Summary

NEOTS represent a rare group of ovarian tumours that predominantly affect young women and can usually be managed using fertility-conserving approaches. Because of their rarity and the need to better define prognostic subgroups to refine management and improve survival outcomes, they may be best managed through centralised care pathways like the ones established for gestational trophoblastic neoplasia (GTN) and MOGCT.

Gestational Trophoblastic Disease

Gestational trophoblastic disease (GTD) consists of a spectrum of disorders:

- Pre-malignant GTD – including complete hydatidiform (CHM) and partial hydatidiform (PHM) moles
- Malignant GTD – including invasive mole, gestational choriocarcinoma, placental-site trophoblastic tumour (PSTT) and epithelioid trophoblastic tumour (ETT).

The malignant tumours are also known as gestational trophoblastic tumours (GTTs) or GTN and PSTT/ETT are often described together as they appear to behave clinically in a similar fashion. Both CHM and PHM can develop into invasive moles, choriocarcinoma and PSTT/ETT, but the latter three cancers can also develop after any type of pregnancy including term delivery, miscarriage and an ectopic implantation. More recently, atypical placental-site nodules have also been added to the GTD spectrum as these can also develop or be associated with PSTT/ETT in up to 15% of cases. GTN remains an important disorder for the gynaecologist and other clinicians to recognise, because it is always nearly curable, with preservation of fertility, if treated appropriately.

hCG Tests in GTD and Other hCG Secreting Cancers

β-hCG assays – The family of pituitary/placental glycoprotein hormones includes hCG, follicle-stimulating hormone (FSH), luteinising hormone (LH) and thyroid-stimulating hormone (TSH). Each hormone comprises an α-subunit, which is common between the family members, and a distinct β-subunit. Consequently, assays to measure hCG are directed against the β-subunit. Many different β-hCG assays are available. Some detect intact β-hCG and others are either selective for individual fragments or detect various combinations of fragments. In pregnancy, hCG is usually intact, and fragments of β-hCG are not produced. However, in cancer, β-hCG may circulate in many different forms that can vary in their glycosylation status. Therefore, assays used in patients with GTD and cancer need to be able to detect all forms of β-hCG equally well thereby reducing the risk of false negative results. Moreover, the assay should not produce false positive results, as this is well recognised to be associated with unnecessary medical interventions and potentially life-threatening complications.

β-hCG as a Tumour Marker

hCG has a half-life of 24–36 hours and is the most sensitive and specific marker for trophoblastic tissue. However, hCG production is not confined to pregnancy and GTD. Indeed, hCG is produced by any trophoblastic tissue found, for example, in germ cell tumours and in up to 15% of epithelial malignancies. The hCG levels in such cases can be just as high as those seen in GTD or in pregnancy. Therefore, measurements of hCG do not reliably discriminate between pregnancy, GTD or non-GTTs. However, serial measurements of hCG have revolutionised the management of GTD for several reasons. The amount of hCG produced correlates with tumour volume (except for PSTT/ETT) so that a serum hCG of 5 IU/l corresponds to approximately 10^4–10^5 viable tumour cells. Consequently, these assays are several orders of magnitude more sensitive than the best imaging modalities available today. In addition, hCG levels can be used to determine prognosis. Serial

measurements allow progress of the disease or response to therapy to be monitored. Development of drug resistance can be detected at an early stage, which facilitates appropriate changes in management. Estimates may be made of the time for which chemotherapy should be continued after hCG levels are undetectable in serum to reduce the tumour volume to zero. For these reasons hCG is the best tumour marker known.

> **TIP**
> Serial hCG is an extremely sensitive tumour marker in GTD, and is far superior than imaging.

Hydatidiform Moles

Epidemiology, Origin and Pathology

The commonest form of GTD is the hydatidiform mole, which occurs in approximately 1–3:1000 pregnancies in the United Kingdom. Both CHM and PHM are more common in women who become pregnant below 16 years or above 40 years. Hydatidiform moles are also more common in women who have had previous molar pregnancies; the incidence rises to about 1:100 with one previous mole, and to 1: 6.5 with two previous moles. Most of this risk resides with CHM rather than PHM.

CHM typically arises when an ovum devoid of maternal nuclear DNA is fertilised either by two sperms or by a single sperm which duplicates its chromosomes to give a diploid complement of DNA (an androgenetic CHM). However, patients with a history of three or more CHM may rarely have retained an apparent normal genetic phenotype with both maternal and paternal chromosomes present. In these cases, 75% are linked to mutations/truncations in a gene called NLRP7 and another 5–10% in KHD3CL mutations. Recognition of this rare variant is important as it is most unlikely that such affected women can have a normal pregnancy and the risk of malignancy is just as high as for androgenetic CHM. These patients may have children via in vitro fertilisation of eggs from an unaffected donor. In contrast to CHM, PHMs arise when two sperms fertilise an ovum that has retained its nuclear DNA, forming a triploid conceptus. These proliferate into abnormal trophoblast with variable amounts of foetal tissue. The trophoblast forms hydropic villi, which are most obvious in complete moles and macroscopically resemble a bunch of grapes. Microscopically, the dilated villi consist of hyperplastic syncytio- and cytotrophoblast that initially lines oedematous mesenchyme. This breaks down with increasing gestational age to form cisterns. In PHMs these changes are milder and focal, and consequently the diagnosis of PHM may not be immediately apparent at the time of spontaneous miscarriage. Therefore, the true incidence of PHM has been underestimated. A vast increase in maternal blood vessel formation is also triggered by molar tissue, resulting in large arteriovenous shunts that facilitate the metastatic spread of the disease. The ability to synthesise hCG is preserved in molar tissue, enabling it to be used as an extremely sensitive tumour marker.

TIP
Complete hydatidiform moles are diploid, containing no maternal chromosomes and a diploid (double) complement of paternal chromosomes. Partial hydatidiform moles are triploid and contain a normal complement of maternal chromosomes and a double complement of paternal chromosomes.

Clinical Presentation

Presenting symptoms may include:

- Vaginal bleeding or miscarriage in early pregnancy
- Intraperitoneal bleeding (which may be catastrophic)
- Symptoms related to very high hCG levels: toxaemia, hyperemesis, hyperthyroidism and theca luteal cysts
- Excessively large uterus for dates
- Symptoms related to pulmonary, vaginal or cervical metastases.

The commonest presentations of CHM and PHM are threatened or missed miscarriages, usually at the end of the first trimester, with CHM usually presenting earlier than PHM. Symptoms related to metastasis can also occur, although these may spontaneously disappear following evacuation of the mole. Trophoblastic embolisation and disseminated intravascular coagulation are now rarely seen.

Investigations

Patients with a suspected molar pregnancy should undergo:

- Pelvic ultrasound
- hCG estimation in serum and/or urine
- Chest radiography if clinically indicated.

In CHM, the classical ultrasound appearance is described as a snowstorm, although this is not often seen until the second trimester of pregnancy. In PHM, occasionally foetal parts may be identified on ultrasound, in association with an abnormal placenta. In both CHM and PHM vascular flow abnormalities indicative of arteriovenous malformations, with or without endometrial encroachment, are frequently seen with modern colour power Doppler. The chest radiograph may be normal, or show evidence of tumour metastases.

Management

The primary treatment for molar pregnancy is prompt evacuation of the uterine contents using gentle suction dilation and curettage (D&C). Prostanoids to ripen a nulliparous cervix are not recommended as this may induce uterine contractions and trigger trophoblastic embolisation. The latter can be fatal and is probably also the explanation for why there is a higher risk of needing subsequent chemotherapy if medical or other surgical methods are used to evacuate the uterus.

Key practice point: Do not administer prostanoids to ripen the cervix prior to surgical evacuation in women with suspected molar pregnancy.

Registration with GTD centre – In the United Kingdom, all women diagnosed as having GTD are registered with one of three centres located in Dundee, Sheffield, and the Charing Cross Hospital in London, which together form the UK GTD national follow-up service. These patients and their gynaecologists then receive an information pack and the histological slides are requested for central review. All patients then send two-weekly blood and urine samples to one of the three centres for serial hCG estimations.

Serial hCG monitoring – In the majority of cases any residual molar tissue regresses and the hCG levels return to normal (≤ 4 IU/l). In PHM once the hCG is normal a single confirmatory normal value is all that is required before attempting a further pregnancy. The risk of missing disease is only 1:3,000. However, for CHM, the rate of fall of hCG after surgical uterine evacuation can predict the likelihood of subsequently developing a trophoblastic tumour. If the hCG has fallen to normal within 8 weeks of evacuation then marker follow-up for CHM is only required for 6 months from the date of evacuation. However, in women with CHM whose hCG levels are still elevated beyond 8 weeks from the date of evacuation, follow-up is currently continued until there are 6 months of normal values. This protocol results in only 1:1,400 women being missed with malignant change in their CHM.

The failure of hCG to normalise following molar evacuation heralds the development of GTN. A second suction evacuation of the uterus may be helpful in selected cases but should only be performed after consultation with a GTD centre as in most patients it will not prevent the need for chemotherapy. Moreover, each uterine evacuation carries a risk of uterine perforation, introducing infection and triggering major haemorrhage.

Chemotherapy for GTN

Overall, approximately 16% of CHMs and 0.5–1% of PHMs require chemotherapy. The indications for chemotherapy in patients with suspected GTN are shown in Box 15.1.

Box 15.1 Indications for treatment with chemotherapy in GTN

1. Plateaued or rising hCG value over 3 or 2 consecutive values, respectively
2. Histological evidence of choriocarcinoma
3. Evidence of metastases in brain, liver or gastrointestinal tract, or radiological opacities >2 cm on chest radiograph
4. Raised hCG 6 months after evacuation even if still falling
5. Bleeding requiring transfusion (UK specific)
6. Serum hCG >20,000 IU/l more than four weeks after evacuation, because of the risk of uterine perforation (UK specific)
7. Pulmonary, vulval or vaginal metastases unless hCG falling (no longer seen in isolation of other indications)

The first four indications are widely used by most centres and covered by International Federation of Gynecology and Obstetrics (FIGO) recommendations. However, the fourth recommendation has now been shown to be unnecessary as all patients with a raised but falling hCG level 6 months post molar evacuation will spontaneously normalise and this will usually happen within the following 6 months. The remaining recommendations are UK-specific. Approximately 1% of patients have significant bleeding requiring transfusion which interferes with normal life despite a falling hCG. Starting chemotherapy in such individuals helps

to prevent further blood loss. Approximately 2–5% of patients will have an hCG value >20,000 IU/l 4 weeks after evacuation of their mole or rising values in this range at an earlier stage. This is linked to an increased risk of GTN, uterine perforation or severe haemorrhage. These complications can be life-threatening and the risk can be reduced by starting chemotherapy. The final indication has not been seen by the authors in more than 20 years of practice in over 2,500 patients.

Chemotherapy Work-Up

- Bloods – routine bloods including full blood count, coagulation screen, group and save, urea, glucose, creatinine and electrolytes, liver function, thyroid function tests and viral screen for hepatitis and human immunodeficiency virus
- Pelvic ultrasound with Doppler (Figure 15.1) to determine the uterine volume and vascularity chest X-ray to look for pulmonary metastases.
- Brain imaging (CT or preferably MRI) – in high-risk disease or clinical suspicion of CNS involvement; pulmonary lesions on chest radiograph (CXR); or the patient's prognostic score predicts high-risk disease (see below). Subsequently, no intracranial metastases are identified, and cerebrospinal fluid (CSF) is obtained for hCG estimation (an hCG ratio of >1:60 CSF:blood indicates CNS involvement).

The information from these staging investigations is then used in the FIGO scoring system (Table 15.2) to determine the risk of disease becoming resistant to single-agent chemotherapy with either methotrexate or actinomycin D.

Chemotherapy Administration

Low-risk disease – About two-thirds of women who score low risk (<7 FIGO score) can expect to be cured with methotrexate alone. Methotrexate is given intramuscularly, alternating daily with oral folinic acid for 1 week followed by a week of rest prior to recommencing treatment. Chemotherapy shrinks the disease rapidly predisposing the patient to an increased risk of tumour haemorrhage which can be severe in about 1:50 cases. In addition, about 2% of patients experience mucosal ulceration, conjunctivitis and occasionally serositis. For these reasons, patients remain in hospital for the first week of treatment. Overall, methotrexate therapy is very well tolerated, does not induce alopecia and

Pre-treatment   Post-treatment

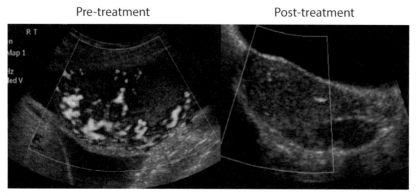

Figure 15.1 Pelvic ultrasound showing a large vascular GTT developed after a molar pregnancy before (left panel) and after (right panel) chemotherapy

Table 15.2 FIGO prognostic scoring system for GTN

Prognostic factor	Score[a]			
	0	1	2	4
Age (years)	<40	≥40	–	–
Antecedent pregnancy (AP)	Mole	Abortion	Term	–
Interval (end of AP to chemotherapy in months)	<4	4–6	7–13	>13
hCG (IU/l)	$<10^3$	10^3-10^4	10^4-10^5	$>10^5$
No. of metastases	0	1–4	5–8	>8
Site of metastases	Lung	Spleen, kidney	Gastrointestinal tract	Brain, liver
Largest tumour mass (cm)		3–5	>5	
Prior chemotherapy			Single drug	≥2 drugs

[a]The total score for a patient is obtained by adding the individual scores for each prognostic factor. Low risk, 0–6; high risk, ≥7.

can be completed at a local health centre. In about one third of women, the tumour becomes resistant to methotrexate and, if this occurs when the hCG is <300 IU/l, then most can be salvaged by switching to single-agent therapy with actinomycin D given intravenously daily for 5 days every 2 weeks. This treatment is sometimes used as a first-line agent in other countries and from nonrandomised data appears to be at least as effective as methotrexate. However, it is more toxic, inducing some alopecia, oral ulceration, nausea, vomiting and myelosuppression. If the hCG is >300 IU/l when resistance develops, then patients are switched to our multi-agent chemotherapy regimen used for high-risk disease.

High-risk disease – Patients scoring ≥7 FIGO score receive 'high-risk' intravenous combination chemotherapy comprising etoposide, methotrexate and actinomycin D (EMA) alternating weekly with cyclophosphamide and vincristine (CO). Acute side effects

include myelosuppression, alopecia, peripheral neuropathy and those associated with single-agent methotrexate therapy. This treatment requires an overnight stay in hospital every 2 weeks and most patients require granulocyte colony-stimulating factor injections to help maintain a sufficient neutrophil count and treatment intensity.

Treatment with either low- or high-risk regimens is continued until the hCG has been normal for 6 weeks. During this time the serum hCG is measured twice a week, so that the tumour response can be closely monitored and appropriate treatment changes made promptly (Figure 15.2).

Choriocarcinoma

Epidemiology, Origin and Pathology

The incidence of choriocarcinoma following term delivery without a history of CHM is approximately

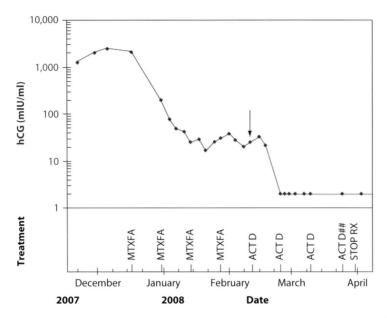

Figure 15.2 Graph of hCG in a patient with low-risk disease who was initially treated with methotrexate (MTX) and folinic acid (FA) but was subsequently changed to actinomycin D (ACTD; arrow) due the development of drug resistance, as indicated by the plateau in hCG levels. RX, treatment

1:50,000. Although choriocarcinoma can arise following any type of pregnancy, CHM is probably the most common antecedent, with an estimated 3% of CHMs developing into choriocarcinomas. In contrast to CHM there are no clear geographical trends in the incidence of choriocarcinoma, but the effect of age remains important. Choriocarcinoma is a highly malignant tumour, which appears as a soft, purple, largely haemorrhagic mass. Microscopically, it mimics the appearances of an early implanting blastocyst, with central cores of mononuclear cytotrophoblast surrounded by a rim of multinucleated syncytiotrophoblast and a distinct absence of chorionic villi. The surrounding areas are usually necrotic and haemorrhagic and tumour is frequently seen within venous sinuses. Genetic analysis frequently demonstrates multiple karyotype anomalies, but none as yet are specific for choriocarcinoma.

Clinical Presentation

Choriocarcinoma following an apparently normal pregnancy or non-molar abortion usually presents within a year of delivery. The presenting features may be similar to hydatidiform moles, with vaginal bleeding, abdominal pain, pelvic mass and symptoms due to a high serum hCG. However, one third of all patients with choriocarcinomas present without gynaecological features, and instead manifest symptoms and signs associated with metastases. Pulmonary, cerebral (Figure 15.3) and hepatic deposits are most frequent but any site may be involved, including the cauda equina and skin.

TIP
Lives can be saved by remembering to include choriocarcinoma in the differential diagnosis of metastatic malignancy presenting in a woman of childbearing age.

Investigations – All women with choriocarcinoma should have a CT whole body, MRI brain and pelvis all with contrast together with a Doppler ultrasound pelvis. Although these tumours are highly vascular, excision biopsy of a metastasis should be considered where it can be safely achieved. This not only enables histological confirmation of the diagnosis but also permits genetic analysis to prove the gestational nature of the tumour. Thus, if there are only maternal genes and no paternal genes present, the patient has a non-gestational tumour, e.g. an ovarian choriocarcinoma or more rarely an epithelial tumour which has

161

Pre-treatment
Post-treatment

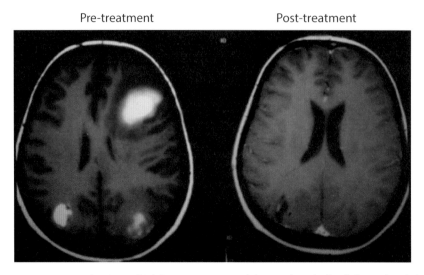

Figure 15.3 Magnetic resonance scan showing multiple brain metastases with haemorrhage before (left panel) and after CNS modified etoposide, methotrexate and actinomycin D/cyclophosphamide and vincristine (EMA/CO) chemotherapy (right panel) in an 18-year-old patient with choriocarcinoma

differentiated into choriocarcinoma. Frequently, however, biopsy is not possible and the diagnosis is made on the clinical history and other investigation findings. Fortunately, very recent data has shown that in some circumstances circulating free tumour DNA in patient blood can be used to distinguish gestational from non-gestational cancers.

Management – Patients are scored and treated as described for molar disease. Thus, a low-risk choriocarcinoma can be safely started on single-agent therapy which will be curative in approximately 40% of cases. Occasionally, the choriocarcinoma will have been completely resected as part of the initial investigations and such cases can be managed by observation and may avoid the need for chemotherapy altogether. While most high-risk choriocarcinomas can be successfully treated with EMA/CO, their management does require a little more consideration. Patients who present with very advanced disease in the lungs or with brain and/or liver metastasis and/or a FIGO score more than 12 should be considered as ultrahigh risk for both early death within the first 4 weeks of admission and/or late death from drug-resistant disease. These patients should receive gentle induction chemotherapy with low-dose etoposide and cisplatin every week until their condition permits normal dose chemotherapy which itself may need adjustment (see section below on management of specific complications of GTN).

Placental-Site and Epithelioid Trophoblastic Tumour

PSTT/ETT can develop following any type of pregnancy including term delivery, non-molar miscarriage, CHM and PHM. They may also be associated with, or develop after, atypical placenta site nodules so are no longer considered to be a benign condition. There are currently about 360 recorded cases of PSTT and <40 ETT in the literature and so estimates of their incidence are inaccurate. However, a UK-wide analysis of all PSTTs diagnosed up to 2007 has demonstrated that PSTTs comprise about 0.2% of all GTD in the United Kingdom and ETT is much less frequent. PSTT/ETTs are usually diploid, and may be biparental or androgenetic in origin but, if they follow a PHM, they are triploid. PSTT/ETT are the malignant equivalent of extravillous, interstitial implantation site-like trophoblast and form uterine lesions with less haemorrhage and necrosis, and lower hCG concentrations than does choriocarcinoma. ETT exhibits a distinctive hyalinisation pattern compared to PSTT. Both tumours usually spread by local infiltration, with distant metastasis occurring late via the lymphatics and blood. The behaviour of PSTT/ETT is thus quite different from other forms of GTN and they are often relatively chemoresistant. Consequently, the mainstay of treatment is hysterectomy when the disease is localised to the uterus. When metastatic disease is present, individual patients can respond and be apparently cured by multi-agent chemotherapy either alone or in combination with surgery. The key prognostic factors predicting outcome on multivariate analysis of both the United Kingdom and world data sets appears to be advanced stage and the interval between the antecedent-causative pregnancy and starting therapy. Thus, in our earlier 62-women series from the United Kingdom, 100% of the 13 women treated greater than 4 years following pregnancy died. In contrast, 98% (48/49) of those treated within 4 years survived. Consequently, new treatments are needed for patients who present more than 4 years out from their last known and likely causative pregnancy. Indeed, we have now introduced tandem high-dose chemotherapy with autologous peripheral stem cell support and early data from our latest analysis in 124 women suggest survival rates have improved for these poor risk patients but follow-up is still too short to be certain.

Management of Specific Complications of GTN

Haemorrhage – This usually responds to bed-rest and chemotherapy, along with adequate blood transfusion. However on occasion uterine packs, selective embolisation or laparotomy may be necessary; hysterectomy is rarely required.

Respiratory failure – This can be multifactorial due to parenchymal tumour deposits and/or tumour or clot embolisation. In the majority of patients respiratory failure can be adequately managed by increasing the inspired oxygen concentration and early chemotherapy. When embolism is suspected, the patient should also be anticoagulated with unfractionated heparin. The administration of dexamethasone (8 mg once every eight hours) may prevent deterioration associated with tumour necrosis and oedema. If possible, mechanical ventilation should be avoided as the high airway pressures can trigger fatal pulmonary haemorrhage from metastases.

Cerebral and liver metastasis – Following low-dose induction etoposide and cisplatin death may occur secondary to haemorrhage and/or oedema. To avoid this risk, women with overt cerebral metastases require a modified EMA-CO regime, in which the methotrexate in the EMA is increased to achieve CNS penetration and intrathecal methotrexate is given after each CO assuming it is safe to do so. Patients will require high-dose dexamethasone to reduce cerebral oedema and may need emergency neurosurgery to remove bleeding metastasis and/or raise a skull flap to relieve intracranial pressure. Patients with lung metastases are at high risk of brain metastases, and therefore these will also receive three prophylactic doses of intrathecal methotrexate. This is given at the start of courses of low-risk treatment, or with the CO element of high-risk therapy. Patients presenting with liver metastases, with or without brain metastases, have a particularly poor prognosis, and after treatment with low-dose induction of etoposide and cisplatin seem to achieve high cure rates if managed with modified EMA on an alternative weekly basis, in which the day 2 of etoposide and actinomycin D are omitted (EP-EMA).

Drug-resistant disease – In the case of low-risk patients treated with single-agent methotrexate, resistance can be overcome in all cases by changing to the high-risk EMA-CO regimen, or single-agent actinomycin D in some patients. Patients who become resistant to EMA-CO may be salvaged with EP-EMA, or with paclitaxel and cisplatin alternating every 2 weeks with paclitaxel and etoposide (TP-TE). The latter regimen is much less toxic than EP-EMA, but a randomised trial is required to determine whether it is as effective. Selected patients may benefit from high-dose chemotherapy with autologous bone marrow or peripheral stem cell rescue. A number of other agents such as pemetrexed and germ cell tumour regimens are also active but their 3 weekly cycles may allow too much tumour regrowth to be as effective. New anti-cancer agents such as checkpoint immunotherapies and anti-endoglin antibodies with or without bevacizumab (Avastin) are also under evaluation in GTN. A strategy of debulking surgery in an attempt to excise drug-resistant tissue, followed by chemotherapy for residual disease, may also salvage some patients. In this context tumour localisation may be aided by whole-body CT or MRI, and by novel imaging techniques such as fluorine-18-fluoro-2-deoxy-D-glucose positron-emission tomography (PET)-CT/MRI.

Twin pregnancies – Twin pregnancies comprising a CHM and healthy co-twin are rare and raise concerns for both the mother and her unborn baby's health. Fortunately, our latest analysis in over 90 cases has supported our earlier analysis in 77 affected women showing that early termination of pregnancy does not reduce the risk of needing chemotherapy, and that continuing such pregnancies are associated with an approximately 50% chance of a healthy baby. Moreover, although there is a slightly increased risk of pre-eclampsia/toxaemia, this can be managed in the usual way and there were no cases of uterine perforation or maternal deaths. Therefore, it seems reasonable to allow women to continue their pregnancy if this is what they desire.

Infantile choriocarcinoma – This is an extremely rare condition with about 60 reported cases worldwide. Usually the disease presents in the baby within weeks of delivery and is not always coexistent in the mother. The outcome in these infants is often very poor, possibly due to delayed diagnosis, although some have been saved with chemotherapy. We currently advise checking the urine hCG on at least one occasion in all infants born to mothers with choriocarcinoma and conversely to check the mother's hCG in infants presenting with choriocarcinoma.

Patient Follow-Up and Prognosis

On completion of their chemotherapy, women are advised to:

- avoid pregnancy for 1 year;
- use adequate sun-block to minimise the effect of therapy-induced skin photosensitivity; and
- remain on hCG follow-up for life to confirm that their disease is in remission.

In addition, women with PSTT/ETT may be reviewed regularly in clinic with MRI imaging of the abdomen and pelvis for at least 4 years after the completion of treatment, as hCG is not as reliable a marker in PSTT.

Approximately 4% of low- and high-risk patients will relapse. In our experience all low-risk patients have been salvaged with further chemotherapy (EMA/CO or alternative regimens) and this group has a close to 100% cure rate. Following the introduction of low-dose etoposide and cisplatin induction chemotherapy to eliminate early deaths, and a genetics service to exclude non-gestational disease, high-risk patients have an overall 94% 5-year survival rate. Deaths in this group now usually occur due to drug resistance in very advanced disease. It is hoped that the introduction of new salvage therapies will eliminate the last few women who die. These new therapies will also hopefully impact positively on the poor risk PSTT/ETT patient cohort.

Low-risk chemotherapy with methotrexate is not associated with any long-term toxicity. However,

combination agent chemotherapy such as EMA/CO therapy may expedite the menopause by an average of 3 years. Fortunately, with more than 30,000 patient years of follow-up this chemotherapy does not appear to increase the overall risk of second cancers provided the duration of treatment is kept to within 6 months. Importantly, low- or high-risk treatment does not affect fertility or increase rates of foetal abnormality in subsequent pregnancies.

Summary of Gestational Trophoblastic Disease

GTD forms a spectrum of illness, from the borderline malignancy of hydatidiform moles to the highly aggressive behaviour of choriocarcinoma, which were fatal in the past. However, in the past 55 years we have learnt much about the biology, pathology and natural history of GTD. Furthermore, accurate diagnostic and monitoring methods have been developed together with effective treatment regimens. As a result, the management of GTD is one of the modern success stories in oncology. Today, with an integrated approach to management, nearly all women are cured from their trophoblastic tumours, with their fertility intact.

Further Reading

Brown J, Friedlander M, Backes FJ et al. Gynecologic Cancer Intergroup (GCIG) consensus review for ovarian germ cell tumours. *Int J Gynecol Cancer.* 2014 November; 24(9 Suppl 3): S48–54.

Fotopoulou C, Savvatis K, Braicu EI et al. Adult granulosa cell tumours of the ovary: tumour dissemination pattern at primary and recurrent situation, surgical outcome. *Gynecol Oncol.* 2010 November; 119(2): 285–90. doi: 10.1016/j.ygyno.2010.06.031. Epub 2010 Jul 15.

Shah SP, Köbel M, Senz J et al. Mutation of FOXL2 in granulosa-cell tumours of the ovary. *N Engl J Med.* 2009 June 25; 360(26): 2719–29. doi: 10.1056/NEJMoa0902542. Epub 2009 Jun 10.

Seckl MJ, Sebire NJ, Berkowitz R. Gestational trophoblastic disease. *Lancet.* 2010 August 28; 376(9742): 717–29.

Seckl MJ, Sebire NJ, Fisher RA et al. ESMO Guidelines Working Group Gestational trophoblastic disease: ESMO Clinical Practice Guidelines for diagnosis, treatment and follow-up. *Ann Oncol.* 2013 October; 24(Suppl 6): vi39–50.

Chapter 16

Palliative Care

Sara Booth and Mary McGregor

Introduction

Palliative and supportive care is integral to providing excellent care of patients with any life-threatening or life-altering disease. Patients and families now expect that they will receive attention that centres on their human as well as their medical needs. They expect that the emotional and psychological aspects of care will be recognised and addressed.

Palliative care, similar to comprehensive cancer care, is always a team effort as one clinician cannot answer the complex needs of someone at a time of crisis such as life-threatening illness.

The absolute ideal is to have palliative care specialists or a member of the gynae-oncology team with a special interest in palliative care, available from the inception of treatment, whatever the individual's prognosis. Some people will require minimal input from palliative care, while some will benefit from intense periods of input from palliative care specialists at specific points in their treatment. Others will require no direct intervention at all from specialist care. Additionally, some may benefit from discussion with the specialist palliative care team, although they will not need to be seen by them.

There is some confusion over the definitions of the terms palliative care, supportive care and end-of-life or terminal care, although they are widely used. This uncertainty can lead clinicians to wonder whether their patient is 'ready for palliative care' or 'at that stage yet'. Patients themselves often share this confusion, and this may be particularly problematic in young people who are highly symptomatic but want to go on having life-prolonging treatment. They may fear that accepting palliative care is accepting psychological defeat leading to inevitable death and the end of their 'active treatment'. This is a great shame as effective symptom control, alleviation of psychosocial distress and other problems (related to, but not necessarily caused by, the direct effects of the tumour) will provide a better quality of life, and possibly an improved prognosis.

Standard Definitions

Palliative Care

It was first defined by the WHO (1967) as 'the *active, total* care of patients when the disease is no longer curable and the prognosis is short'. The complete opposite is 'there is nothing we can do'. It involves meticulous symptom control as well as care of the patient and their family.

The WHO expanded this definition in 2012 to specify that palliative care aims to:

- Provide relief from pain and other distressing symptoms
- Neither hasten nor postpone death
- Integrate the psychological and spiritual aspects of palliative care
- Offer a support system to help patients live as actively as possible until death
- Use a team approach to address the needs of patients and their families including bereavement counselling, if indicated
- Enhance quality of life (this may also positively influence the course of the illness).

This definition also makes it clear that palliative care is applicable *early* in the course of the illness, in conjunction with other therapies that are intended to prolong life such as chemotherapy and radiation therapy, and includes those investigations needed to better understand and manage distressing clinical complications.

Supportive Care

It is defined by the National Cancer Institute (NCI) as 'Care given to improve the quality of life of patients who have a serious or life-threatening disease. The goal of supportive care is to prevent or treat as early as possible the symptoms of a disease; side effects caused by treatment of a disease; and psychological, social and spiritual problems related to a disease or its treatment'.

The NCI then uses the terms palliative care and symptom control as synonymous with this, which is not generally agreed. Everyone in a gynae-oncology team will be providing supportive care and everyone needs to be trained to be able to provide *general palliative care* (see Table 16.1). Palliative care meshes with supportive care. It includes those aspects of care that are additional to 'disease management' but essential if patients are to have the best chance of engaging with their treatment and obtaining the best outcome from it.

End-of-Life Care/Terminal Care

This is the care of people in their last weeks, days or hours of life when death is inevitable. Confusingly, the 'UK End-of-Life Care Strategy' considers the end-of-life phase to be the last year of life.

It is better not to be too concerned about these terms but to give patients the care they require whatever the stage of their illness. Anyone with severe symptoms, even if they have a curable illness and are receiving intensive treatment, may be helped by seeing a specialist palliative care clinician.

At the end of life, routine symptom control combined with a caring supportive attitude to the patient and their family is the remit of all hospital and primary care teams whatever their specialty. This will often offer the best option for patients who would prefer to be cared for by their gynae-oncology team who have known them for some years and in whom they have great trust.

Principles of Symptom Control

Whatever the symptom, the most effective treatment will be found most quickly if a systematic approach is taken to diagnosis and therapy. The general principles of symptom management in palliative care are set as follows:

- Make the best diagnosis possible of the cause(s) and ensure that the patient understands what treatment you are going to follow.
- Symptoms are often multifactorial in advanced disease, and symptom control often involves incremental improvement in a number of causative factors to bring about significant relief. A good history of the problem is essential.
- The patient's wishes and her prognosis are central to decisions about appropriate investigation and treatment. For example, it is usually not in the patient's best interests to treat refractory malignant hypercalcaemia repeatedly with intravenous bisphosphonates or perform major surgery in someone with widely disseminated disease, nor is it right to pressurise someone into a course of action which they are unwilling to undertake, even if it is the acknowledged 'next step' on a care pathway or protocol.
- Document your findings with a quantitative assessment of symptom severity to allow treatment responses to be monitored. Complex regimens, built up incrementally, are often necessary to manage symptoms in advanced disease.
- Recognise and manage any precipitating or exacerbating factors, such as fear, fever, underlying metabolic problems and other symptoms (e.g. pain exacerbating dyspnoea). Helping patients and families manage their anxiety associated with life-threatening diseases is always essential and will be more successful if anxiety is acknowledged and addressed at diagnosis.
- Assess and reassess the effectiveness of your symptom control regimen regularly. If the disease is advancing, treatment strategies may need frequent revision.
- Ensure that you have explained and discussed your assessment and plans with the patient in detail so that her goals and ideas guide management. When management of symptoms is difficult, this becomes even more important. The patient needs to understand and agree with your reasoning and choice of the next possible line of treatment available if initial approaches fail.
- Be prepared to re-evaluate your initial diagnoses if your management plan is not working.
- Be aware of the psychosocial context of the symptom. For example, vulval pain has different connotations and meaning from arm pain. Malodorous, fungating wounds have an immense impact on a woman's social existence and view of herself.
- Get specialist help earlier, rather than later, when a symptom or situation is not improving. For difficult symptoms or psychosocial distress contact the palliative care team.
- Make sure everyone involved in the patient's care keeps communicating so that the patient and her family do not get mixed messages or confusing or even contradictory picture of what is going

Table 16.1 Outline of generalist and specialist care aspects of problems typical of those occurring in women with gynaecological malignancies[a]

Problem	Generalist aspects	Specialist aspects
Pain	Recognising that the patients have pain that requires treatment, and ability to take a full pain history. Knowledge of common pain syndromes in gynaecological malignancy. Begin pain therapy using WHO pain ladder for guidance. Recognising when the pain needs immediate specialist help or when it develops into a specialist palliative care problem, e.g. neuropathic features not responding to initial therapy.	Will take detailed pain history and initiate treatment with specialist analgesic drugs and/or combinations of drugs and/or doses outside guidelines, e.g. anticonvulsants, 2nd/3rd line opioids, antidepressants. Recognition of when referral needed to specialist pain services, e.g. regional pain blockade.
Breathlessness	Eliciting that patient has breathlessness causing them distress or difficulty. Recognising if end of life very near (days or weeks). Taking basic breathlessness history and rating with basic outcome measures. Initiating basic therapy by encouraging activity and use of hand-held fan. Referring/discussing with specialist palliative care services.	Recognise and elicit the wide-ranging effects of respiratory symptoms and their impact on patient and family. Initiation of complex interventions encompassing a range of non-pharmacological and pharmacological interventions.
Distressed patient or family	Ability to listen, elicit worries, fears and concerns about illness or its wider effects on patient and their family. Ability to reassure honestly (i.e. about what and where possible), giving appropriate information as the patient wishes or needs to know. Ability to show empathetic concern. Recognising when specialist psychological, psychiatric, psychosexual or palliative care is needed and helping patient to accept this help.	Helping a patient who is persistently depressed/anxious/worried despite extra support and in partnership with other specialist colleagues. Recognising and initiating treatment (pharmacological and non-pharmacological) for depression and anxiety as necessary within multidisciplinary team or with colleagues in psychological care specialties.
Bowel obstruction	Skilled in predicting when partial bowel obstruction (PBO) is likely to occur and in diagnosing on clinical grounds. With seniority, ability to recognise when surgery may be a helpful option or the possibility of a venting gastrostomy. Initiating medical therapy for symptomatic relief of PBO and giving helpful basic dietary advice and information on prognosis.	Able to diagnose PBO and instigate treatment when it has not responded to initial therapy. Take part in discussions when surgery is possible but probably not appropriate or where patient or gynae-oncology team is concerned. Managing refractory obstruction (including faeculant vomiting, giving advice regarding venting gastrostomies frozen pelvis). Supporting complex, or highly symptomatic end-of-life care on ward or in community.
Extensive and/or malodorous discharge and/or malodorous or distressing wounds or tumours	Ability to anticipate when difficult wound is likely to develop as complication of advanced disease or treatment. Provide initial counselling and advice regarding treatment (e.g. diagnosis and treatment of infection). Recognising when specialist help is necessary (e.g. specialist nursing, plastic surgery and radiotherapy). If experienced or undertaken specialist training may cross-over with specialist palliative care team input.	Recognising when specialist palliative care nursing assessment and treatment may be needed. Hospices may offer frequent dressing of complex wounds for patients, particularly for frail patients living alone. Arranging specialist psychological help if needed for patient and family. Hospices may also have access to specialist treatments that may help disguise/reduce odour and may offer symptom control admissions for particularly complex wounds or end-of-life care, when this cannot be managed at home. Can also help to train the family how to manage the wound or odour at home and provide ongoing support. Offer help with topical analgesia and management of friable or bleeding wounds.
Chronic haemorrhage	Ability to anticipate when difficult bleeding may be a problem and, with seniority, develop the knowledge and ability to use surgical options, other local treatments (e.g. radiotherapy) and supportive care (e.g. transfusions).	Stepping in when local treatment and supportive care (e.g. transfusions) no longer helpful, although early referral important for general assessment if cause not treatable. Helping with end-of-life care issues.

[a]The generalist palliative care problems are those which every clinician needs to be able to manage.

on. Make sure everyone (patient, family and professionals) understands and agrees to the goals of care.

- Women may find it more acceptable to be referred to specialist palliative care services for a difficult symptom than for psychosocial support. If patients find palliative care helpful they may then be more willing to use their skills for other needs.

At any stage of illness if the patient or family are greatly distressed or symptomatic, or if young children or other dependants are involved, do not hesitate to contact palliative care for advice, if not referral, even if you consider the patient is still on a treatment regimen leading to cure.

> **TIP**
> Symptoms are often multifactorial and taking a good history is essential.

Managing Pain

Pain remains the most feared symptom for many patients. It is frequently under-diagnosed and under-treated for many reasons, including patients' reluctance to complain and failure of healthcare professionals to ask about pain and treat it systematically. It is estimated that if the WHO analgesic pain ladder is used to guide therapy, then approximately 80% of pain accompanying advanced cancer could be controlled on simple, oral, drug treatment alone (Figure 16.1).

To control the patient's pain optimally, the following approach is recommended:

1. A full pain history is essential for excellent management. Many patients have more than one pain and a good history is needed for each one. If someone is in severe pain when you first see them, a complete pain history for each pain may have to wait until the patient is more comfortable. Obtain enough initial information (previous notes, GP notes and letters, online records and from family if the patient is too distressed) to be able to make a 'good enough' diagnosis of pain. Start appropriate analgesics – then complete the pain history as soon as possible so that other necessary investigations can be carried out.
2. Establish the causes of the pain using special investigations where needed. An increase in pain may often be due to disease progression, requiring both oncological treatment and more analgesia.
3. Assess and record the initial level of pain to facilitate continuing assessment of the effect of the therapeutic strategy adopted. For example, a short numerical rating scale (NRS) may be used.
4. Start treatment using the WHO pain ladder at the step nearest the patient's pain level, e.g. if the patient is in severe pain start with strong analgesic and non-steroidal anti-inflammatory drugs (NSAIDs) in combination. That is, start at step 3. The oral route is preferable, with transdermal or subcutaneous routes as first alternatives. However, when someone is in severe pain then a subcutaneous or intravenous route, provide rapid relief. Intestinal absorption is even slower when someone is stressed and useless when someone is vomiting.
5. Morphine is still the strong opioid of first choice. Change to transdermal fentanyl (particularly, if constipation or sedation are the major problems), or oxycodone, hydromorphone or buprenorphine if adverse effects cannot be managed. Discuss this with your palliative care service as switching between opioids can be complex. When initiating pain control it is usual to use short-acting/immediate release morphine (with a half-life of approximately 3–4 hours), switching to modified-release preparations for greater convenience when the pain is controlled, and the 24-hour dose requirements can be calculated. The patient will continue to need an immediate release/short-acting preparation, to take as required for breakthrough pain episodes.
6. Reassess treatment effectiveness at least daily when titrating analgesics, and more frequently if the pain is severe.
7. Adjust the regimen to control pain for example by increasing the dose of your chosen drug, adding co-analgesics, adjuvants changing analgesics or route of drug administration when necessary.
8. Anticipate, prevent or, where necessary, treat adverse effects of the analgesics prescribed, e.g. anti-emetics. If pain does not respond to standard treatment or is recognised as difficult pain, e.g. neuropathic pain, bone pain or where there is extreme psychological distress, get immediate help from the specialist palliative care team. The patient with uncontrolled pain will lose

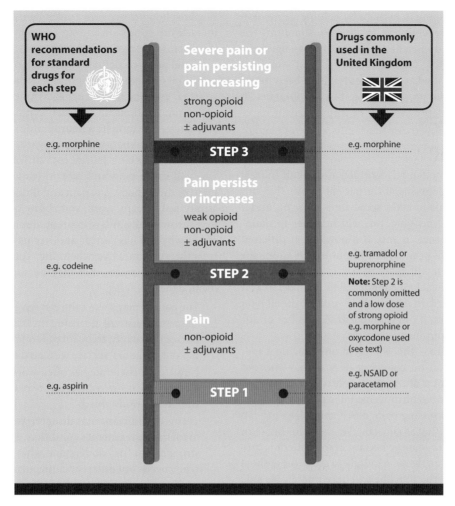

Figure 16.1 WHO – Pain ladder. It is frequent now not to use a separate drug for step 2 but to use a lower dose of your strong opioid of choice, e.g. low dose morphine or lower dose oxycodone. Codeine is a very unpleasant drug for many people with a high incidence of nausea, vomiting, sedation and constipation and rather than starting with a weak opioid, it may be better and easier to titrate moving on to the stronger opioids first.

confidence as well as suffer enormously and may develop intractable pain. Intervene early to get the best pain relief.

9. Make direct contact with the GP, district nurse team, nursing home or other community team where the patient is discharged to discuss the diagnosis, to inform them fully of any drugs or treatments being used, their indications and how they need to be continued and any follow-up arrangements that have been planned.

10. Ensure all other teams involved in the community or hospital are aware of what the patient has been instructed to do. For example, which team they

have been advised to contact in case of pain crisis or other emergency.

11. Give pain relief for chronic pain regularly and not 'as required'. Prescribe any necessary adjuvant drugs to prevent known adverse effects at the time of analgesic prescription (e.g. anti-emetics) and prescribe 'as required' doses of the regular analgesic to be taken for 'breakthrough' pain.

12. If the patient suffers from regular breakthrough pain, prescribe an increased dose of the regular analgesic.

Adjuvants – These are drugs that are not marketed as, or considered to be, pain medication but may be helpful in managing it, perhaps by helping depression or anxiety or preventing or treating constipation. The word is also used interchangeably with co-analgesics.

Co-analgesics – These are drugs that were not originally described as analgesics but have been found to have analgesic properties, e.g. bisphosphonates in bone pain, antidepressants for neuropathic pain.

Difficult Pains

Some pains can often be identified as difficult to treat at the time of diagnosis. If the patient knows that this sort of pain usually takes some time to bring under the best control possible, this will help her to maintain her confidence in you. If a number of different approaches have been tried without explanation, she may think that it will never be controlled and anxiety will be added to lack of confidence to the pain mix. If the drugs prescribed initially have only a limited pain killing effect then it can lead to fear. A number of difficult pains are outlined as follows.

Incident pain – This is present only during a specific activity (e.g. on coughing or walking) and not when the patient is at rest. Pain control is satisfactory most of the time, but on movement the patient has overwhelmingly distressing pain, albeit short-lived. It can be as incapacitating as constant, severe pain. Incident pain is difficult to manage because if the patient is prescribed enough analgesic regularly to cover these short but severe exacerbations she will have intolerable side effects, as she will be relatively overdosed most of the time. Investigate for a specific cause and refer to the specialist palliative care team early. A pain block, surgery for a pathological fracture, radiotherapy, rapid-release analgesic such as a fentanyl lozenge or intranasal preparation may be needed for pain control.

Neuropathic pain – It is caused by damage to the central or peripheral nervous system. It is usually only partially responsive to opioids and co-analgesics such as anticonvulsants and antidepressants. It may be helped by additional non-pharmacological techniques such as transcutaneous electrical nerve stimulations (TENS) or other specialist interventions. Neuropathic pain can usually be identified on history and clinical diagnosis; however, specialist investigations may also help, e.g. nerve invasion identified on MRI.

Bone pain – It is very common in malignancy, and often quite resistant to treatment even when adequate doses of radiotherapy, opioids and NSAIDs are used. Addition of co-analgesics may be helpful.

Bisphosphonates are now routinely used in the treatment of this condition and surgery may be appropriate if pathological fracture is anticipated.

Total pain – is defined as the suffering that encompasses all of a person's physical, psychological, social, spiritual and practical struggles. This definition articulates the relationship between physical and mental suffering. For example, a neuropathic lower limb pain resulting in weakness will also cause disability, will stop the patient working (social loss of role and income) and will cause pain and anxiety about the advancement of the tumour. The pain and illness will affect her family, self-esteem, work, and ability to be a parent. It may throw up all kinds of existential spiritual questions about why she has cancer and her psychological distress then becomes overwhelming. Total pain is rarely obvious, but features that may be suggestive of this include the following:

- The patient may seem calm but have behaviours suggesting distress, e.g. using the buzzer to call the nurses frequently, frequent presentations to A&E or the 'out-of-hours' service with no discernible cause.
- New treatment strategies often work well for a short time initially then severe pain returns, sometimes re-doubled.
- Teams of clinicians may disagree about how to manage the patient's condition, each feeling strongly that they understand what the patient really needs but different clinicians may be understanding different things from the patient.

It is easy for healthcare professionals to feel 'angry' with patients (although often difficult to acknowledge), when pain does not respond to carefully thought out treatment. It is crucial to get help from specialist palliative care, as soon as you perceive that the pain is not going to be managed by first line treatments or if there is significant underlying psychological distress, apparent or not.

> **TIP**
> Pain medication for chronic pain is given regularly to get best relief.

Nausea and Vomiting

First distinguish whether the patient has:

- Nausea *or* vomiting, or
- Nausea *and* vomiting

and which of these is most distressing.

Partial Bowel Obstruction (Avoid the Term Sub-acute Obstruction)

This is a very common problem in gynaecological malignancy, particularly in advanced ovarian carcinoma. This may be caused by tumour occluding or narrowing the bowel, which may or may not be resectable depending on the patient's wishes, stage of illness, the presence of other metastatic disease and the patient's general condition. Multiple tumours or extensive adhesions cannot be resected. Partial obstruction is often due to dysmotility, as a result of infiltration of the nerve plexuses innervating the bowel by small-volume disease, which may not always be visible on scans, leading to gut dysfunction.

Features in the history indicating obstruction include:

- Vomiting after meals, sometimes hours after, producing undigested food
- Colicky abdominal pain
- Borborygmi audible by patient
- Infrequent stools or diarrhoea
- Abdominal distension with ascites or tumour
- Constipation with failure to pass flatus.

The general principles of management are:

- Stop all prokinetic drugs (e.g. metoclopramide).
- Use only faecal softeners rather than stimulants.
- Advise a low residue diet, i.e. one without much fibre and refer the patient to a specialist dietician.
- Consider surgical options if there is a single site of occlusion and the patient is willing to have surgery. These patients usually present with abdominal distension. This is in contrast to those with 'stuck down' bowel, as this cannot distend. The decision to proceed with surgery requires a highly individualised approach.

Palliative care clinicians rarely advise 'drip and suck' with nasogastric tube and intravenous fluids, preferring:

- A continuous subcutaneous infusion (CSCI), via syringe driver, of an anti-emetic (e.g. cyclizine or haloperidol) with analgesia (e.g. diamorphine or morphine)
- Adding hyoscine butylbromide (60–120 mg, buscopan) to CSCI if colicky pain is present
- A separate CSCI of octreotide (or other somatostatin analogue) was once routinely used (evidence is being reviewed currently) to reduce the volume of bowel secretions if there is insufficient response to hyoscine butylbromide (indicated by continuing large volume vomits or nasogastric aspirates).

Nasogastric tubes are needed when there is upper gastrointestinal obstruction. Metoclopramide can be prescribed if there is certainty that there is dysmotility and no physical blockage, but it should be stopped immediately if the patient develops colicky pain or an exacerbation of her symptoms. Sometimes patients who recover quickly on a CSCI are sent home from the hospital, but they return with obstruction within a few days. It is often better to discharge the patient on the CSCI on medium to longer term; she will be able to take fluids and light foods and this may protect her from frequent readmissions which are demoralising. It is much more important for the patient to be at home with well-controlled symptoms with on or off a CSCI.

Other causes of nausea and vomiting include:

- Adverse effects of drugs, e.g. NSAIDS, opioids, antibiotics (particularly metronidazole)
- Hypercalcaemia
- 'Squashed stomach' from large intra-abdominal masses
- Raised intracranial pressures
- Massive ascites.

This list is not exhaustive and careful diagnosis is required. Several causes for nausea and vomiting may co-exist.

Anti-emetics

Prescribe anti-emetics systematically. They act in different ways. Prescribe on the basis of known or likely diagnoses and manage exacerbating factors such as fear, anxiety and fever.

A typical prescription for an opioid-naive patient with PBO would be: 5 mg haloperidol (anti-emetic), 10 mg diamorphine if in pain (titrated from individual's analgesics need orally, this would be equivalent to 30 mg oral morphine daily dose) and 120 mg hyoscine butyl bromide (reduces abdominal secretions and colic) in 24 hours by CSCI.

1. Start with your 'best guess' anti-emetic, e.g. haloperidol , given subcutaneously as an 'as needed' dose.
2. Review after one hour to assess impact.
3. If the patient is improved start a CSCI with haloperidol +/– other appropriate drugs.

Commonly used anti-emetics in palliative care

It is essential to check all drugs before use as guidance changes rapidly.

Consult unit and hospital policies and pharmacy information where unsure.

Local palliative care policies and BNF have specific guidance for palliative care or Palliative Care Formulary (online).

Check contra-indications and cross-reactivity between drugs.

Prokinetic Anti-emetics

For dysmotility – functional bowel obstruction (peristaltic failure), gastritis, gastric stasis, 'opioid bowel'

e.g. metoclopramide 10 mg PO tds, or used SC by continuous subcutaneous infusion (CSCI) from a syringe driver.

Anti-emetics Acting Principally in Chemoreceptor Trigger Zone (CTZ) in the CNS also Called 'Centrally Acting'

For most biochemical causes of nausea and vomiting from drugs (e.g. morphine, chemotherapy) or metabolic abnormalities, e.g. renal failure or hypercalcaemia.

Haloperidol 1.5–3.0 mg PO stat and then bd/tds and 2.5–10 mg/24 hours CSCI.

Metoclopramide has some central activity.

Antispasmodic and Antisecretory Anti-emetics

Used for bowel colic/pain control and reduce bowel secretions.

Hyoscine butyl bromide 20 mg SC stat. 60–120 mg in 24 hours CSCI (higher doses on specialist advice only): can be used 20 mg up to qds PRN.

Anti-emetic Acting Principally in the Vomiting Centre in CNS

For raised intracranial pressure (with dexamethasone), motion sickness, and in partial bowel obstruction (PBO).

Cyclizine 50 mg PO stat and then bd to qds or 50 mg SC stat and 150 mg/24 hours CSCI.

Anti-emetic Acting on Serotonin Receptors

For use when bowel cells damaged and releasing serotonin, e.g. chemotherapy, abdominal radiotherapy or direct bowel injury.

Ondansetron 4–8 mg PO/SC bd-tds, 8–16 mg over 24 hours in CSCI.

Broad-Spectrum Anti-emetics Working in a Number of Ways

Used when other anti-emetics/combinations of anti-emetics have failed, may be useful in bowel obstruction.

Levomepromazine 6.0–12.5 mg PO/SC stat, then up to qds PRN. NB long-acting drug therefore no need to use in CSCI, but sometimes more convenient

Dexamethasone

Rarely used on its own though sometimes in specialist hands, when others fail, specifically for raised ICP, and synergistic effect with $5HT_3$ antagonists, most commonly used orally. Discuss with specialist before use outside standard chemotherapy regimens due to wide range of adverse effects.

Abbreviations

PRN, as needed; PO, orally; SC, subcutaneously; CSCI, continuous subcutaneous infusion; qds, four times daily; bd, twice a day; tds, three times a day; and stat, immediately.

4. Prescribe second-line anti-emetic (with a different mode of action) on PRN section of chart.
5. Move to or add second-line drug if first approach is ineffective.

Constipation

Bowel habit is very individual, so it is the change (passage of stools uncomfortable, infrequent or incomplete) rather than the absolute frequency of stool that characterises constipation. It is often an embarrassing subject for many people so direct questions on bowel symptoms are very important, especially in women who have pelvic disease, which is a risk factor in itself. Even if their disease is not apparently extensive, infiltration of the neural plexuses can cause dysmotility.

Severe constipation is both painful and disabling as patients are unable to enjoy anything because their bowel problems overwhelm everything else and they may spend hours in the lavatory. This can lead to social isolation and extreme anxiety in both the patient and her family. Constipation can mimic bowel obstruction or herald it. It can cause rectal and abdominal pain as well as nausea and vomiting.

Prevention:

- Encourage patients to remain mobile and to keep up an adequate fluid intake. This is also helpful for general fitness and preventing DVT.
- Start laxatives when starting opioids, and adjust the dose to keep the bowel habit comfortable (which may be very different from patient's previous habit). The dose range can be very wide. Patients on opioids need a bowel stimulant (e.g. senna) and a stool softener (such as Movicol, docusate). Co-danthrusate is a combination of softener and stimulant in one preparation but only available for short-term use or for patients with life-limiting illness. There are few trials and therefore a poor evidence base for the management of constipation in people with advanced disease.
- Mitigate the effects of a number of risks factors; for example, if the patient is taking a 5HT3 antagonist and receives a drug with an anti-cholinergic effect (e.g. amitriptyline or cyclizine) and an opioid, she will be at risk of severe constipation. The drug therapy combined with the effects of the disease may contribute to the risk of developing PBO, particularly if she is immobile and dehydrated. Think about drug combinations; other drugs that

can precipitate constipation are carboplatin, iron, some antacids and calcium channel blockers.

- Many patients dislike opening their bowels on a ward on a commode; it is inhibiting. It is important to offer the patient the chance to go to the lavatory in a wheelchair.
- Anticipate (to prevent) constipation in all patients with neurological problems affecting the pelvis.

Local pain will inhibit bowel activity, so actively prevent constipation in those with perineal wounds or scars, anal fissures, haemorrhoids or other incidental bowel conditions. Treat metabolic and electrolyte abnormalities such as hypercalcaemia.

Diagnosis

The diagnosis of constipation is made on history and examination, including careful abdominal examination and digital rectal examinations. Special investigations are rarely necessary but if faecal impaction develops, patients may have faecal leakage or diarrhoea (leaking from above the faeces which have become impacted in the rectum). A plain abdominal film will reveal faecal loading. If a CT/MRI is carried out for disease staging, evaluate the images for signs of developing constipation.

Treatment

All preventative measures outlined above should be commenced and will need to be continued once the immediate problem has been solved. Faecal impaction requires oral pharmacological treatment to prevent continuation of the problem. Immediate measures to manage an established problem include:

- Glycerol suppositories (softening also stimulates peristaltic action).
- Retention enemas used over-night (arachis/peanut oil) contraindicated in peanut allergy – be certain to ask specifically.
- Stimulant suppositories such as bisacodyl; these have a more marked peristaltic action.
- Manual removal of faeces (under sedation and analgesia) and/or high enemas. These techniques are rarely needed particularly with modern care. Specialist advice should be sought from gastrointestinal specialists and/or palliative care physicians before considering them.

  Oral treatment:
- If routine laxative treatment, e.g. co-danthrusate is not working consider macrogol 1–3 sachets

daily until the bowel starts to work. Patients with life-limiting illness may remain on macrogol for a longer term, provided electrolytes are monitored regularly.

Hypercalcaemia

Hypercalcaemia (corrected calcium > 2.6 mmol/L) can be a life-threatening condition and is linked to poor prognosis even when it responds to treatment. It affects approximately 30% of patients in advanced malignancies, especially those with bone metastases. Symptoms are multi-system and include renal impairment, confusion, constipation and increased pain.

Diagnosis

Although hypercalcaemia is not particularly common in gynaecological malignancies, it should be suspected in any patients with new-onset, refractory or progressive:

- Nausea
- Vomiting
- Fatigue
- Constipation
- Confusion
- Sedation.

Treatment

The treatment of choice is intravenous bisphosphonate therapy and intravenous rehydration, with the dose directed by the calcium level and renal function. Symptomatic hypercalcaemia (particularly with levels of Ca^{2+} above 3.0 mmol/L) requires very active rehydration with normal 0.9% saline and potassium. The monoclonal antibody denosumab is now being used as a second-line treatment for hypercalcaemia resistant to bisphosphonates. It has a longer duration of action than bisphosphonates but does cause more symptomatic hypocalcaemia.

Cautions

The dose of bisphosphonate must be reduced in patients with renal failure.

Given hypercalcaemia is associated with advanced cancer and is, in itself, a poor prognostic feature, careful consideration should be given as to whether attempts to reverse it are appropriate. Many symptoms of hypercalcaemia can also be present in the dying phase, and aggressive fluid resuscitation and intravenous treatments may not be in the patient's best interests. If possible, and especially when the hypercalcaemia is recurrent, sensitive discussions should be held with the patient and their carers about their future wishes. This enables the patient to participate fully and thus avoid having to make an 'emergency decision'. At such times the patient will certainly be less well and a doctor or even clinical team may have to carry out the difficult discussion about 'not treating' aggressively.

Complex Fungating and Malodorous Wounds

Complex, fungating and malodorous wounds occur when tumour erodes through the skin or other epithelial layers, and thus prevents healing. It is always more common in advanced disease because of the other factors that prevent healing such as poor performance status, reduced nutrition (often signalled by low albumin) and anaemia. This problem can be devastating for a woman and her family and is frequently difficult to manage. It is important to be honest and advise the patient that the wound may never fully heal nor the smell go away completely, while being clear that you are committed to continue working on the problem. Explain that, as a team, you will be making cumulative, small improvements to make life as good as possible for the woman living with, potentially pain, discomfort, discharge and an unpleasant smell. It is important to make, and be seen to make, every effort to mitigate the effects of an unhealed, and particularly a smelly, wound. The distress for the individual, the impact on her psychological state and relationships with friends and family can overwhelm the last few months of her life with shame and fear, leaving painful memories for survivors.

In gynaecological oncology, the wound may be deep, inaccessible and affect the sexual organs or structures associated with excretion. The problem may seem so personal that the patient may even conceal its extent until it becomes obvious to everyone because of the smell.

The general principles of management are listed below:

- Support the woman, finding out her goals for care, approach the smell in a matter of fact way; being very 'sympathetic' in an emotional way without offering practical help may only make her feel the problem is even more obvious than it seems already.
- Use sophisticated imaging to investigate the extent of the wound; biopsy may be necessary to distinguish between tumour, radiation necrosis or infection. Often it is more important to investigate the aetiology of the wound than to try and repair it, which is likely to be difficult. Knowing the aetiology may help with management.
- Local treatment for cancer, such as radiotherapy, may help to palliate the wound by reducing bleeding or slowing disease progression.
- Try to isolate the organism, but treat infection without waiting for the results. Whenever there is a smell, infection is always present. Topical metronidazole may be helpful as well as intravenous or oral metronidazole.
- Careful wound management is essential (irrigation). The patient may need pain relief to do this successfully and it will often need to be repeated over a long period of time. Many women will die with their wounds unhealed.
- Frequent dressings, several times a day, are sometimes required. Patients may dread dressing changes, which may inhibit those carrying out the dressings if they are very painful.
- Do use opioids, where needed, before dressing changes. Specialist advice may be helpful. Short-acting opioids, such as fentanyl lozenges which act as rapidly as intravenous opioids, may be helpful. However, tolerance may well develop so seek help. Sometimes women find nitrous oxide/oxygen mix (Entonox) effective.
- Seek expert help in wound dressing. Most hospitals now have specialist nurses who are expert in tissue viability/wound healing, or a plastic surgery opinion may be helpful. A huge range of dressings are now available and options are constantly evolving. Stoma bags can be helpful to contain exudates and tampons can be used on internal wounds.
- A consultation with an interventional radiologist may be beneficial, particularly if there is frequent haemorrhage or any uncertainty about the origins of the wound.
- If the patient is at home and requires frequent changing of complex dressings, this may be possible at a hospice and may help to build trust for end-of-life care.

Breathlessness

Breathlessness is one of the most common symptoms of advanced cancer of all aetiologies. It can occur even when patients have no known disease affecting the chest. Breathlessness is not easy to palliate but it is easy to overlook its presence. It is rarely volunteered unless asked about directly, and yet causes very severe distress not only to the sufferer, but also to those closest to them. This is the symptom that may be most helped by specialist advice from the palliative care service.

Ensure that reversible conditions are adequately and appropriately treated, for example pleural effusions, pulmonary emboli and infections. Help the patient to start the simple initial measures unless the patient is severely breathless or very distressed. These women need specialist palliative care urgently and probably the initiation of oral opioids to manage the symptom effectively.

Anxiety and Depression

A supportive approach to cancer management from the time of diagnosis will both help to reduce unnecessary anxiety and ensure that contact with the hospital will not exacerbate the fear inevitable with the diagnosis. If left unaddressed, one anxiety may compound others and patients can spiral into a state of high arousal: it is important to build and support the natural resilience that most women possess rather than unwillingly exacerbating fear. Most patients stress that a lack of communication about their disease and its treatment is one of the major difficulties they face.

She needs time and a supportive, easily accessible oncology team to replenish her personal resources and find a new balance.

Practical Issues

When you take a history, as well as accumulating the necessary facts, demonstrate empathy with the feelings in the story she is telling. Acknowledge what the patient is saying. For example, the patient may say, 'I kept going back to the doctor but they could not find anything wrong'.

So you might say:

- 'that must have been very frustrating for you'.
- 'It was probably initially reassuring for you, but then it must have got a bit frightening'.

These are all empathetic statements and, depending on the patient's response, will help you form an idea of their mental state without letting feelings escalate out of control.

A major cause of anxiety for patients is not being heard. This can be helped by summarising what you hear as you take the history. For example:

- 'Can I just recap to make sure I have understood you correctly: you have had some nausea throughout your treatment in spite of a number of different drugs being tried'.
- 'Metoclopramide has been the most helpful drug so far'.

Ideally, when it feels that a clinical situation is becoming rapidly worse, try to make a space to listen to, rather than talk to, the patient (plus anyone else they choose for support) to reach an understanding of what she feels are the major problems. Before such a meeting in clinic or on the ward:

- Make sure that you are as up to date as possible on what has been going on (and that the multidisciplinary team's decision on treatment is clear) read the notes and talk to the GP beforehand so you understand any longstanding psychosocial issues.
- Start with an open-ended question such as 'Can you tell me what is the worst thing for you at the moment?' The difficulties which emerge may not be the ones that you are qualified to manage (e.g. difficult pain, family strife, financial problems) but the patient will have been heard and you can start referrals or discussion which may help.
- Do not forget to screen for depression at different points in the disease course – approximately 45% of patients with cancer have significant anxiety or depression at some point in the illness. The most common points are at diagnosis and when metastatic disease is first diagnosed.
- Look out for low mood, self-blame and someone who looks sad and burdened.
- Ask 'What gives you pleasure at the moment?' If there is nothing, the patient is likely to have anhedonia and maybe clinically depressed.
- Depression is treatable and anxiety can be helped. Talk to the GP, the liaison psychiatry and the palliative care service to organise a treatment plan. Medication, social support and psychological

treatments (as well as exercise and activity, see below) can all improve psychological problems.

Psychosocial Issues in Advanced Disease

Anger and distress are common feelings in advanced disease, and sometimes this becomes enmeshed with feelings about care, leading to conflicts. Mistakes and poor communication can occur, in even exceptional departments.

When you recognise that psychological issues (such as distress, anxiety, depression) may be exacerbating the physical aspects of a symptom, take a detailed symptom history. Such 'therapeutic listening' may be helpful in itself. Explain at the outset that it may take some time for symptoms to come under control. This should prevent the patient from feeling that everything is going wrong, or that the team do not know what they are doing. When symptoms are difficult to control, then reassess for their aetiology and reassure the patient that you have not given up on understanding or managing their symptoms. Specialist psychological care may be required for some patients, and they should be advised that such care is an important part of general medical care and very important in cancer medicine.

Carer Distress and Exhaustion

Carers often experience distress when they are supporting a loved one through cancer. If this becomes extreme it is likely to affect the medical outcomes of the patient and it may be at the root of unhelpful (for the patient) emergency admissions. Too little help is given to carers and it is important to do what you can for them. A focus on the carer's individual needs and health is important. Help may come from carer support services, primary care or specialist psychological support. Carers should be encouraged to look after their own needs and will also benefit from the 'five ways to wellbeing'. Carer exhaustion should be anticipated and prevented. This can be achieved by early control of patient's symptoms, advising the carer of resources and support available, and advising them of the importance of looking after their own physical and mental well-being.

The situation becomes difficult if the carer is clearly distressed, and needs help but will not accept it. A distressed carer is unlikely to be able to offer support to an unwell patient.

Patient Feels Alienated from Doctors or the Clinical System

For reasons related to their care, their distress about their illness or any other aspect of life, the patient may feel totally disenchanted or even distrustful of their care. A psychologically informed approach is particularly important in these circumstances, i.e. thinking about the impact of the illness on the woman's life and self as a whole and that it is important to engage with her emotions and ideas about the illness. The most important initial response is to empathise with the patient. You may offer to liaise with their healthcare team or urge her to talk directly with the team about her difficulties.

Anger at Failure of Therapeutic Interventions

Whenever patients or carers are angry when interventions fail, listen to them, and do not try to damp down the anger, but do not encourage it. Demonstrate that you empathise with their situation. Try to understand who is the angriest, the patient or carer, and therefore who needs more attention in this area. Ensure you have clear, consistent plans. Seek help from specialist teams, such as the palliative care team. Remember that anger at the lack of success of therapeutic interventions can often be anger about the illness itself.

If Relationships Break Down

Treating women with gynaecological malignancy is often highly charged and may take place over a protracted period of time, with many ups and downs. Even with the very best treatment, there may be periods when the patient seems to lose trust in her team. It is very important at times like this not to back away from contact with that individual and their family but actually to engage more strongly. It is particularly important not to feel defensive or to take the patient's dissatisfaction personally. This may be the time to bring in extra help both for your team so they can continue to function effectively – often distressed patients lead to distressed and split teams. Such teams then become ineffective for the patient.

If relationships with the patient or family are coming under strain, even if symptom control does not lie at its root, it may be very helpful to involve the specialist palliative care team to help with distress and difficulty.

It is also important to be prepared to offer, rather than wait to be asked for, a second specialist gynaecological opinion perhaps with another consultant, or at another cancer centre.

Improving General Health and Well-Being of Women Living with Gynaecological Malignancy 'Supportive Care'

Many women now live with gynaecological malignancy for years. A simple focus on their disease can leave some with constant feelings of anxiety and distress, albeit low level. If women do not get access to clinicians who can take a psychologically informed approach from the time of diagnosis, even those who are cured can go on to live more limited lives. There are some simple, health-promoting measures that everyone can use, even those whose lives are going to end in the near future. The 'five ways to wellbeing' is a simple, evidence-based framework aimed at everyone, to give the best chance of achieving the best psychological and physical health. It is applicable in both health and disease, so carers and patients can use it together, taking an individual path.

The 'five ways to wellbeing' are (Figure 16.2):

- Connect – with people to develop social relationships
- Be active – physically, in whatever way is possible
- Take notice – be mindful and be more aware of the present moment
- Keep learning – learning new skills can increase confidence and optimism
- Give to others – acts of kindness, time or volunteering (for example taking part in research).

Entering the End-of-Life Phase

When patients enter the stage where everyone acknowledges that cure is no longer possible, even if they have months, or possibly years to live, it is important to find out the choices the individual would like to make about their future care. Research shows that patients expect health care professionals to start discussions about treatment options. Introducing the idea of palliative

Connect ...
Connect with the people around you. With family, friends, colleagues and neighbours. At home, work, school or in your local community. Think of these as the cornerstones of your life and invest time in developing them. Building these connections will support and enrich you every day.

Be active ...
Go for a walk or run. Step outside. Cycle, play a game, garden, dance. Exercising makes you feel good. Most importantly, discover a physical activity you enjoy and one that suits your level of mobility and fitness.

Take notice ...
Be curious. Catch sight of the beautiful. Remark on the unusual. Notice the changing seasons. Savour the moment, whether you are walking to work, eating lunch or talking to friends. Be aware of the world around you and what you are feeling. Reflecting on your experiences will help you appreciate what matters to you.

Keep learning ...
Try something new. Rediscover an old interest. Sign up for that course. Take on a different responsibility at work. Fix a bike. Learn to play an instrument or how to cook your favourite food. Set a challenge you will enjoy achieving. Learning new things will make you more confident as well as being fun.

Give ...
Do something nice for a friend, or a stranger. Thank someone. Smile. Volunteer your time. Join a community group. Look out, as well as in. Seeing yourself, and your happiness, linked to the wider community can be incredibly rewarding and creates connections with the people around you.

Figure 16.2 Five ways to wellbeing

care early, perhaps by an initial consultation with the hospital support team, may help women feel in control of their contact with these services, and not feel they are associated with certain death imminently, but with improving quality of life.

Younger women may want to continue to embark on chemotherapy knowing it has small chance of success, certainly of cure and even of palliation.

If the tumour does not respond to treatment, you will need to gently raise the possibility of treatment not working and find out what she would want if this were to happen. Would she like to continue treatment however small the chance of cure? Would her main focus be on improving quality of life? Find out about her experience of treatment thus far. Focusing on excellent symptom control is likely to extend rather than shorten life. Introducing the concept of palliation makes discussion about stopping chemotherapy or surgery or finding out where the patient would like to be cared for when she is dying, a gradually evolving one rather than a sudden occurrence. This can be very frightening and can shut any sort of conversation down for some time. The patient then may die in hospital when she would have preferred to be at home. She may continue to have treatment that the gynae-oncologist does not feel helps and may even harm her. Support communication in the family by seeing the patient and her 'significant other' together (always with her consent) particularly when the illness enters a palliative or end-of-life phase, putting the emphasis on the quality of life rather than focusing solely on disease management at any personal cost.

Key points

- Palliative care is a multidisciplinary approach to improving quality of life in patients with life-limiting and life-altering disease, particularly those with life-limiting disease.
- It addresses the medical, psychological, social and spiritual aspects of illness with equal vigour.
- Symptom control is an important part of helping patients with gynaecological malignancy to achieve the best outcomes.

- Psychological status is becoming recognised as a predictor of recovery from physical illness and successful medical outcomes.
- Gynaecological malignancy presents particularly complex psychosocial and psychosexual issues for patients: these need to be addressed actively.
- Specialist palliative care services are there to help: telephone advice is always available.

Further Reading

Akhmatova A, Saliev T, Allan IU et al. Comprehensive review of topical odor-controlling treatment options for chronic wounds. *J Wound Ostomy Continence Nurs.* 2016; 43(6): 598–609.

MacDonald M, Palmer J. Palliative care in gynaecological oncology. *Obstet Gynaecol Reprod Med.* 2014; 24(12): 365–70.

Metz T, Klein C, Uebach B et al. Fungating wounds – multidimensional challenge in palliative care. *Breast Care* 2011; 6: 21–4.

Noble S, Prout H, Nelson A. Patients' Experiences of LIving with CANcer: the PELICAN study. *Patient Prefer Adherence* 2015; 9: 337–45.

O'Brien C. Malignant wounds. Managing odour *Can Med J.* 2012; 58: 272–4.

Quill TE, Abernethy A. Generalist plus specialist palliative care – creating a more sustainable model *N Engl J Med.* 2013; 368(13): 1173–5.

The 'Five Ways to Wellbeing Cards' were designed by the New Economics Foundation and are free to use without copyright infringement.

Chapter 1

Living with Cancer

Andy Nordin and Manas Chakrabarti

Living with Gynaecological Cancer

As oncological treatments for gynaecological malig-nancy have improved over the decades, associated with improved 1-, 3- and 5-year survival and a reduction in mortality, there has been an increased focus on the impact of disease and treatment modalities on quality of life (QOL). QOL is now a standard secondary out-come measure for all oncology clinical trials, recognis-ing the balance of quantity and quality of the lives of cancer sufferers.

A number of clinical and research domains have evolved in response to this challenge, and it is impor-tant for specialist trainees in gynaecology to under-stand the basic principles, research fields and the medico-political agenda that have evolved during the past few decades.

In the United Kingdom, the Independent Cancer Taskforce was established in January 2015 by NHS England to develop a 5-year strategy for cancer ser-vices. The political importance of 'living with cancer' domain is evidenced by the Taskforce report (July 2015), detailing 96 recommendations for cancer ser-vices in England. One of the principal objectives for the NHS was to transform its approach to support people living with and beyond cancer, with a recommendation for national rollout of stratified follow-up pathways and the Recovery Package. The Recovery Package is an initiative championed by the cancer charity Macmillan, with the following four main interventions:

1. Holistic Needs Assessment and Care Planning
2. Treatment Summary
3. Cancer Care Review
4. Health and Well-being Events.

These elements form a part of an overall support and self-management package for people affected by cancer – physical activity as part of a healthy lifestyle, managing consequences of treatment, information, financial and work support. The Taskforce also rec-ommended that a national QOL measure should be developed to ensure that the NHS is able to monitor and learn lessons to support people better in living well after the completion of treatment.

In this chapter we will cover the following topics:

- QOL as a multidimensional construct
- Measurement of QOL in clinical trials
- Cancer survivorship
- Patient reported outcome measures (PROMS) and survivorship
- Holistic care
- Sexuality
- Lymphoedema
- Fertility issues after gynaecological cancer treatment.

QOL as a Multidimensional Construct

Cancer and its treatment have a major impact on all facets of patients' lives, frequently leading to difficul-ties in fulfilling family roles, the ability to work or par-ticipating in common social activities. The underlying factors are complex and multiple, relating to impact on symptoms of disease, side effects and morbidity during treatment, long-term late effects from disease and treatment side effects, and complex psychosocial and psychosexual issues. QOL is a complex multi-dimensional concept in medicine. The World Health Organisation (WHO) Quality of Life Group defined it as 'individuals' perception of their position in life in the context of the culture and value systems in which they live and in relation to their goals, expectations, standards and concerns. It is a broad-ranging con-cept affected in a complex way by the persons' physi-cal health, psychological state, level of independence, social relationships and their relationship to salient features of their environment'.

Traditionally, the focus of cancer therapy related to tumour response and survival, but over recent decades QOL has become a major determinant of efficacy of can-cer management. The focus on QOL in cancer care over recent decades has been the driving force behind innovations in medical treatments including chemotherapy, radiation oncology and surgery. Gynaecological oncology is no exception, with a recent history of innovative treatment modalities with the motivation to improve quality-of-life outcomes as prominent as their aim for effective cancer treatment and improved survival. Targeted cancer therapies with lower morbidity than conventional chemotherapy are the focus of extensive research. Intensity modulated radiation therapy (IMRT) was developed to reduce morbidity from radiotherapy, and minimal access and robotic surgery achieve effective oncological outcomes with markedly reduced surgical morbidity and complications. QOL issues of gynaecological malignancy patients are compounded with complexities relating to body image, fertility and sexuality. There is also a recently emerging focus on QOL impacts of screening and genetic testing for prevention or early diagnosis of gynaecological cancers, with reference to patients and their family members.

> **TIP**
> QOL is a complex multidimensional concept in medicine.

Measurement of QOL in Clinical Trials

To compare the effects of different cancer treatments on QOL in clinical trials, it is essential to be able to objectively assess QOL as a trial endpoint. Since QOL assessment requires capture of information from the patient perspective, patient self-reporting is the standard approach for assessment. Based on this theoretical framework, researchers have developed reliable and valid instruments. However, currently there is no uniformly accepted gold standard for QOL measurement.

In cancer care, the need for QOL assessment led to a new discipline of quantitative psychology instrument (questionnaire) development for cancer clinical trials. In Europe, this has been led by the European Organization for Research in Treatment of Cancer (EORTC) Quality of Life Group, established in 1980. There are now more than 15 European countries, including others, such as Australia, Canada, the United States, Taiwan, Brazil and India, represented within the group. The group incorporates a broad range of professionals, including oncologists, radiotherapists, surgeons, psychiatrists, psychologists, palliative care specialists, nurses, social workers, epidemiologists and

research methodologists. The instrument development protocol includes a systematic literature review, qualitative research with patients and healthcare professionals and a structured psychometric analysis of a provisional questionnaire before validation testing.

The core questionnaire, known as the EORTC QLQ-C30, is the most commonly utilised standard QOL measure employed in pharmacological, radiotherapy and surgical cancer clinical trials. In addition to two general questions about QOL and general health, the QLQ-C30 includes a further 28 questions pertaining to functioning and specific symptoms commonly expressed by many cancer patients, including lethargy, shortness of breath, nausea, vomiting and constipation. Patients report their responses on a simple 4-point Likert scale, with responses ranging from 'not at all' to 'very much'. It has been demonstrated to be a valid and reliable self-administered tool in a range of languages and cultural settings.

Additional questionnaires have been developed that are specific to a disease, population, function or condition. This is because general tools lack the sensitivity to demonstrate potentially clinically important QOL issues relating to specific types of cancers and cancer treatments. The EORTC Quality of Life Group therefore embarked on a programme of module development, with disease-specific modules developed under the same guidelines to assess QOL issues identified by patients and healthcare professionals as relevant for specific tumour sites. The gynaecological group of the EORTC Quality of Life Group has subsequently developed modules for ovarian cancer (OV28), cervix cancer (CX24) and uterine cancer (EN24), and the group is about to embark on the phase 4 validation study for a vulval cancer-specific module. Each self-administered module is designed to be completed in conjunction with the core questionnaire (QLQ-C30), and additionally covers issues such as pain, bleeding, bowel and bladder dysfunction, lymphoedema, body image and sexuality which are relevant to women undergoing treatment for these gynaecological malignancies.

A similar process of instrument development has run concurrently in the United States in the 'FACT' (Functional Assessment of Cancer Therapy) group, now known as 'FACIT' (Functional Assessment of Chronic Illness Therapy). This group has also developed core and disease-specific questionnaires. While EORTC instruments are most commonly utilised in European and international studies, FACT instruments are particularly common in North American research.

While QOL is generally a secondary endpoint in clinical trials, there are several types of trials where QOL assessments are a relevant primary endpoint. These include trials in which a new treatment is expected to have only a small impact on clinical endpoints such as survival, cure or response, and equivalence trials where the disease course in both arms is expected to be similar but the QOL benefits or morbidity are expected to be different. In trials of palliative treatments, specifically intended to improve QOL or symptom control in end of life care, QOL is almost always the primary endpoint. For patients with advanced or recurrent disease, shorter instruments are appropriate as these minimise the burden of self-reporting. The EORTC QLQ-C15-PAL, a 15-item 'core questionnaire' for palliative care, was specifically developed for this purpose.

It is important to recognise that the EORTC and FACT instruments were developed for use in clinical trials, generally comparing two different treatment modalities for QOL differences. There is a move towards validation of these tools for use in clinical practice, but unless formal validation studies are conducted within a specific clinical cohort, caution should be used in implementing these instruments for any purpose outside the clinical trial setting.

Cancer Survivorship

Macmillan Cancer Support is a UK charity who works to improve the lives of cancer-affected patients. Their definition of a cancer survivor is anyone who is living with, or after, a cancer diagnosis. It embraces a holistic definition, covering the physical, psychosocial and economic issues of cancer, from the time of diagnosis until the end of life. It focuses on the health and life of a person with cancer beyond the diagnosis and treatment phases. Survivorship includes issues related to the ability to get health care and follow-up treatment, late effects of treatment, cancer recurrence, and QOL. Family members, friends and caregivers are also part of the survivorship experience.

The survivorship pathway starts at the point of diagnosis. The holistic and all-encompassing nature means that multiple aspects of peoples' lives need to be addressed within the survivorship umbrella, including work, finance, personal relationships and managing pain and fatigue. Survivorship also includes making positive lifestyle changes, such as promotion of a healthy diet and physical activity.

In the United Kingdom, Macmillan and the National Cancer Intelligence Network (NCIN) performed a detailed analysis of 85,000 patients diagnosed with cancer in 2004, incorporating data in the National Cancer Data Repository (NCDR) with inpatient Hospital Episode Statistics (HES) data. These data sources were used to map patients' long-term journeys from cancer diagnoses through to a set of clinically defined and meaningful outcomes, defining a 'survivorship outcome framework'. The cancers included in the analysis were breast, lung, prostate and central nervous system tumours, but unfortunately gynaecological cancers have yet to benefit from this analysis. Notwithstanding, the work has provided an extremely useful model on which to analyse cancer survivorship pathways, and is equally relevant to all gynaecological malignancies.

In the simplest construct, cancers fall into one of three groups. A proportion of cancers progress very quickly, with patients succumbing to the disease within a short period of time. This group includes the 31% of epithelial ovarian cancer patients who die within 12 months of diagnosis. Another group comprises patients who present with curable disease, and undergo effective curative treatment without disease relapse. In between these two, there is a heterogeneous group of cancer patients who have persistent disease or experience remission and relapse, some of whom will eventually succumb to the disease and many of whom will experience cancer as a chronic illness with ongoing disease and treatment-related morbidity.

The Macmillan/NCIN simplified survivorship outcome framework takes this concept a step further, outlining a series of survivorship pathways which designate all cancer patients into one of the eight distinct groups. The model applies a consistent set of four principles across all cancers to describe the length and complexity of survival:

1. Survival is the overwhelming priority in cancer.
2. Early in survivorship, the cancer itself is the priority.
3. Later in survivorship, morbidities are more impactful.
4. Wherever possible, it is important to describe factors that may have a bearing on QOL.

To plot the pathway for an individual cancer patient, it is essential to identify whether there are any cancer complications (including metastases and disease recurrence), and whether the patient has other morbidities,

Table 17.1 Macmillan/NCIN simplified survivorship outcome framework (used with permission)

Identifying the simplified survivorship outcomes groups			
A	**B**	**C**	**D**
Survival	*Cancer complications*	*Other inpatient morbidities*	*No other inpatient morbidities*
Limited	Group 1 • 0–12 months • Limited survival		
	Group 2 • 1–5 years • More aggressive complications and recurrence	Group 3 • 1–7 years • Patient with survival limited by other morbidities	Group 4 • 1–7 years • Limited intervention
Moderate	Group 5 • 5–7 years • Less aggressive complications and recurrence		
Ongoing	Group 6 • 7+ years • Cancer as a chronic disease	Group 7 • 7+ years • Living with or beyond cancer with other morbidities	Group 8 • 7+ years • Living beyond cancer

either at the time of diagnosis or developing later. This model is illustrated in Table 17.1. It defined survivorship pathways into eight distinct groups, which covered the full spectrum of survivorship over a 7-year period of the study:

1. Aggressive disease, limited survival 0–12 months
2. Cancer complications, limited survival 1–5 years
3. More aggressive cancer complications/recurrence, limited survival 1–7 years
4. Patients with survival limited by other morbidities, survival 1–7 years
5. Cancer complications, moderate survival 5–7 years
6. Less aggressive cancer complications/recurrence: living with cancer as a chronic disease, ongoing survival 7+ years
7. Living beyond cancer with other morbidities (may include late effects of cancer treatment), survival 7+ years
8. Living beyond cancer, no recurrence or cancer complications, no other significant morbidities, survival 7+ years.

An assessment of the proportion of patients with each gynaecological cancer falling into these survivorship cohorts in the future will aid effective concentration of resources appropriately for each tumour site.

The UK NHS National Cancer Survivorship Initiative (2010)

This sets out a framework for survivorship in five steps:

1. Information and support from the point of diagnosis
2. Promoting recovery
3. Sustaining recovery
4. Managing the consequences of treatment
5. Supporting people with active and advanced disease.

It recognised that the decisions taken about treatment options may impact upon QOL long after the completion of treatment. Therefore, clinical teams should offer patients support in making the decisions that best reflect their individual priorities.

The Cancer Recovery Package

In 2015 the Independent Cancer Taskforce published a strategy for achieving world-class outcomes for England 2015–2020. Among the recommendations, was the implementation of the 'Cancer Recovery Package' for all cancer survivors. This includes four main interventions:

1. Holistic Needs Assessment and Care Planning
2. A Treatment Summary
3. Cancer Care Review
4. Health and Well-being Events (a patient education and support event).

The cornerstone of the Cancer Recovery Package is the Holistic Needs Assessment (HNA). This is a simple questionnaire filled in by cancer patients as soon as possible after diagnosis, and at key stages on their cancer pathway. It allows them to highlight the most important issues at that time, and can inform the development of a care and support plan with their clinical nurse specialist (CNS) or key worker. The HNA ensures that people's physical, practical, emotional, spiritual and social needs are met in a timely and appropriate way, and that resources are targeted to those who need them most.

Evidence has shown providing effective individual HNA, and care and support planning can contribute to better identification of patient's concerns. It also enables early intervention and diagnosis of side effects or consequences of treatment.

A person's holistic needs are likely to change at key points in their cancer journey, signifying different priorities and needs at the time of diagnosis compared to the end of treatment. It is recommended that the information gathered from an HNA can be shared with the multidisciplinary team (MDT) and GP, to improve management and care. Such data could also be used to influence service developments and the commissioning of future services.

PROMS and Survivorship

By definition, any questionnaire that is completed by patients and seeks to document their thoughts, views, feelings, well-being or experience is a PROM. As such, the HNA is an example of a PROM in routine clinical practice in the United Kingdom, which is principally focused at improving care and support for the individual patient.

On a service level basis, patient's well-being is an important outcome measure in addition to mortality and survival, and may be a valid assessment to discriminate between service providers and assess quality of care. The NHS Cancer Patient Experience Survey has been designed to monitor national progress on cancer care, to provide information to drive local quality improvements, to assist commissioners and providers of cancer care, and to inform the work of the various charities and stakeholder groups supporting cancer patients. The NHS administers this survey on a regular basis. However, it is largely restricted to an evaluation of the service from a user perspective.

There are currently no validated PROMS for use in cancer follow-up in a gynaecological oncology survivorship population. Survivorship questionnaires must recognise that it is a much broader concept than QOL and encompasses all aspects of an individual's life and experience, including the health-related QOL issues but also incorporating social roles and functioning, relationships, sexuality, fertility, social and financial security. Many of these issues will be generic and relate to many different cancer types, but some are disease-specific. Therefore, sensitive PROM questionnaires are required to capture these important issues. In the United Kingdom, Public Health England and NHS England, in collaboration with the British Gynaecological Cancer Society, conducted a series of PROMS pilot studies for gynaecological cancers. The impact of the diagnosis of gynaecological cancer and late effects of treatments such as radiotherapy, chemotherapy and surgery were reflected in the findings of these pilot studies. Respondents reported issues such as anxiety and depression, impact on body image, urinary and sexual problems. For example, cervical cancer patients reported difficulties concerning body image (47%), sexual matters (38%), domestic chores (35%), finances (33%), communicating with those closest to them (31%) along with feelings of isolation (41%). It should be stressed that normative data do not exist for non-cancer survivors against which these data can be benchmarked. Three quarters of respondents, all treated between 1 and 5 years previously, said that they either agreed or strongly agreed with the statement 'I have fears about my cancer coming back'. Patients from all three disease groups also frequently reported that they had experienced a lack of good information and advice during and after completion of treatment.

The Independent Cancer Taskforce recommended the use of PROMs to create a national metric for QOL for people living with and beyond cancer. The metric should be suitable for use at various levels of the system, including by commissioners and providers. The UK Gynaecological Oncology PROMS Pilot demonstrated that it is feasible to administer a postal self-completed questionnaire to women who have previously been treated for gynaecological cancer, with satisfactory levels of acceptability and response. However, such a detailed questionnaire has limited utility in a routine clinical setting, and an abridged user-friendly gynaecological cancer PROM is required for incorporation into routine clinical practice. Work is ongoing as a collaboration between quality-of-life researchers, Macmillan and NHS England, to identify a select group of highly informative and sensitive items to assess issues affecting well-being for cancer survivors. Administration would be necessary on a user-friendly platform, providing contemporaneous data available not only to healthcare administrators but to clinicians and their teams. Potentially these data could be used to modernise cancer follow-up, with PROMS data identifying patients with symptoms of disease recurrence or late effects of treatment who require formal face-to-face assessment.

Holistic Care

Holistic medicine has been defined as 'the art and science of healing that addresses the whole person – body, mind, and spirit'. It recognises that healing of disease encompasses various complex, interrelated, non-linear cause and effect producing factors such as social, psychological and spiritual needs, aiming to achieve optimal health and wellness. This definition echoes the concept of 'health' published by the WHO.

The concept of holistic care has now become incorporated into cancer services in the NHS in a formalised process, namely the HNA. However, the concept should extend beyond a patient self-reported questionnaire and interaction with her CNS. The MDT has the potential to be a powerful tool in providing holistic care and maximising clinical effectiveness. This has been underlined by The NHS Cancer Plan and The Policy Frameworks for Commissioning Cancer Services. The MDT not only encompasses the so-called core medical members (gynaecological oncologists, clinical oncologists, medical oncologists, histopathologists, cytologists and radiologists) but also the representatives from local palliative care services, surgical and oncology nurses, CNSs and indirectly patient group representatives.

Spirituality is an important aspect in gynaecological cancer, like any chronic or life-threatening disease. Patient's spirituality is an important component of QOL, and increasingly patients desire that their physicians discuss spirituality during their medical assessments. Recognising patients' spiritual values help them maintain a sense of human coherence. For patients and family who may not understand technical aspects of their diagnosis and treatment, religion can provide an important internal locus of control. However, understanding the sense of spirituality can be incongruous

between patients and doctors. In a study to reveal the role of faith in decision-making in cancer treatment, it was concluded while patients ranked faith in God second only to advice of doctors, oncologists ranked it as least important in decision-making. Studies specifically involving gynaecological cancer patients showed religious commitment was an important factor in coping with disease, optimising family support and achieving a more significant improvement in social activities after treatment.

TIP
Holistic care is an integral part of cancer services.

Sexuality

Various physical, psychological and social effects resulting from diagnosis and treatment of cancer can impact on a person's sexuality. Sexuality involves multiple aspects including the sexual response cycle, body image, sexual relationships and a person's sexual role, and as such is a complex concept. Sexual health (SH) is defined by the WHO as a state of physical, emotional, mental and social well-being relating to sexuality, and is not merely the absence of disease, dysfunction or infirmity. Sexual dysfunction, in contrast, is more specifically defined as dysfunction of one of the four phases of the sexual response cycle, or pain during intercourse. In 2014, the National Cancer Institute at the National Institutes of Health in the United States published data revealing that 40–100% of persons diagnosed with cancer experience some form of sexual dysfunction. Diminished sexual desire and painful intercourse are common issues of sexual dysfunction among cancer patients.

For gynaecological cancer survivors, sexuality is a heterogeneous experience which varies throughout different stages of their lives. For many women, sexual satisfaction equates with the expression of intimacy and sensuality above coital aspects. Intimacy can be considered a process in which one person expresses important self-relevant feelings and information to another and, as a result of the other's response, comes to feel understood, validated, and cared for. Following a cancer diagnosis, intimacy can decline in association with a reduction in sexual activity, or become an alternative to sexual activity. Sometimes increased intimacy as a result of a cancer diagnosis may lead to increases in sexual activity.

In cancer patients, the impact on sexuality not only persists during the treatment phase, but also frequently extends into the follow-up period, influencing survivorship. Some evidence suggests increasing sexual morbidity after completion of cancer treatment, as time from completion of treatment increases, negatively influencing QOL. In one study, 78% of female patients reported a decline in their sexual activity after cancer, as did 76% of males.

In order to comprehensively understand and adequately determine the impact of cancer on a patient's SH, it is crucial to conceptualise SH as a multidimensional construct. There is a need for validated, cross-cultural, site-specific PROMS, applicable to female and male cancer patients, which can help in research and shaping patient care. Existing instruments mainly focus on physical sexual functioning, neglecting psychosexual and socio-behavioural issues. The most widely utilised sexual function and satisfaction questionnaire for cancer patients is the United States National Institutes of Health (NIH) PROMIS® questionnaire, but this instrument lacks site specificity and has limited multi-cultural applicability. The EORTC Quality of Life Group is currently performing a validation study for an SH questionnaire for cancer patients, which reflects the multi-faceted concept of SH. This instrument will be validated for use in clinical trials and in survivorship patient cohorts.

Lymphoedema

Lymphoedema is caused by mechanical destruction of lymphatic vessels and innervation of blood vessels and may be associated with radiation or surgery. Both of these factors can increase hydrostatic pressure, leading to accumulation of extracellular fluid in the limbs resulting in lymphoedema. Occasionally lymphoedema can result directly from disease-causing pelvic lymphatic obstruction by cervical or vulval cancer. Regardless of the cause, lymphoedema is challenging to manage. In most cases lymphoedema cannot be cured, as the causes are mostly irreversible. The condition can however be managed to an acceptable limit if treatment is implemented early. If management is implemented late, it frequently becomes a chronic health concern, with important health, QOL, body image and financial implications.

There is no universally agreed standard definition for lymphoedema leading to use of various approaches. Leg volume measurements enable an objective reproducible diagnosis, with lymphoedema diagnosed as a 5% or more increase in volume in the limb. Looser definitions include a patient reported swelling which is confirmed by lymphoedema specialist, or simply swelling or oedema.

A significant number of gynaecological cancer survivors develop lower limb lymphoedema after their treatment. Across gynaecological malignancies, the lowest incidence is seen after treatment for ovarian cancer (4–7%), and highest in women treated for vulval cancer (36–47%). The quoted incidence of lymphoedema after cervical cancer treatment ranges from 1.6% to 41.0%. Approximately three quarters of cases are diagnosed within the first year after the treatment with a further 20% in the second year following treatment.

Several risk factors for lymphoedema development have been reported, including lymphadenectomy, radiotherapy, the number of lymph nodes removed, patient's age and body mass index. Triggering factors for lower limb lymphoedema include infection, prolonged standing, hot weather and long-haul travel. However, there is generally a lack of strong evidence pertaining to aetiology.

Lymphoedema itself is an incurable and morbid condition, with a significant impact on QOL. Consequently, the risk of lymphoedema is an important consideration when tailoring treatment modalities. Before treatment commences patients should be adequately counselled regarding the risk of developing lymphoedema.

In selected cases sentinel lymph node assessment may achieve adequate information regarding lymph node involvement, but with a markedly reduced incidence of post-treatment lymphoedema. This particularly applies to small vulval carcinomas, where sentinel lymph node evaluation can frequently avoid a highly morbid systematic inguinofemoral lymphadenectomy. In selected cases of cervical and endometrial cancer the role of sentinel node sampling is under evaluation. There is a synergistic effect of multimodal systematic lymphadenectomy and radiotherapy, producing an increased risk of lymphoedema. Therefore, multidisciplinary case review and treatment planning is important in order to minimise the need for these treatments in combination.

In cases of lymphoedema, education of clinicians and patients can achieve early detection. Prescription of support hosiery, manual lymphatic drainage massage, appropriate skin care, and protection of the extremity from infection or trauma will reduce the

---

severity of the condition, minimising the symptoms and related impact on QOL. Patients will benefit from referral to specialist lymphoedema clinics.

Fertility

Most gynaecologic cancers are managed by single or multimodality treatment with radical surgery, chemotherapy or radiotherapy, and infertility is a common consequence of treatment in younger patients. Additionally, as women extend their reproductive lives into their thirties and forties, more pregnancies will be complicated by co-morbidities of premalignant and malignant diseases of the genital tract. Treatment-related infertility can be psychologically devastating, including to some who had previously considered that they had completed their families. The impact on psychological health, relationships, and overall QOL can be extreme for women planning future pregnancies, particularly those who are nulliparous at the time of diagnosis.

There has been a cautiously progressive trend towards fertility-preserving management of gynaecological malignancies. This decision-making can be complex for both patients and their care providers, and a team approach is required to ensure proposed treatment pathways are optimised from both the oncology and fertility perspectives, and to assess and manage psychological distress. Healthcare providers caring for young patients must be aware of fertility preservation options (surgical and non-surgical) which patients may be suitable for these procedures, and the potential options for fertility treatment with assisted reproductive technology. This may require coordination between surgical and clinical oncologists, reproductive gynaecologists and endocrinologists, and the expanded multidisciplinary team including nurse specialists, in order to facilitate optimal outcomes. Synchronising such approaches can be challenging, and there may be a need for a centralised specialised service model to improve outcomes for these women.

International guidelines and expert recommendations for fertility preservation are available, supporting access to fertility preservation for young patients. In particular they promote the use of routine established assisted reproductive methods, such as cryopreservation of oocytes or embryos after emergency in vitro fertilisation. For successful embryo or oocyte cryopreservation, chemotherapy or irradiation may need to be postponed by several weeks or longer. At present,

the most effective technique for patients experiencing loss of ovarian function as a result of oncology treatment is the cryopreservation of fertilised embryos. These embryos may be transferred at a later date, either to the patient if her uterus has been conserved, or to a surrogate. Embryo preservation requires that the patient is in a relationship with a partner willing to undergo IVF, or has access to donor sperm. At present cryopreservation of ovarian tissue is the only available option for prepubertal girls. Research is ongoing into futuristic approaches including agents slowing follicle loss, in vitro maturation of non-antral follicles and generation of follicles from oogonial stem cells. These methodologies remain at research level currently, as does uterine transplant for patients having had previous hysterectomy.

In screened populations cervical cancer is primarily a disease of young women. In FIGO 1A2 and 1B1 disease, fertility-preserving treatment is often feasible (if desired) by the use of conisation or radical trachelectomy. Treatment planning depends on the accurate assessment of disease dimensions, and risk factors with the support of high quality histopathology, imaging and review by the MDT. Although these options do preserve fertility, there is an associated increased risk of adverse obstetric outcomes. The psychological and QOL impacts of fertility sparing surgery are complex and should not be underestimated.

While endometrial cancer is mostly a disease of post-menopausal women, approximately 7% of cases occur in women under the age of 45 years. In early stage type 1 endometrial cancer, high-dose oral progesterone, locally delivered progesterone (levonorgestrel releasing intrauterine device) or their combination have been utilised with a 72% positive response rate. In view of frequent relapses (up to 50%) after conservative treatment, strict vigilance including hysteroscopy and endometrial sampling should be undertaken, and recommendation for definitive conventional treatment when fertility is no longer desired.

Twelve per cent of ovarian cancer patients are below 44 years of age. Fertility preservation may be an option for highly selected patients with stage IA epithelial ovarian cancer, following full surgical staging with omentectomy, peritoneal biopsies, pelvic and para-aortic lymphadenectomy. This will require conservation of the uterus and contralateral healthy ovary. After completion of her family, the patient may opt to have excision of the retained ovary. Following unilateral oophorectomy, gonadotropic hormone–stimulated egg retrieval can be an option to further safeguard fertility via cryopreservation of embryos or oocytes. Young women with ovarian tumours of borderline malignant potential face similar dilemmas. Fertility sparing surgery is advised for a young woman with a borderline tumour who has not completed her family, but fertility sparing management options are limited if the disease involves both ovaries.

Malignant ovarian germ cell tumours are the most common ovarian tumours in women below 20 years of age, and are commonly FIGO stage I at diagnosis. Survival rates and outcome of fertility sparing surgery are encouraging. Fertility preservation is frequently feasible even for higher stage disease, and surgery should be planned as part of a coordinated treatment pathway under the guidance of a specialist malignant germ cell tumour multidisciplinary team in order to optimise outcome.

Further Reading

DH, Macmillan Cancer Support, NHS Improvement. Living with and beyond cancer: taking action to improve outcomes. In: *Department of Health*. London: National Cancer Survivorship Initiative; 2013.

Independent Cancer Taskforce NE. Achieving World-Class Cancer Outcomes a Strategy for England 2015–2020. 2015 [cited 2017 January]; Available from: www.cancerresearchuk.org/sites/default/files/achieving_world-class_cancer_outcomes-a_strategy_for_england_2015-2020.pdf

Macmillan Cancer Support. Recovery Package [cited 2017 January]. Available from: www.macmillan.org.uk/about-us/health-professionals/programmes-and-services/recovery-package-297633

NHS England. Cancer Patient Experience Survey. 2015 [cited 2017 January]. Available from: www.england.nhs.uk/statistics/statistical-work-areas/cancer-patient-experience-survey/

Public Health England. *Living with and Beyond Cervical Cancer. A Descriptive Summary of Responses to a Pilot of Patient Reported Outcome Measures for Gynaecological Cancer.* London: Public Health England; 2015.

Communication in Gynaecological Oncology

Nicholas Wood and Georgios Theophilou

Introduction

The ability to communicate effectively is at the core of delivering effective and safe clinical care. This applies to healthcare professionals during patient and carer interactions, as well as to discussions between healthcare professionals. As a consequence, there is a plethora of academic and operational literature defining optimal communication and decision-making frameworks (for example, multidisciplinary team meetings, MDTMs) and the methodology for 'breaking bad news'. Effective communication with patients, relatives and carers is a fundamental aspect of medicine. The spectrum of patients presenting with gynaecological cancer ranges from young, healthy, asymptomatic patients with screen detected disease and a high chance of cure to elderly, co-morbid, symptomatic patients with a poor performance status who are only suitable for best supportive care. Each will present challenges relevant to their disease state and treatment options.

This chapter focuses on frameworks and guidance for the delivery of gynaecological cancer care in the United Kingdom, and also includes reference to international evidence and guidelines.

The Multidisciplinary Team

The concept of the multidisciplinary team (MDT) meeting may have been pioneered in cancer care; however, it has now been adopted in many aspects of obstetrics and gynaecology. The primary challenge is to define and resource the membership of an MDT. Ideally this should be justified with a firm evidence-base. The mechanics of an MDT meeting are reliant on the venue, technology and communication skills of its membership. These issues will be explored in greater depth.

The MDT: Communication and Clinical Management Decisions

The contemporary structure of gynaecology oncology services in the United Kingdom was developed following the 'Calman–Hine Report' (1995) and the subsequent publication 'Improving Outcomes in Gynaecological Cancers (1999)'. A collection of 'Improving Outcomes' documents were produced by what came to be known as the National Cancer Advisory Group to implement the recommendations of the Calman–Hine Report. These documents and recommendations determined that, due to the relatively low incidence of gynaecological cancers compared to more common cancers (breast, colorectal, lung), treatment quality and outcomes would improve with the centralisation of services. There is now compelling evidence to support the principle of centralisation and sub-specialisation of gynaecological oncology services with regard to both patient experience and cancer outcomes. This is particularly evident with the management of ovarian cancer.

In the NHS, the membership and role of the MDT was originally defined through the National Cancer Action Team (NCAT), followed by the widespread implementation of well-constructed cancer treatment networks that included local cancer units, diagnostic services and cancer centres. The implementation was driven by the NHS Cancer Peer Review Process and supervised by the NCAT.

The underlying principle of an MDT meeting (MDTM) is that better clinical decisions will be made about patient care if those decisions are made by a team of clinicians representing all clinical specialties involved in cancer care. In addition to case discussion and management decision-making, the MDTM also has an administrative function of capturing the decisions and other metrics important for demonstrating cancer outcomes (the Cancer Outcomes and Services Dataset and the National Cancer Registry and Analysis Service). It is common for MDTMs to utilise video-conference technology to circumvent the need for clinicians to travel long distances. The use of this technology presents a number of difficulties to an effective MDTM process that are both technical and human. However, the economic and ecological benefits of effective tele-medicine to support MDTMs working across a large geographic area have been demonstrated. An effective MDTM requires clear governance with regard to 'terms of reference', roles and responsibilities. This will include the MDTM referral criteria to ensure that only appropriate patients are reviewed, and that all the required and necessary information is readily available for the MDT discussion.

The key components of an effective MDT are summarised in Box 18.1.

The role of the MDTM in the United Kingdom is comparable to what is referred to as the Tumour Board in North America (USA and Canada). However, there is no regulation in these countries to ensure that all cancer patients are discussed at Tumour Board prior to management decisions. The Tumour Board tends to be reserved for the discussion of complex cases. There is conflicting evidence on the objective benefit of MDTM with regard to care quality or cancer outcomes. A recent report published by Cancer Research UK has identified the challenges to the existing MDTM format in UK cancer care and made suggestions for improvement in efficiency and quality, summarised in Box 18.2.

Box 18.1 Categorisation of MDT characteristics

The team
  Membership
  Attendance
  Leadership
  Team working and culture
  Personal development and training
Infrastructure for meetings
  Physical environment of meeting venue
  Technology and equipment (availability and use)
Meeting Organisation and Logistics
  Scheduling of MDT meetings
  Preparation prior to MDT meetings
  Organisation/administration during MDT meetings
  Post MDT meeting /co-ordination of service
Patient-centred clinical decision-making
  Who to discuss?
  Patient-centred care
  Clinical decision-making process
Team governance
  Organisational support
  Data collection, analysis and audit of outcomes
  Clinical governance

Box 18.2 Improving the effectiveness of MDTMs in cancer services

- The United Kingdom's health services should work with NICE and SIGN to identify where a protocolised treatment pathway could be applied, and develop a set of treatment recommendations for each of these to be implemented. Every Cancer Alliance or devolved cancer network should develop their own approach based on these central recommendations. These treatment protocols should be reviewed regularly.
- MDTs for tumour types for which a protocolised approach has been developed should agree and document their approach to administering protocols. This could include a 'pre-MDT triage meeting'. The implementation and outcomes of these protocols should be audited and reviewed by the full MDT in an operational meeting.
- National requirements for individual minimum attendance should be reviewed and amended where necessary, with an emphasis on ensuring all required specialties are present at a meeting. NHS England should run a series of pilots to determine optimal percentage attendance requirements. The success of these pilots should be evaluated and national guidance changed as appropriate.
- The United Kingdom's health services should lead the development of national proforma templates to be refined by MDTs. MDTs should require incoming cases and referrals to have a completed proforma with all information ready before discussion at a meeting. The proforma could include:
  - Patient demographics
  - Diagnostic information
  - Patient fitness and co-morbidities, history of previous malignancies
  - Results from a Holistic Needs Assessment (if available)
  - The patient's preferences (if known)
  - The rationale for requiring MDT discussion
  - Whether there were known treatment protocols for the specific tumour type
  - Whether the patient is suitable for any current clinical trials.

  The MDT should have the power to bypass this requirement in exceptional circumstances.
- MDTs should use a database or proforma to enable documentation of recommendations in real time. Ideally this should be projected so that it is visible to team members; if this is not possible there should be a named clinical individual responsible for ensuring the information is accurate. Hospital Trusts and boards should ensure that MDTs are given sufficient resource to do this.
- Each MDT should ensure that they have mortality and morbidity process to ensure all adverse outcomes can be discussed by the whole MDT and learned from, rather than discussed in silos. The operational meeting should either be a quarterly or biannual. Time for quarterly operational meetings should be included in attendees' job plans. There should be oversight from national MDT assessment programmes.

Informed Consent

Informed consent is defined in the Oxford English Dictionary as 'a granted permission in full knowledge of possible consequences'. A legal definition of consent is an 'assent to permit an occurrence, such as surgery that is based on a complete disclosure of facts needed to make the decision intelligently, such as knowledge of the risks entailed or alternatives'. Informed consent safeguards patients' autonomy by considering health intervention options and opting for those that are acceptable for the individual. Consent validity is subject to ethical, legal, historical and resource considerations that pose conceptual and regulatory limitations. In the United Kingdom doctors are bound to professional duties, and these are regulated by the General Medical Council.

Obtaining informed consent in a gynaecological oncology setting can be particularly challenging as it may involve decisions that affect fertility or impact on health options for family members. This may involve decisions on prevention, screening, diagnosis, treatment, follow-up and participation in research. The Royal College of Obstetricians and Gynaecologists and the General Medical Council provide specific guidance on obtaining valid consent.

Several pre-requisites have to be present for consent to be achieved satisfactorily. A framework to achieve this may include:

1. Appropriate expertise
2. Patient's capacity
3. Rapport
4. Information exchange
5. Absence of conflict.

Each element of the consent procedure can harbour pitfalls, which should be avoided by exercising good communication with both patients and other health professionals.

Appropriate Expertise

The person providing information on a proposed medical intervention must have adequate knowledge of the specifics that the intervention involves. Such persons include doctors who will be undertaking proposed procedures or personnel specifically trained in discussing consent in relation to those procedures. Training in advanced communication skills is desirable.

The options that are available to the patient must be discussed. These should include doing nothing, initiating investigations, watchful waiting and providing treatment. These options may have been discussed in advance at the MDT meeting, so it is prudent that this is kept in mind and discussed with patients.

There is a risk that only options discussed at MDT meetings are made available to the patient. Appropriate knowledge of other potential treatment modalities is important for patients who want to explore all avenues available to them.

There are two complications that must be considered in the case of gynaecological cancer:

1. The complexity of discussion regarding the prognosis for each type and stage of cancer when opting for each of the options above
2. The lack of general consensus on the management modalities and the variability in management in relation to different cancers.

To counteract these challenges it is suggested that healthcare professionals make use of a matrix containing available options for each type and stage of cancer along with the morbidity and mortality rates for each option. Such a matrix cannot be provided in this writing due to the variability in practice between cancer centres. Such protocolled management can be locally agreed and with time become robust national or international guidance.

Patient's Capacity

Capacity to consent to treatment should be presumed until proven otherwise. A patient may be judged as lacking capacity when they cannot understand, retain, use or weigh-up information needed to make relevant decisions, despite support to do so. The assessment of capacity needs to be guided by the specific type of decision that needs to be made, and performed at the time consent is taken. In these cases it is important to provide appropriate support to encourage their involvement in making care decisions. This can be achieved by:

- Correct timing of the discussions as lack of capacity can be temporary.
- Involving family members, carers or advocates to provide psychological support and assistance with explanations as they may have deeper understanding of communication avenues with the patient.
- Providing written or recorded information that can be reviewed by the patient in their own time and environment and re-discussing them

in person at a later stage. This is particularly important in cases where the problem is retention of information.

- Involving other healthcare professionals in identifying the best way to communicate with the patient.

Making treatment decisions for patients who lack capacity to consent is governed by the 'Mental Capacity Act 2005' in England and Wales and by 'Adults with Incapacity Act 2000' in Scotland. These decisions should be made with the involvement of other health professionals and, where appropriate, the patient's family. They should always be made with respect to dignity and for the overall benefit of the patient. The patient's previous wishes should be considered and where there is an advanced statement or an advocate they should be consulted. A holistic approach, taking into account the patient's values and beliefs, should be used.

In gynaecological oncology surgery, taking consent has several specific complexities. Many treatments for younger women have an impact on fertility, and discussion regarding family plans can be challenging. For example, in early cervical cancer there is currently insufficient evidence regarding the use of large loop excisions versus trachelectomy, and in early ovarian cancer where several fertility sparing options exist including incomplete staging, oocyte/embryo freezing, etc.

Other pitfalls may arise in the setting of acute surgery where the patient is already anaesthetised, for example, and a gynaecological oncology surgeon is called to review an ovarian mass that looks malignant. Lack of information other than initial imaging and view at surgery may complicate the decision on the extent of surgery to be undertaken if at all.

Dialogue

Healthcare professionals have a duty to establish an effective dialogue with their patients to facilitate effective communication. This relationship is based on exploring and understanding each other's views, feelings and beliefs and determining the goals of their collaboration. As long as the patient and their family identify that healthcare professionals involved are genuinely concerned about the patient's well-being, the relationship will usually be based on mutual trust and respect. This is not a single event, rather an ongoing process that starts with the first encounter and continues through the patient's journey. This process entails

detailed discussions on the overall care and includes prognosis, risks and complications to be expected when choosing any of the management options presented. Detailed explanation of what is to be expected informs the patient and allows active involvement in decision-making, rather than just acceptance of recommendations. This promotes a better experience even when complications arise. A comprehensive consent process requires a greater investment of time and effort on the provider's part. However, it has also been noted that better communication, afforded by tools employed during the informed consent process, may be key to reducing a physician's risk of litigation.

In gynaecological oncology surgery, patients are usually seen after the MDT discussion has taken place and recommendations have been given. This should not restrict the discussion to the management options recommended, but all options should be explained to the patient taking into account their own views. In the case that the patient does not agree with any of the recommended options their views can be brought back to the team meeting to be re-discussed.

Information Exchange

Information exchange in relation to consent has two meanings. It involves information exchange with the patient to allow an informed consent. It also involves taking patients' consent to exchange information with other health professionals to facilitate decision-making and organise management.

Providing adequate information on all options available to the patient is of paramount importance. These options should always include a discussion of the option of 'doing nothing', especially in the setting of palliative interventions. Patients' beliefs about cancer vary significantly; therefore very detailed and specific information about their disease and the options available to them in the particular hospital setting are paramount. An 'aide memoire' used to explain the different options along with their relative prognosis and complication rates can be valuable. Some patients will appreciate written or recorded information and a further appointment to re-discuss their options after they have done their own research and considered their options. Some patients may also seek information on alternative treatments such as homeopathy. It is important to provide further information on the effectiveness of these treatments where available, or direct the patient to health professionals who have expertise on these matters. It is important not to be dismissive to options explored by the patient in order to maintain effective dialogue during decision-making.

With regard to consenting to sharing information with other health professionals, this is usually assumed when the patient engages with health services. Explaining to the patient why their information is shared with other professionals encourages rapid establishment of rapport with those involved with their care.

Absence of Conflict

Medical intervention is permissible only with a patient's consent. It is possible that conflict arises when a health professional and a patient have different views on the management options best suited to the condition. The medical practitioner may act in accordance to their duty of care and propose what they feel is in the patient's best interests. A patient may consent or refuse management, which may lead to a decline of their health or progression of their cancer. In these cases, the general principle is that informed consent – in a competent patient – takes priority and every effort is made to resolve conflict and acquire appropriate consent. Although attempts to resolve such conflict may initially appear paternalistic, they may be necessary to morally safeguard the patient's well-being. Where there is such a conflict that cannot be resolved, assistance may be helpful by agreeing to obtain a second opinion.

These situations become increasingly complicated when fertility is at stake, or when hereditary cancers are diagnosed. This is because the patient may experience an internal conflict between what they feel is best for them and best for their family. Exploration of these ideas and their burden on the patient and their family is important as it may help identify management avenues that are acceptable to the patient and allow consent. Input from a genetic counsellor, psychosexual counsellor and subfertility specialist in these cases may prove valuable.

In conclusion consent is central to everyday practice and should not be taken lightly. There are several pitfalls that can be encountered and understanding of the mechanisms involved in consenting is important. When difficulties are encountered sharing the weight of assessing capacity and resolving conflict are central to safeguarding patient wellbeing and preventing litigation.

> **TIP**
> Taking informed consent is a complex but vital aspect of a patients' care.

Communication Skills Training in Gynaecological Oncology

There is evidence to demonstrate that the implementation of structured training in communication skills for oncologists provides measurable benefit in terms of their emotional support, setting up a supportive environment and ability to deliver information. Moreover, oncologists who have received specialised communication training express greater confidence with their consultations and their patients have significantly reduced scores in measures on anxiety and depression.

Breaking Bad News

Most patients attending a tertiary cancer centre will already know their cancer diagnosis. Breaking bad news in this setting rarely involves informing the patient that they have cancer. It is more frequent that breaking bad news involves talking about inability to cure, complications occurring as a result of treatment and cancer recurrence or progression despite treatment. Nevertheless, breaking bad news is a difficult task but an essential part of professional practice. Bad news has been defined as 'any information which adversely and seriously affects an individual's view of his or her future'. Such information often drastically alters patients' perceptions about their future and may cause them to enter the five stages of grief:

- Denial
- Anger
- Bargaining
- Depression
- Acceptance.

Good communication skills when breaking bad news can improve patients' emotional adjustment through these stages and improve compliance with potential treatments. There is also an ethical and legal perspective that mandates doctors to be open and honest with their patients about the extent and gravity of their condition.

In general, two tools are recommended for providing some structure to breaking bad news: the Baile/SPIKES model and the ABCDE mnemonic (Boxes 18.3 and 18.4).

Box 18.3 SPIKES model for breaking bad news

Setting up
- Arrange for privacy
- Involve significant others
- Sit down
- Make connection with the patient
- Manage time constrains and interruptions

Perception assessment
- Ask questions to assess patient's understanding of the situation so far
- Correct any misinformation

Invitation to disclose information
- Ask what and how much information the patient wants
- Separate information about test results and proposed treatments

Knowledge giving
- Warn patient that you have bad news
- Disclose bad news without using any jargon
- Check patients understanding at regular intervals
- Allow for taking-in time
- Be empathetic

Emotions
- Observe and identify emotion verbally so that the patient knows you are paying attention
- Identify the reason for their emotions

Summary
- Create plan for the future
- Initiate a discussion on consenting for management

Box 18.4 ABCDE mnemonic for breaking bad news

Advance preparation
- Arrange for adequate time, privacy and no interruptions (turn pager off or to silent mode)
- Review relevant clinical information
- Mentally rehearse, identify words or phrases to use and avoid
- Prepare yourself emotionally

Build a therapeutic environment/relationship
- Determine what and how much the patient wants to know
- Have family or support persons present
- Introduce yourself to everyone
- Warn the patient that bad news is coming
- Use touch when appropriate
- Schedule follow-up appointments

Communicate well
- Ask what the patient or family already knows
- Be frank but compassionate; avoid euphemisms and medical jargon
- Allow for silence and tears; proceed at the patient's pace
- Have the patient describe his or her understanding of the news; repeat this information at subsequent visits
- Allow time to answer questions; write things down and provide written information
- Conclude each visit with a summary and follow-up plan

Deal with patient and family reactions
- Assess and respond to the patient and the family's emotional reaction; repeat at each visit
- Be empathetic
- Do not argue with or criticise colleagues

Encourage and validate emotions
- Explore what the news meant to the patient
- Offer realistic hope according to the patient's goals
- Use interdisciplinary resources
- Take care of your own needs; be attuned to the needs of involved house staff and office or hospital personnel

It is essential to offer a follow-up consultation to the patient and family after breaking bad news. This is preferably done by the person breaking the bad news but can be taken over by a cancer nurse specialist or the general practitioner. Therefore, close communication with those caring for the patient is important.

There are several pitfalls when breaking bad news that can make an uncomfortable situation worse. Common faults that can cause a break in communication are:

- Not picking up cues, verbal or non-verbal
- Not being completely open and honest and 'hiding' the extent of the problem
- Being overly optimistic or pessimistic
- Using jargon or lengthy and overly medicalised answers
- Trying to identify with the patient's situation: 'I know exactly how you feel'.

There is no right or wrong way to break bad news, but the above general suggestions may help develop individual techniques to treat patients and families with sensitivity and respect during these difficult situations. Reflection will assist continuing development of communication approaches to deal with breaking bad news.

Patient Reported Communication Needs and Information Requirements

Patient communication needs and information requirements have been assessed in England since 2010 through the National Cancer Patient Experience Survey. In addition, there are numerous peer-review publications relating to cancer patients in general but also the specific needs of gynaecological cancer patients.

The National Cancer Patient Experience Survey includes all adult patients with a confirmed primary diagnosis of cancer who have been discharged from an NHS Trust following an inpatient or day case attendance for cancer-related treatment during a 3-month period. The last iteration was published in 2015. Communication and information needs are assessed in a number of parts of the survey. The survey has consistently highlighted specific information needs:

- Forty-five per cent of patients did not get adequate information regarding financial help or benefits that they might be entitled to
- Nineteen per cent of patients were not given written information following their initial diagnosis
- Ten per cent of patients were given written information that was difficult to understand
- Sixty-seven per cent of patients had not received a care plan (a document that '... sets out your needs and goals for caring for your cancer ...').

The information needs of patients are complex and variable. The concerns and anxieties of patients do not always reflect the nature and stage of their cancer diagnosis. In a recent pilot of collecting Patient Reported Outcome Measures in patients treated for gynaecological cancers in NHS England, the fear of disease recurrence was disproportionately increased with respect to actual prognosis in women diagnosed with cervix cancer compared to women with ovarian cancer.

Communication at the End-of-Life

Barriers to effective communication about the end of life have been examined in cancer care as well as other life-limiting diseases. This aspect of communication has been reported by clinicians as one of the most stressful parts of cancer care. Poor doctor-patient communication in late-stage cancer care can lead to extra or unnecessary, and even futile treatment. The majority of patients receiving palliative chemotherapy for colorectal and lung cancer believe that there is still a chance of their cancer being cured. Evidence shows that most cancer patients wish to be told 'all possible information' with a minority who do not want to hear bad news (Box 18.5).

The oncology community have accepted the need for improved communication with regard to end-of-life discussions and the involvement of palliative care

Box 18.5 Benefits of timely and appropriate outpatient end-of-life care discussions

- Lower incidence of chemotherapy in last 14 days of life
- Lower incidence of admission to acute hospital in the last 30 days of life
- Lower incidence of ICU admission in last 30 days of life
- Lower incidence of dying in acute setting
- Greater use of hospice care
- Lower incidence of being admitted to hospice within 3 days of death

Box 18.6 Aids to discussing transitions from curative to palliative care

- Discuss anticancer treatment failure in a timely manner
- Use bad news recommendations to establish shared understanding of clinical situation
- Be prepared to acknowledge and grieve losses
- Explore hopes other than cure, support realistic hopes
- Allow patients to hold private hopes and avoid dismissing these hopes
- Emphasise what can be done for the patient and family
- Reaffirm commitment to the patient and family

Box 18.7 Aids to communicating evidence for decision-making about anticancer therapy in the palliative setting

- Offer to discuss treatment options, impact on survival and quality of life to patients considering palliative chemotherapy
- When discussing treatment options, explicitly mention the option of supportive care without anticancer therapy
- For patients considering clinical trials, explicitly discuss the purpose of the trial, risks and benefits, and the patient's ability to withdraw at any time
- After your discussion, check patient understanding

teams. Appropriate end-of-life care provides improvement in symptoms, quality of life, patient satisfaction, reduced caregiver burden, more appropriate referral and use of hospice, reduced use of futile intensive care and other invasive care and even improved survival (Boxes 18.6 and 18.7).

According to the General Medical Council's 'Treatment and care towards the end of life: good practice in decision-making' document, patients are defined as approaching the end of life when they are likely to die within the next 12 months. This includes those with advanced, progressive and incurable

Box 18.8 Barriers in diagnosing 'dying'

- Hope that the patient may get better
- No definitive diagnosis
- Pursuance of unrealistic or futile interventions
- Disagreement about the patient's condition
- Failure to recognise key symptoms and signs
- Lack of knowledge about how to prescribe
- Poor ability to communicate with the family and patient
- Concerns about withdrawing or withholding treatment
- Fear of foreshortening life
- Concerns about resuscitation
- Cultural and spiritual barriers
- Medicolegal issues

conditions and those that are at risk of dying for an acute crisis in their condition. Patients with high-stage gynaecological cancers may fall into one of these categories at some point. Some patients may have a diagnosis of incurable cancer but a prognosis of longer than one year. Discussions regarding prognosis are valuable in this setting and end-of-life discussions may prove important in cases where complications leading to death are expected. Being honest and open is central to such discussions. There are several ethical issues surrounding decisions to treat, especially when treatment may improve patient's quality of life without necessarily prolonging it.

The first step in discussing end of life is to diagnose 'dying'. Recognising this phase is difficult especially in a hospital setting where the focus is on intervention. There are several barriers in diagnosing dying (Box 18.8).

Inability to diagnose or communicate dying has adverse consequences including loss of rapport with patient and family when deterioration in condition is not expected, uncontrolled symptoms causing distress, inappropriate cardiopulmonary resuscitation attempts leading to loss of dignity and unmet cultural and spiritual needs. This series of events may lead to dissatisfaction of the patient or family, and result in complaints about care.

There is a shift in the needs of the patient and family that should be appreciated by the caring team. Therefore discussions about care take a more holistic angle, as they involve physical, psychological, social and spiritual aspects to end-of-life care. Therefore a multidisciplinary approach, engaging specialists in different areas of care may be useful.

The autonomy of patients should always be respected. End-of-life discussions should be had at a time where capacity to consent to treatment or to establish advance directives is optimal. Patients often wish to have family members as proxies in end-of-life decisions. Other reasons for involving families in end-of-life discussions include the contrast between the obligation that family members feel for caring for their loved one, and the patient's concerns about burdening loved ones. The focus during these discussions should not be treatments or outcomes, but the patient's own wishes and models of end-of-life planning. Patients' perspectives of end-of-life planning may be more aligned with their valued activities and expectations of quality of life rather than aggressive medicalised approaches to achieve life prolongation or complication reduction. Active treatment need not stop when end-of-life discussions happen. It is preferable to have these discussions early to avoid situations where patients' preferences are not adequately discussed. This should not jeopardise patient-doctor rapport or result in withdrawal of consent to treatment when done well. Discussions regarding end-of-life care planning pose similar difficulties as breaking bad news, so similar models of communication can be applied such as SPIKES or ABCDE. Difficult questions can be asked in this setting, including ones that are challenging to answer, for example: 'how long have I got?' Other challenges may include language, cultural and spiritual differences. It is important to breach any gaps in communication that may arise using active listening, appropriate silences, acknowledgement, clarification and empathy. It can be easy to avoid tackling major concerns by repeatedly questioning patients, turning attention to families, or simply by excessive information giving. Therefore a structured approach is preferable.

Communication between healthcare and social-care professionals for matters concerning end-of-life care is paramount. It can be challenging to lead the care of such patients from a tertiary hospital setting. Involving the MDT including palliative care specialists and general practitioners in verbal and written communication is helpful. Such information may include preferred place of death, individual needs and concerns of the patient and/or their family and advance directives that may include resuscitation decisions. Providing patients with written material about their care-plan and direct contact information in cases that they experience problems ensures a level of safety.

195

Follow-up, independent of need for active intervention, may also be appreciated by patients and families and assist in the provision of care by other professionals who may be introduced in this setting.

Communication does not stop when the patient's life has ended. It is important to ensure continuing support for the bereaved family. Good communication between the MDT will ensure a proactive approach to identify and support carers who may be at risk of various morbidities including post-traumatic stress disorder or depression.

Conclusion

The effective clinical management of patients with gynaecological cancer provides many communication challenges. Effective communication enhances clinical care through cohesive MDT working and shared decision-making with patients and their carers.

Knowledge, empathy and clarity are all features of good human clinical interactions.

Further Reading

Department of Health. *Reference Guide to Consent for Examination or Treatment*. London: Department of Health. 2012; 11.

Department of Health, Department for Constitutional Affairs, Welsh Assembly Government. *Mental Capacity Act 2005 Summary*. October 2007.

General Medical Council. *Consent: Patients and Doctors Making Decisions Together the duties of a Doctor Registered with the General Medical Council*. London: General Medical Council. 2008; 34.

Treatment and Care towards the End of Life: Decision Making. London: General Medical Council. 2010.

Morris E. *Obtaining Valid Consent (Clinical Governance Advice No. 6)*. London: British Medical Association. 2015.

Appendix

WHO Performance Status Classification

Performance status is frequently used to quantify cancer patients' well-being and often used to indicate whether or not a patient can tolerate certain treatment such as chemotherapy. Other uses include dose reduction, use in trial and quality of life.

Grade	Explanation of activity
0:	Able to carry out all normal activity without restriction
1:	Restricted in physically strenuous activity, but ambulatory and able to carry out light work
2:	Ambulatory and capable of all self-care, but unable to carry out work; up and about more than 50% of waking hours
3:	Capable only of limited self-care; confined to bed more than 50% of waking hours
4:	Completely disabled; cannot carry out any self-care; totally confined to bed or chair

Criteria of chemotherapy response (WHO)

- Complete response (CR) – resolution of all measureable or evaluable disease
- Partial response (PR) – ≥50% reduction in measureable or evaluable disease in the absence of progression in any particular disease site
- Stable disease (SD) – <50% decrease or <25% increase in measureable or evaluable disease
- Progressive disease (PD) – >25% increase in measureable or evaluable disease or development of a new lesion

Clinical Trials and Drug Development

Clinical trials are divided into different stages, called phases. The earliest phase trials may look at drug safety or side-effect profile and tolerability. A later phase trial aims to test whether a new treatment is better than existing treatments.

There are three main phases of clinical trials – phases I to III. But some trials have an earlier stage called phase 0, and there are some phase IV trials done after a drug has been licensed.

Phase 0 Trials

Phase 0 trials are aimed to find out whether the behaviour of the drug *in vivo* is as expected from laboratory studies.

Phase I

Aim is to establish human toxicity of new drug; to establish the safe dose at which to start further trials and to measure the pharmacokinetics of the drug.

Phase II

Aim is to establish the anti-tumour activity of the drug against a particular tumour in patients where no curative therapy is possible; further information on toxicity is obtained. Phase II studies are usually non-randomised.

Phase III

Aim is to compare the new drug with the conventional best therapy. Trials are prospective, randomised and controlled. Large number of patients required to show effect.

Phase IV

Aim is to establish efficacy of drugs in adjuvant trials; determine long-term toxicity of drug.

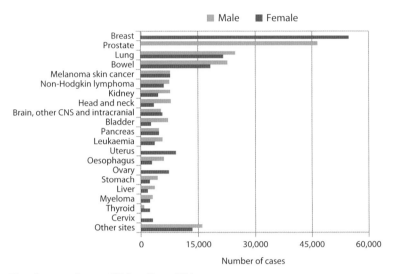

Figure A.1 The Twenty Most Common Cancers, UK, New Cases: 2014

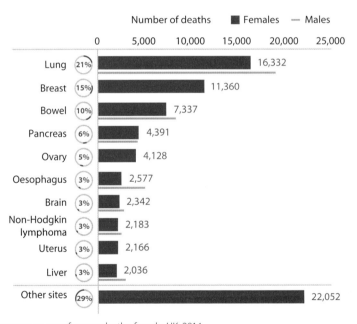

Figure A.2 The 10 most common causes of cancer deaths, female, UK, 2014

Breast cancer is by far the commonest cancer for women in the United Kingdom. Of the gynaecological cancers, uterus has become the most common and the incidence continues to increase in the United Kingdom. Cervix cancer incidence continues to decrease in the United Kingdom.

There has been a significant increase in uterus cancer, while the incidence of ovary and particularly cervix cancer has decreased.

There has been an increase in age-standardised mortality due to uterus cancer. However, ovary and cervical cancers have seen a decrease in mortality rates.

Rules for FIGO Clinical Staging

The main purpose of staging systems is twofolds: to provide standard terminology that allows comparison of patients between centres, and to assign patients and their tumours to prognostic groups requiring specific treatments.

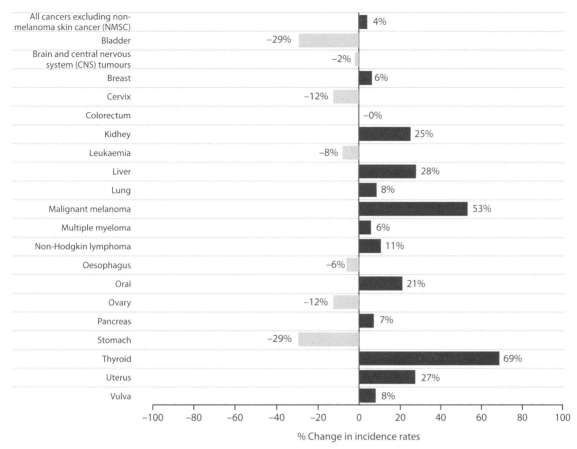

Figure A.3 Percentage changes in European age-standardised 3-year average incidence rates, main cancers, female, UK, 1997–9 to 2006–8

Clinical staging should be based on careful examination and should be performed before any definitive therapy. It is desirable that the examination be performed by an experienced examiner and under anaesthesia when appropriate.

Surgical-pathologic findings are adapted for staging of uterus, ovary, fallopian tube, and vulva cancers, and for gestational trophoblastic disease. Cervix cancer is staged clinically.

The clinical stage, under no circumstances, must be changed on the basis of subsequent findings.

When it is doubtful to which stage a particular case should be allotted, the case must be referred to the earlier stage.

For clinical staging purposes the following examination methods are permitted: palpation, inspection, colposcopy, endocervical curettage, hysteroscopy, cystoscopy, proctoscopy, intravenous urography and X-ray examination of the lungs and skeleton. Suspected bladder or rectal involvement should be confirmed by biopsy and histologic evidence.

Findings by examinations, such as computed tomography, magnetic resonance imaging, lymphangiography, arteriography, venography and laparoscopy, are of value for the planning of therapy, but, because these are not available easily world-wide and also the interpretation of results is variable, the findings of such studies should not be the basis for changing the clinical staging.

The staging for endometrial, cervical and vulval carcinoma was revised by FIGO in 2014 and is included in this appendix. Uterine sarcomas are staged separately in this revision and are detailed.

TNM Staging System

The TNM system is one of the most commonly used staging systems. This system has been accepted by the International Union against Cancer (UICC) and the American Joint Committee on Cancer (AJCC). Most

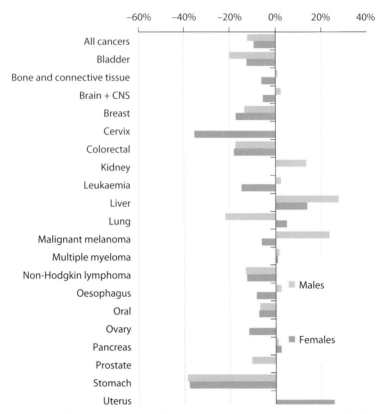

Figure A.4 Percentage change in the European age-standardised mortality rates, by sex, major cancers, UK, 1997–2006

Table A.1 Primary tumour (T)

TX	Primary tumour cannot be evaluated
T0	No evidence of primary tumour
Tis	Carcinoma in situ (early cancer that has not spread to neighbouring tissue)
T1, T2, T3, T4	Size and/or extent of the primary tumour

Table A.3 Distant metastasis (M)

MX	Distant metastasis cannot be evaluated
M0	No distant metastasis (cancer has not spread to other parts of the body)
M1	Distant metastasis (cancer has spread to distant parts of the body)

Table A.2 Regional lymph nodes (N)

NX	Regional lymph nodes cannot be evaluated
N0	No regional lymph node involvement (no cancer found in the lymph nodes)
N1, N2, N3	Involvement of regional lymph nodes (number and/or extent of spread)

medical facilities use the TNM system as well as the FIGO staging for cancer reporting.

The TNM system is based on the extent of the tumour (T), the extent of spread to the lymph nodes (N) and the presence of metastasis (M). A number is added to each letter to indicate the size or extent of the tumour and the extent of spread.

FIGO Staging for Carcinoma of the Ovary

Staging of ovarian carcinoma is based on findings at clinical examination and by surgical exploration. The histologic findings are to be considered in the staging, as are the cytologic findings as far as effusions are concerned. It is desirable that a biopsy be taken from

Table A.4 FiGO staging of carcinoma of the ovary

Stage 0	No evidence of primary tumour
Stage I	Tumour confined to ovaries or fallopian tube(s)
Stage IA T1a N0 M0	Tumour limited to 1 ovary (capsule intact) or fallopian tube; no tumour on ovarian or fallopian tube surface; no malignant cells in the ascites or peritoneal washings
Stage IB T1b N0 M0	Tumour limited to both ovaries (capsules intact) or fallopian tubes; no tumour on ovarian or fallopian tube surface; no malignant cells in the ascites or peritoneal washings
Stage IC T1c N0 M0	Tumour limited to one or both ovaries or fallopian tubes, with any of the following:
Stage IC1 T1c1 N0 M0	Surgical spill
Stage IC2 T1c2 N0 M0	Capsule ruptured before surgery or tumour on ovarian of fallopian tube surface
Stage IC3 T1c3 N0 M0	Malignant cells in the ascites or peritoneal washings
Stage II T2 N0 Mo	Tumour involves one or both ovaries or fallopian tubes with pelvic extension (below pelvic brim) or primary peritoneal cancer
Stage IIA T2a N0 M0	Extension and/or implants on uterus and/or fallopian tubes and/ or ovaries
Stage IIB T2b N0 M0	Extension to other pelvic intraperitoneal tissues
Stage IIC T2c N0 M0	Either Stage IIA or IIB but with tumour on the surface of one of both ovaries; or with capsule(s) ruptured; or with ascites containing malignant cells present or with positive peritoneal washings
Stage III T1/T2 N1 M0	Tumour involving one or both ovaries with peritoneal implants outside the pelvis and/or positive retroperitoneal or inguinal nodes; superficial liver metastasis equals Stage III; tumour is limited to the true pelvis but with histologically proven malignant extension to small bowel or omentum
Stage IIIA1 T3a N0 M0	IIIA1: Positive retroperitoneal lymph nodes only (cytologically or histologically proven): IIIA(i) Metastasis up to 10 mm in greatest dimension IIIA1(ii) Metastasis >10 mm in greatest dimension
Stage IIIA2 T3a2 N0/N1 M0	Microscopic extrapelvic (above the pelvic brim) peritoneal involvement with or without positive retroperitoneal lymph nodes
Stage IIIB T3b N0/N1 M0	Macroscopic peritoneal metastasis beyond the pelvis up to 2 cm in greatest dimension, with or without metastasis to the retroperitoneal lymph nodes
Stage IIIC T3c N0 M0 Any T N1 M0	Macroscopic peritoneal metastasis beyond the pelvis >2 cm in greatest dimension, with or without metastasis to the retroperitoneal lymph nodes (includes extension of tumour to capsule of liver and spleen without parenchymal involvement of either organ)
Stage IV Any T Any N M1	Growth involving one or both ovaries, with distant metastases. If pleural effusion is present, there must be positive cytologic findings to allot a case to Stage IV; parenchymal liver metastasis equals Stage IV Stage IVA: Pleural effusion with positive cytology Stage IVB: Parenchymal metastases and metastases to extra-abdominal organs (including inguinal lymph nodes and lymph nodes outside of the abdominal cavity)

Table A.5 FIGO staging for carcinoma of the corpus uteri

Stage 0 TIS	Carcinoma in situ (preinvasive carcinoma)
Stage I	Tumour confined to the corpus uteri
Stage IA T1a N0 M0	Tumour limited to endometrium or invades less than one half of the myometrium
Stage IB T1b N0 M0	Tumour invades one half or more of the myometrium
Stage II T2 N0 M0	Cervical stromal invasion, but not beyond uterus[a]
Stage III	
Stage IIIA T3a N0 M0	Tumour invades serosa or adnexa[b]
Stage IIIB T3b N0 M0	Vaginal and/or parametrial involvement[b]
Stage IIIC	Metastases to pelvic and/or para-aortic lymph nodes[b]
Stage IIIC1 T1–3b N1 M0	Positive pelvic lymph nodes
Stage IIIC2 T1–3b N2 M0	Positive para-aortic lymph nodes with or without positive pelvic lymph nodes
Stage IV	Tumour invades bladder and/or bowel mucosa, and/or distant metastases
Stage IVA T4 Any N M0	Tumour invasion of bladder and/or bowel mucosa
Stage IVB Any T Any N M1	Distant metastases including abdominal metastases and/or inguinal lymph nodes

Any stage can be G1, G2, G3.
[a]Endocervical glandular involvement only should be considered as Stage I and no longer as Stage II.
[b]Positive cytology has to be reported separately without changing the stage.

suspicious areas outside pelvis. Primary peritoneal cancer and primary fallopian tube cancer share many similarities with ovarian cancer. Clinically, these three cancers are managed in a similar manner.

Histopathology – Degree of Differentiation

Cases of carcinoma of the corpus should be classified (or graded) according to the degree of histologic differentiation as follows:

Grade 1 = ≤5% of a nonsquamous or nonmorular solid growth pattern

Grade 2 = 6–50% of a nonsquamous or nonmorular solid growth pattern

Grade 3 = >50% of a nonsquamous or nonmorular solid growth pattern

Notes on pathological grading:

1. Notable nuclear atypia, inappropriate for the architectural grade, raises the grade of a Grade 1 or Grade 2 tumour by 1.
2. In serous adenocarcinoma, clear-cell adenocarcinomas, and squamous-cell carcinomas, nuclear grading takes precedence.
3. Adenocarcinomas with benign squamous differentiation are graded according to the nuclear grade of the glandular component.

Rules related to staging:

1. Because uterine cancer is now staged surgically, procedures previously used for determination of stages are no longer applicable (e.g. findings from fractional D&C to differentiate between Stage I and Stage II).

Table A.6 FIGO staging for uterine sarcomas (leiomyosarcomas, endometrial stromal sarcomas, adenosarcomas and carcinosarcomas)

(1)	**Leiomyosarcomas**
Stage I	Tumour limited to uterus
Stage IA	<5 cm
Stage IB	>5 cm
Stage II	Tumour extends to the pelvis
Stage IIA	Adnexal involvement
Stage IIB	Tumour extends to extrauterine pelvic tissue
Stage III	Tumour invades abdominal tissues (not just protruding into the abdomen)
Stage IIIA	One site
Stage IIIB	More than one site
Stage IIIC	Metastases to pelvic and/or para-aortic lymph nodes
Stage IV	Tumour invades bladder and/or rectum, and/or distant metastases
Stage IVA	Tumour invades bladder and/or rectum
Stage IVB	Distant metastasis
(2)	**Endometrial stromal sarcomas (ESS) and adenosarcomas**[a]
Stage I	Tumour limited to uterus
Stage IA	Tumour limited to endometrium/endocervix with no myometrial invasion
Stage IB	Less than or equal to half myometrial invasion
Stage IC	More than half myometrial invasion
Stage II	Tumour extends to the pelvis
Stage IIA	Adnexal involvement
Stage IIB	Tumour extends to extrauterine pelvic tissue
Stage III	Tumour invades abdominal tissues (not just protruding into the abdomen)
Stage IIIA	One site
Stage IIIB	More than one site
Stage IIIC	Metastases to pelvic and/or para-aortic lymph nodes
Stage IV	Tumour invades bladder and/or rectum, and/or distant metastases
Stage IVA	Tumour invades bladder and/or rectum
Stage IVB	Distant metastasis
(3)	**Carcinosarcomas**

Carcinosarcomas should be staged as carcinomas of the endometrium.

[a]Simultaneous tumours of the uterine corpus and ovary/pelvis in association with ovarian/pelvic endometriosis should be classified as independent primary tumours.

2. It is appreciated that there may be a small number of patients with uterine cancer who will be treated primarily with radiation therapy. If that is the case, the clinical staging adopted by FIGO in 1971 still would apply, but designation of that staging system would be noted.

3. Ideally, width of the myometrium should be measured along with the width of tumour invasion.

Table A.7 FIGO staging for carcinoma of the cervix

Stage 0 TIS	Carcinoma in situ, intraepithelial carcinoma
Stage I	The carcinoma is strictly confined to the cervix (extension to the corpus should be disregarded)
Stage IA	Invasive carcinoma which can be identified only by microscopy, with deepest invasion ≤5 mm and largest extension ≤7 mm
Stage IA1 T1a1 N0 M0	Measured stromal invasion of ≤3.0 mm in depth and extension of ≤7.0 mm
Stage IA2 T1a2 N0 M0	Measured stromal invasion of >3.0 mm and not >5.0 mm with an extension of not >7.0 mm
Stage IB	Clinically visible lesions limited to the cervix uteri or preclinical cancers greater than IA[a]
Stage IB1 T1b1 N0 M0	Clinically visible lesion ≤4.0 cm in greatest dimension
Stage IB2 T1b2 N0 M0	Clinically visible lesion >4.0 cm in greatest dimension
Stage II	Cervical carcinoma invades beyond the uterus, but not to the pelvic wall or to the lower third of the vagina
Stage IIA	Without parametrial invasion
Stage IIA1 T2a1 N0 M0	Clinically visible lesion ≤4.0 cm in greatest dimension
Stage IIA2 T2a2 N0 M0	Clinically visible lesion >4.0 cm in greatest dimension
Stage IIB T2b N0 M0	With obvious parametrial invasion
Stage III	The tumour extends to the pelvic wall and/or involves the lower third of the vagina and/or causes hydronephrosis or non-functioning kidney[b]
Stage IIIA T3a N0 M0	Tumour involves lower third of the vagina, with no extension to the pelvic wall
Stage IIIB T1 N1 M0 T2 N1 M0 T3a N1 M0 T3b Any N M0	Extension to the pelvic wall and/or hydronephrosis or non-functioning kidney
Stage IV	The carcinoma has extended beyond the true pelvis or has involved (biopsy proven) the mucosa of the bladder or rectum. A bullous oedema, as such, does not permit a case to be allotted to Stage IV
Stage IVA T4 Any N M0	Spread of the growth to adjacent organs
Stage IVB Any T Any N M1	Spread to distant organs

[a]All macroscopically visible lesions – even with superficial invasion – fall under stage IB carcinomas. Invasion is limited to a measured stromal invasion with a maximal depth of 5.0 mm and a horizontal extension of not >7.0 mm. Depth of invasion should not be >5.0 mm and a horizontal extension of not >7.0 mm. Depth of invasion should not be >5.0 mm taken from the base of the epithelium of the original tissue – superficial or glandular. The depth of invasion should always be reported in mm, even in those cases with "early (minimal) stromal invasion" (~1 mm). The involvement of vascular/lymphatic spaces should not change the stage allotment.
[b]On rectal examination, there is no cancer-free space between the tumour and the pelvic wall. All cases with hydronephrosis or non-functioning kidney are included, unless they are known to be due to another cause.

Table A.8 FIGO staging for carcinoma of the vagina

Stage 0	
TIS	Carcinoma in situ, intraepithelial carcinoma
Stage I	
T1 N0 M0	The carcinoma is limited to the vaginal wall
Stage II	
T2 N0 M0	The carcinoma has involved the subvaginal tissue but has not extended on to the pelvic wall
Stage III	
T1 N1 M0	The carcinoma has extended on to the pelvic wall
T2 N1 M0	
T3 N0 M0	
T3 N1 M0	
Stage IV	The carcinoma has extended beyond the true pelvis or has clinically involved the mucosa of the bladder or rectum. Bullous oedema as such does not permit a case to be allotted to Stage IV
Stage IVA	
T4 Any N M0	Spread to adjacent organs and/or direct extension beyond the true pelvis
Stage IVB	
Any T Any N M1	Spread to distant organs

Table A.9 FIGO staging for carcinoma of the vulva

Stage 0	Carcinoma in situ; intraepithelial carcinoma
Stage I	Tumour confined to the vulva
Stage IA	Lesions ≤2 cm in size, confined to the vulva or perineum and with stromal invasion ≤1.0 mm,[a] no nodal metastasis
Stage IB	Lesions >2 cm in size or with stromal invasion >1.0 mm,[a] confined to the vulva or perineum, with negative nodes
Stage II	Tumour of any size with extension to adjacent perineal structures (1/3 lower urethra, 1/3 lower vagina, anus) with negative nodes
Stage III	Tumour of any size with or without extension to adjacent perineal structures (1/3 lower urethra, 1/3 lower vagina, anus) with positive inguino-femoral lymph nodes
Stage IIIA	(i) With 1 lymph node metastasis (≥5 mm), or (ii) 1–2 lymph node metastasis(es) (<5 mm)
Stage IIIB	(i) With 2 or more lymph node metastases (≥5 mm), or (ii) 3 or more lymph node metastases (<5 mm)
Stage IIIC	With positive nodes with extracapsular spread
Stage IV	Tumour invades other regional (2/3 upper urethra, 2/3 upper vagina), or distant structures
Stage IVA	Tumour invades any of the following: (i) Upper urethral and/or vaginal mucosa, bladder mucosa, rectal mucosa, or fixed to pelvic bone, or (ii) Fixed or ulcerated inguino-femoral lymph nodes
Stage IVB	Any distant metastasis including pelvic lymph nodes

[a]The depth of invasion is defined as the measurement of the tumour from the epithelial-stromal junction of the adjacent most superficial dermal papilla to the deepest point of invasion.

Table A.10 FIGO staging for trophoblastic tumour

Stage I	Disease confined to uterus
Stage IA	Disease confined to uterus with no risk factors
Stage IB	Disease confined to uterus with one risk factor
Stage IC	Disease confined to uterus with two risk factors
Stage II	Gestational trophoblastic tumour extending outside uterus but limited to genital structures (adnexa, vagina, broad ligament)
Stage IIA	Gestational trophoblastic tumour involving genital structures without risk factors
Stage IIB	Gestational trophoblastic tumour extending outside uterus but limited to genital structures with one risk factor
Stage IIC	Gestational trophoblastic tumour extending outside uterus but limited to genital structures with two risk factors
Stage III	Gestational trophoblastic tumour extending to lungs with or without known genital tract involvement
Stage IIIA	Gestational trophoblastic tumour extending to lungs with or without genital tract involvement and with no risk factors
Stage IIIB	Gestational trophoblastic tumour extending to lungs with or without genital tract involvement and with one risk factor
Stage IIIC	Gestational trophoblastic tumour extending to lungs with or without genital tract involvement and with two risk factors
Stage IV	All other metastatic sites
Stage IVB	All other metastatic sites with one risk factor
Stage IVC	All other metastatic sites with two risk factors

Risk factors affecting staging include the following: (1) serum human chorionic gonadotropin >100,000 mIU/ml and (2) duration of disease >6 months from termination of antecedent pregnancy.

The following factors should be considered and noted in reporting: (1) Prior chemotherapy has been given for known gestational trophoblastic tumour, (2) placental site tumours should be reported separately and (3) histologic verification of disease is not required.

Index

Note: Page numbers followed by '*b*', '*f*' and '*t*' refer to boxes, figures and tables, respectively.

age-standardised incidence (or morality rate) (ASR), calculation of, 3

body mass index (BMI)
  and endometrial cancer, 118
  and laparoscopic surgery, complications of, 84, 86
  and ultrasound (US) limitations, 23

cancer datasets for cancer staging, patient management and prognosis, 22
cancer of female genital tract
  and endometriosis, 21
  management of by pathologists, 11–13
cancer screening. *See also screening of individual cancers*
  calculation of sensitivity, specificity and predictive value of screening test, 4–5, 5*t*
  definition of, 4
  screening test performance, 4–5
cervical cancer. *See also* cervical intraepithelial neoplasia (CIN)
  aetiology of, 9
  HPV and pre-invasive cervical disease, 63
  HPV as factor in, 9
  incidence and morality of in UK *vs.* world, 8–9
  prevalence of in UK, and developed countries, 127
cervical cancer, diagnosis and investigation of
  baseline blood tests for, 128
  determination of parametrial involvement, 131
  diagnosis by tissue biopsy, 128
  examination of cervix with speculum, 128
  examination under anaesthetic and clinical staging, 129–131
  post-coital bleeding, post-menopausal bleeding as symptoms, 127, 128
  signs and symptoms, 127–128
  squamous epithelium thickness, lack of maturation in, as symptom, 14*f*
  symptoms in late stages, 127
cervical cancer, diagnostic imaging in
  diagnosis by biopsy, CT, 27
  diagnostic imaging in cancer recurrence, modalities used in, 29
  image of MRI cervix and PET/CT of nodal disease, 129*f*
  imaging of lymph nodes, 128–129

magnetic resonance imaging (MRI) and radiotherapy planning, 29
magnetic resonance imaging (MRI) for assessing optimal brachytherapy position, 29
magnetic resonance imaging (MRI) for identifying complications, 29
magnetic resonance imaging (MRI) for staging investigation, 27, 28, 28*f*, 39
pelvic MRI imaging for stage IIb cervical cancer, 28
radiology in staging tumour, 27–29
repeated imaging and chemoradiation in treatment of advanced disease, 29
cervical cancer, pathology of
  histological features of, 127
  spread of cervical cancer to organs, 130
  squamous cell carcinoma, adenocarcinoma, 127
cervical cancer, prevention and screening for
  HPV DNA testing, 63
  HPV testing and cervical cytology, 63
  HR HPV testing, compared to cytology, 63
  MRI for staging investigation, 39
  NHS Cervical Screening Programme (NHSCSP), 63–64
  NHS Cervical Screening Programme (NHSCSP), management guidelines, 63
  prevention of with HPV screening, HPV vaccine, 9
  screening, importance of, 127
cervical cancer, staging of
  clinical staging, 129–131
  diagrammatic representation of staging for cervical cancer, 130*f*
  FIGO staging for carcinoma of the cervix, 204*b*
  5-year survival rates by stage, 44, 136
  magnetic resonance imaging (MRI) for staging investigation, 27, 28, 28*f*, 39
  pelvic MR imaging for stage IIb cervical cancer, 28
  stage I, 28, 43–44
  stage II, 28, 44
  stage III, 26, 44
  stage IVA, local invasion of bladder or bowel, 28, 44
cervical cancer, surgical management of. *See also* cervical cancer, treatment of
  cone biopsy, 131–132
  fertility-sparing surgery, 132

pelvic lymph node dissection, 132
radical hysterectomy, 132
radical trachelectomy, 132
sentinel lymph node mapping in cervical cancer surgery, 132
cervical cancer, treatment by stage. *See also* cervical cancer, treatment of
  adjuvant treatment post-surgery with chemoradiotherapy, for stage IB2 to stage IIIB, stage IV, 131
  combined external beam radiotherapy and brachytherapy as treatment for stage Ib1, small volume IIa, 44
  hysterectomy and lymphadenectomy as treatment for stage Ib1, small volume IIa, 44
  laparoscopic surgery for early-stage disease, 86
  large loop excision of transformation zone (LLETZ) as treatment for Stage Ia1 in younger patients, 43
  radiotherapy with chemotherapy as treatment for stage Ib2, IVa, or locally advanced disease, 44
  stage IA1, 131
  stage IA2, 131
  stage IB1, range of tumours, 131
cervical cancer, treatment of
  adjuvant radiotherapy for women with node-positive disease, 39
  adjuvant radiotherapy, chemoradiotherapy for recurrence, 45
  adjuvant treatment, 133
  cervix brachytherapy, 46*f*
  exenerative surgery for recurrence, 39
  hysterectomy and pelvic lymph node dissection for stage IBI, 39
  laparoscopic surgery for, 95–96
  neoadjuvant chemotherapy, 133
  ovarian transposition, in in vitro fertilization, 133
  palliative care, 39
  pan-aortic radiotherapy, survival rates of, 44
  pelvic radiotherapy, and loss of fertility, 133
  primary chemoradiotherapy, 133
  psychosexual counselling in, 39
  radical radiotherapy and chemo for stage IB2 and above, 39
  radical surgery, 39
  radiotherapy, 39

207

cervical cancer, treatment of (*cont.*)
  radiotherapy, planning of, 40
  recurrence, determining risk of, 45
  superior technique of IMRT allowing
    the dose prescribed to be tightly
    conformed to the target volume, thus
    sparing the organs at risk, 45*f*
  time of completion, importance of with
    radical chemoradiotherapy, 39
cervical intraepithelial neoplasia (CIN)
  classification of, 62–63
  definition of, 62
  grading system of, 62–63
  and HPV, 64
  and progression of oncogenic HPV
    infection, 64
  risk factors of, 62
chemotherapy. See also *Systemic therapy and
    chemotherapy for individual cancers*
  CHORUS (chemotherapy or upfront
    surgery) trial, 60
  cytotoxic chemotherapy, basic
    principles of, 52
  myelosuppression, as side effect of
    chemotherapy, 60
  neoadjuvant chemotherapy (NACT), 60
  post-surgery chemotherapy, 60
  sepsis, risk of from chemotherapy, 60
  toxicities of, 52–53
chemotherapy, specific agents of
  angiogenesis inhibitors, 55–56
  anthracyclines, 54
  anti-metabolites, 55
  anti-microtubule agents (taxanes), 53–54
  anti-tumour antibiotics, 55
  bevacizumab, administration and mode
    of action of, 55–56
  bevacizumab, adverse effects of, 56
  bevacizumab, therapeutic uses of, 56
  biological agents, 55–56
  bleomycin, administration and mode of
    action of, 55
  bleomycin, adverse effects of, 55
  bleomycin, therapeutic use of, 55
  carboplatin and cisplatin, administration
    and mode of action of, 53
  carboplatin and cisplatin, adverse effects
    of, 53
  carboplatin and cisplatin, therapeutic
    uses of, 53
  doxorubicin (adriamycin) and pegylated
    liposomal doxorubicin (PLD),
    administration and mode of
    action of, 54
  doxorubicin (adriamycin) and pegylated
    liposomal doxorubicin (PLD), adverse
    effects of, 54
  doxorubicin (adriamycin) and pegylated
    liposomal doxorubicin (PLD),
    therapeutic uses of, 54
  gemcitabine, administration and mode of
    action of, 55
  gemcitabine, adverse effects of, 55
  gemcitabine, therapeutic uses of, 55
  niraparib and olaparib, administration
    and mode of action of, 56

niraparib and olaparib, adverse effects
  of, 56
niraparib and olaparib, therapeutic uses
  of, 56
paclitaxel and docetaxel, administration
  of and mode of action of, 53
paclitaxel and docetaxel, adverse effects
  of, 53–54
paclitaxel and docetaxel, therapeutic uses
  of, 54
PARP inhibitors, 56
platinum agents of, 53
topoisomerase inhibitors, 54–55
topotecan and etoposide, administration
  of, 55
topotecan and etoposide, adverse effects
  of, 55
topotecan and etoposide, mode of action
  of, 54
topotecan and etoposide, therapeutic
  uses of, 55
choriocarcinoma. See also *gestational
    trophoblastic disease* (GTD)
  epidemiology, origin and pathology of,
    160–161
  symptoms of, 161
choricarcinoma, diagnosis and
    investigation of
  diagnosis and investigation, management
    in, 162
  MRI scan showing multiple brain
    metastases with haemorrhage
    before and after central nervous
    system (CNS)-modified etoposide,
    methotrexate and actinomycin D/
    cyclophosphamide and vincristine
    (EMA/CO) chemotherapy, 162*f*
clinical drug trials
  Phase 0 trials, 197
  Phase I trials, 197
  Phase II, 197
  Phase III, 197
  Phase IV, 197
communication in gynaecological
    oncology
  ABCDE mnemonic for breaking bad
    news, 192, 193*t*
  aids to communicating evidence for
    decision-making about anticancer
    therapy in the palliative setting, 194*b*
  aids to discussing transitions from
    curative to palliative care, 194*b*
  barriers in diagnosing 'dying', 195*b*
  breaking bad news, and five stages of
    grief, 192–193
  breaking bad news, pitfalls of, 193
  breaking bad news, tools for, 192–193
  communication training, 192
  dialogue between doctors, patients, 191
  end-of-life communication, 194–196
  end-of-life communication, desired
    results of, 194*b*
  information exchange between doctors,
    patients, 191–192
  internal conflict of patient, complications
    of, 192

multi-disciplinary teams (MDTs), role of,
  188–189
National Cancer Patient Experience
  Survey on information needs of
  patients, 193
patient-reported communication needs
  and information requests, 193–194
SPIKES model for breaking bad news,
  192, 193*t*
Cowden syndrome (CS)
  in endometrial cancer, 113
cumulative incidence, 3

decision-making in gynaecological
    oncology
  in adjuvant treatment, 36
  decision-making approaches in
    gynaecological oncology, 36, 37*b*
  and genetic testing, 74
  and local *vs.* systemic treatment, 36–37
  in palliative treatment, 36, 109
  in radical/curative treatment, 36
  treatment and patient factors, 37
  tumour factors, as treatment
    consideration, 37
diagnosis and investigation of malignancies.
    See also *diagnosis and investigation of
    individual cancers*
  examination steps, 11–13
  frozen section analysis in, 13
  and lymph node involvement, 12–13
  lymphovascular invasion, examination
    of, 12
  and tumour grade, 12
  and tumour stage, 12
  and tumour types, 12
  vascular invasion, examination of, 12
diagnostic imaging. See also *diagnostic
    imaging for individual cancers*
  computerised tomography, phases of,
    24–25
  for diagnosis, treatment planning and
    follow-up, 23–40
  magnetic resonance imaging (MRI),
    conventional imaging sequences of,
    23–24
  magnetic resonance imaging (MRI),
    limitations of, 24
  positron emission tomography (PET),
    with computerised tomography, 25
  ultrasound (US) limitations in patients
    with large body mass index
    (BMI), 23
disability-adjusted life-years (lost),
    calculation of, 4
doll, Sir Richard, 3

endometrial cancer. See also *endometrial
    hyperplasia*
  aetiology of, 8, 112
  age and risk of recurrence of, 47
  Cancer Genome Atlas (TCGA) project
    classification of, 46
  classification of by World Health
    Organization (WHO), 115, 115*t*
  and Cowden syndrome (CS), 76, 113

criteria to identify high risk families of breast, ovarian cancer/endometrial cancer, 73t
cure rate for, 46
and fertility preservation, 186
GOG definition of high-intermediate risk, 47
as hereditary cancer, 71
high dose oral progesterone and/or locally delivered progesterone for early-stage type I, 186
incidence and mortality rates in UK vs. world, 6
and Lynch syndrome (LS), 76, 112–113
malignant progression of, 112
obesity and diabetes as risks for, 8
oestrogens and progestins, role of in malignant transformation, 8
relapse risk of, 118
in women under 45 years of age, 186
in women under 50 years of age, 113
endometrial cancer, diagnosis and investigation of. See also endometrial cancer, staging of
abnormal non-cervical glandular cells on cervical smear as sign of endometrial abnormality, 113
algorithm for assessment of post-menopausal bleeding, 114f
characteristics of type 1 and type 2 endometrial cancer, 17t
clinical history and examination of, 118
endometrial thickness as diagnosis marker, 25, 114
five-year survival following diagnosis of endometrial cancer, 125t
NICE guidelines, 113
postmenopausal bleeding as warning sign of, 25, 113–114
pre-operative investigation of, 118–120
prognosis factors, 124–125
referral guidelines and diagnostic testing, 113–114
symptoms of, 113
tamoxifen as cause of benign symptoms, 114
trans-vaginal ultrasound scan as initial diagnostic tool, 114
endometrial cancer, diagnostic imaging in computerised tomography (CT), role in advanced disease, 27
CT imaging for patients at high risk of recurrence, 27
diagnosis using high-resolution imaging with transvaginal ultrasound (TVUS), 25
MRI imaging in endometrial cancer, 25–26, 26f
MRI scan for pre-treatment evaluation of endometrial cancer, 120f
pre-operative imaging in management of endometrial cancer, 118–120
endometrial cancer, pathology of haematogenous spread, 116
lymphatic spread to lymph nodes, 116
metastasization, 116

trans-tubal spread to fallopian tubes, 116
type I tumours, in early-stage diagnosis, 115
type II tumours, in higher-stage diagnosis, 115
endometrial cancer, prevention and screening of
population screening for endometrial cancer, in asymptomatic women, 116
risk factors associated with, 8t
risk factors for endometrioid endometrial cancers (EEC), 112
and risk for VTE, 124
risk-reducing surgery for women with genetic predisposition, 116
screening for women with genetic predisposition, history of Lynch syndrome, 116
and smoking as risk factor, 112
endometrial cancer, staging of
AJCC (American Joint Committee on Cancer Tumour, Node, Metastasis System for, 116
FIGO Staging for Carcinoma of the Corpus Uteri, 202b
FIGO System (International Federation of Obstetrics and Gynaecology) for, 116
stage I, 26
stage IIIa, IIIb, IIIc, 26
stage IV, 26–27
staging system for endometrial cancer, 25–27, 48
endometrial cancer, treatment of
adjuvant chemotherapy, 38
adjuvant external beam radiotherapy, dose fractionations for, 49
adjuvant radiotherapy for high-intermediate risk patients, 47
adjuvant radiotherapy for stage II, 38–39
adjuvant therapy for, 47
adjuvant treatment for advanced disease, 123
adjuvant treatment for early-stage disease, 123–124
for advanced disease, 121
chemotherapy agents used in, 124
endometrial ablation, as contraindicated for, 118
external beam radiotherapy with a brachytherapy boost for stage II disease, 47–48
fertility-sparing treatment for, 124
fertility-sparing treatment, inefficacy of, 118
field borders for conformal radiotherapy treatment, 48
high-risk disease, recommendations for treatment, 48
hormonal therapy in palliative treatment for recurrent or advanced disease, 124
hysterectomy for stage II, 38
hysterectomy with bilateral salpingo-oophorectomy, as treatment, 47
intra-operative complications of, 121

laparoscopic surgery for, 96, 121
laparoscopic surgery for early-stage disease, 86
levonorgestrel intrauterine system as fertility-preserving treatment, 118
lymphadenectomy for, 38, 121
modern high dose rate (HDR) brachytherapy for early-stage endometrial cancer, 43
neo-adjuvant chemotherapy for, 124
for obese women, 96
omentectomy/omental biopsy in, 38, 121
out-patient hysterectomy for, 114f
palliative care treatment, 39
palliative treatment for recurrent disease, 124
para-aortic radiotherapy, 49
Post-Operative Radiation Therapy in Endometrial Cancer (PORTEC) criteria for high-intermediate risk, 47
radiotherapy as primary treatment, 46–49
radiotherapy types in treatment of endometrial cancer, 122
radiotherapy, side effects and complications of, 123
radiotherapy/chemotherapy for women with recurrent and advanced disease, 39
removal of uterus, cervix, fallopian tubes and ovaries in, 38
risk of adjuvant treatment, 47
surgery as treatment of low-risk disease, 47
surgical complications in, 121–122
vaginal brachytherapy as sole adjuvant treatment, 49
vaginal brachytherapy for stage IB disease, 47–48
endometrial hyperplasia
algorithm for treatment of atypical endometrial hyperplasia (AH), 119f
classification system for, 68
endometrial hyperplasia with atypia, and risk of developing cancer, 69–70
endometrial hyperplasia with atypia, investigation and treatment of, 69–70
endometrial hyperplasia without atypia, 69
epidemiology of, 68–69
hysterectomy as treatment for, 69
hysterectomy for atypical hyperplasia, 118
management of, 69f, 117–118
epidemiology
description of, 1
in public health, 1

gestational trophoblastic disease (GTD)
β-hCG as tumour marker, 156
CHM diagnosis and investigation, steps for, 158
CHM, PHM and serial hCG monitoring, 158
CHM, PHM symptoms, 157

gestational trophoblastic disease (GTD) (*cont.*)
FIGO staging for trophoblastic tumour, 206*b*
GTD and registration in UK, 158
human chorionic gonadotrophin (hCG) production and GTD, 157
hydatidiform moles (CHM and PHM), epidemiology, origin and pathology of, 157–158
hydatidiform moles, description of, 157
procedures for molar pregnancy, 158
serial hCG and tumour marker for, 157
gestational trophoblastic disease (GTD), treatment of
chemotherapy for, 159
chemotherapy for high-risk disease, 160
chemotherapy for low-risk disease, 159–160
FIGO prognostic scoring system for GTD post-treatment, 160*t*
graph of hCG in patient with low-risk disease, 161*f*
management of specific complication of, 163–164
pelvic ultrasound showing large gestational trophoblastic tumour that developed after molar pregnancy and chemotherapy, 159, 160*f*
prognosis and follow-up of, 164
prognosis of, 163
gynaecological cancer, staging of. *See also staging of individual cancers*
FIGO clinical staging, rules for, 198–199
metastatis, staging of, 201*b*
regional lymph nodes, staging of, 200*b*
TNM system, 199–200
gynaecological cancers. *See also entries for individual cancers*
classification of by International Classification of Diseases for Oncology (ICD-O-3), 2
classification of by International Statistical Classification of Diseases and Related Health Problems, 1
five ways to well-being of women living with long-term disease, 177
incidence rate of, 3
morphological classification of malignant neoplasms of female genital organs, 2*t*
ten most common causes of cancer deaths of women in UK, 2014, 198*f*
treatment approaches in, 34–40
twenty most common cancer in UK in 2014, 198*f*

hereditary gynaecological cancers. *See also Lynch syndrome (LS)*
Cowden syndrome (CS), and breast cancer, endometrial cancer, 76
criteria to identify high risk families of breast, ovarian cancer/endometrial cancer, 73*t*
and determining risk using family history, 71
diagnostic genetic testing compared to predictive genetic testing, 72

diagnostic genetic testing, as advocated by international bodies, 72
genetic evaluation of ovarian tumours, 75
genetic testing and decision-making process, 74
genetic testing for, 71
genetic testing for BRCA1/BRCA2 mutations in Ashkenazi Jews in UK, 72
genetic testing for ovarian cancer in high-risk women, lack of programs for, 74
hereditary breast and/or ovarian cancer syndromes, 72
hereditary ovarian cancers and BRCA and BRCA2 mutations, 72
moderate risk genetic mutations for hereditary ovarian cancers, 73
and percentage of ovarian cancer, endometrial cancer, 71
Peutz-Jeghers Syndrome, 76
risk-reducing salpingo-oophorectomy (RRSO) for risk of ovarian cancer, 74
risk-reducing strategies for hereditary cancers, 74–75
risk-reducing surgery for genetic predisposition for endometrial cancer, 116
summary of hereditary gynaeocological cancers, 72*t*
syndromes of, 71
hormonal therapies for gynaecological cancers
anastrazole and letrozole, administration and mode of action of, 57
anastrazole and letrozole, adverse effects of, 57
anastrazole and letrozole, therapeutic uses of, 57
aromatase inhibitors, 57
medroxyprogesterone acetate and megestrol acetate, administration and mode of action of, 57
medroxyprogesterone acetate and megestrol acetate, adverse effects of, 57
medroxyprogesterone acetate and megestrol acetate, therapeutic uses of, 57
oestrogen receptor modulators, 56–57
progestogens, 174
tamoxifen adverse effects of, 57
tamoxifen, administration and mode of action of, 56
tamoxifen, dosing of, 56
tamoxifen, therapeutic uses of, 57
human papillomavirus (HPV)
and anal intraepithelial neoplasia (AIN), 126
in cervical and vaginal tumours, 126
in cervical cancer, 9, 64
and cervical intraepithelial neoplasia (CIN), 126
and development of CIN, 64
genome comprisal of, 126
HPV testing and cervical cytology, 63
NHSCSP Colposcopy and Programme management guidelines for HPV DNA testing, 63

in pathology of gynaecological cancers, 11
and pre-invasive cervical disease, 62
and smoking, 64
vaccination programme in UK, 64, 127
vaccine and cancer reduction rates, 127
vaccine for, 64
and vaginal cancer, risk of, 49, 126–127, 134
and vaginal intraepithelial neoplaisa (VAIN), 126
vulval cancer and prevalence of HPV infection, 146
and vulval cancer, pathology of, 139–140
and vulval intraepithelial neoplasia (VIN), 126

incidence rate. *See also incidence rates of individual cancers*
definition of, 3
frequency distribution (%) of the 22 most common cancers in women, England 2003–2007, 6*f*
partial (or limited duration) incidence, mathematical equation of, 31
trends in UK, 6
use in gynaecological oncology, 3, 5
informed consent
and multi-disciplinary meetings (MDTMs), 190
patient's capacity for, 190–191
pre-requisites for, 190

laparoscopic surgery
advantages of, 86
and BMI as special consideration, 85–86
and BMI, risk of complications with, 84
for cervical cancer, 95–96
and early-stage endometrial and cervical cancer, 86
electrosurgery devices for, 84*f*
for endometrial cancer, 96
energy devices for minimal access and open surgery, principles of, 84–85
energy devices for, types of, 84–85
energy devices, complications of, 85
entry techniques and incisions, 83
equipment for, 88
ergonomics of setup for, 88
fertility-sparing approaches in gynaecologic oncology, 86*t*
laparoscopy and avoidance of diathermy, 94
laparoscopy and BMI-related complications, 94
laparoscopy and risk of conversion to laparotomy, 90
laparoscopy, anaesthetic considerations for, 92
laparoscopy, avoiding complications and injury from, 93–94
laparoscopy, complications of, 92–94
laparoscopy, energy sources for, 85

laparoscopy, establishment of pneumoperitoneum and primary port placement for, 90–91
laparoscopy, positioning of patient for, 90
laparoscopy, post-operative programme for, 86
laparoscopy, range of equipment for, 91
laparoscopy, rate of complications from, 92
laparoscopy, recovery time from, 92
laparoscopy, special considerations for, 94–95
primary and accessory port site placement in relation to vessels of anterior abdominal wall, 84f
and rate of post-operative adverse events, 86
relationship between bifurcation of aorta and umbilicus in normal body weight and obesity, 86f
vs. robotic surgery, 86
robotically-assisted laparoscopic surgery, 95
role of laparoscopic surgery in gynaecological cancers, 86
transperitoneal para-aortic node dissection, 96f
laparoscopy. See entries under Laparoscopic surgery
living with gynaecological cancer
Cancer Recovery Package, as strategized by Independent Cancer Taskforce, 182–183
cancer survivor, definition of by Macmillan Cancer Support, 181
five-year strategy for cancer services, by Independent Cancer Taskforce in UK, 182
holistic care, as part of cancer services, 184
Holistic Needs Assessment (HNA), role of in management and care, 183
and infertility, 186
Macmillan Cancer Support, role of in UK, 181
Macmillan/NCIN simplified survivorship outcome framework, 181
NHS Recovery Package, as support for individuals living with cancer, 182
Patient Reported Outcome Measures (PROMS) questionnaire, and quality of life, 184
Patient Reported Outcome Measures (PROMS) questionnaire, restrictions of, 183
and quality of life as multidimensional concept, 185
quality of life, measurement of in clinical trials, 185
and sexuality, 184–185
survival, length and complexity of as defined by Macmillan Cancer Support, NCIN, 181
and survivor framework, 182
survivorship pathways, 181–182

lymphoedema
assessment of, 185
incidence of in cancer survivors, 185
management of, 185
and quality of life, 185
Lynch syndrome (LS)
Amsterdam II guidelines for clinical diagnosis of, 113b
in endometrial cancer, 76, 112–113
and hereditary disease, 75–76
in ovarian cancer, 76
revised Bethesda guidelines for identification of patients for whom microsatellite instability (MSI) testing is warranted, 113b
screening for women with genetic predisposition, history of Lynch syndrome, 116

malignant germ cell tumours
in premenopausal, postmenopausal women, 153
tumour types, 153
malignant germ cell tumours, diagnosis and investigation of
symptoms of, 154
tumour markers, 154
malignant germ cell tumours, treatment of
fertility-sparing surgery, 154
follow-up requirements for, 155
neoadjuvant chemotherapy in, 154–155
for relapsed disease, 155
for stage IA/B disease, 154–155
for stage IC and above disease, 155
surgery for complete tumour resection and staging, 154
markers used in diagnosis, management and prognostication of tumours
diagnostic immunohistochemistry (IHC), 22
markers to aid management of tumours, 22
molecular pathology for diagnosis, treatment, prognostication of tumours, 22
metastatic tumours, 20–21
minimal access surgery (MAS). See also laparoscopic surgery
and conversion to laparotomy, risk of complications from, 90
pre-operative factors to consider, 89
molar pregnancy. See gestational trophoblastic disease (GTD)
mortality. See also survival
cancer mortality rates, 4
definition of, 4
multi-disciplinary team (MDT)
clinical management decisions by, 188–189
communication, importance of, 188–189
definition of by NHS, 188
improving the effectiveness of multidisciplinary team meetings in cancer services, 189b
key components of, 189b
MDT meetings (MDTM), role of, 188–189

non-epithelial ovarian tumours, classification of, 153, 153t

ovarian cancer
aetiology of, 6
average number of new cases per year and age-specific incidence rates per 100,000 population in UK, 98f
criteria to identify high risk families of breast, ovarian cancer/endometrial cancer, 73t
early detection of in UK, strategies for, 29
epithelial ovarian cancer (EOC) in women with hereditary nonpolyposis colon cancer (HNPCC) syndrome, 100
epithelial ovarian cancer (EOC), description of, 98
and fertility preservation for patients with stage IA epithelial ovarian cancer, 186–187
genetic evaluation of ovarian tumours, 75
genetic testing in high-risk women, lack of programs for, 74
as hereditary cancer, 71, 99
hereditary ovarian cancer syndromes, 72
hereditary ovarian cancers and BRCA and BRCA2 mutations, 72, 99, 99t
and Lynch syndrome (LS), 76
moderate-risk genetic mutations for hereditary ovarian cancers, 73
protective factors of ovarian cancer, 99t
recurrence, risk of, 32–33, 110
recurrent disease, classification of, 107–108
Risk of Malignancy Index (RMI), 102t
risk rates of, 98
survival rates in UK vs. Canada, Australia, Norway, Sweden, 98
theories on association between ovarian cancer and number of ovulation theory, 98–99
ovarian cancer, diagnosis and investigation of. See also ovarian cancer, staging of
borderline ovarian tumours, clinical presentation and diagnoses of, 109
by computed tomography (CT), 102
flow diagram of investigation and management, 103f
investigation, components of, 101
NICE Guidance recommendation of investigation with tumour marker Caner Antigen 125 (CA125), 101
oral contrast to identify serial disease, 31
RCOG Greentop Guideline 34 recommendations for investigation, 101
tumour markers for diagnosis, 101–102
typical symptoms, 101
ultrasonography, 102
USS classification system to differentiate benign and malignant factors, 102, 102t
ovarian cancer, diagnostic imaging in
computerised tomography (CT), 30–31
computerised tomography (CT), as primary staging method, 31

ovarian cancer, diagnostic imaging in (cont.)
    CT image following administration of
        intravenous contrast medium, 31, 32f
    magnetic resonance imaging (MRI) to
        characterize masses, 31
    pelvic ultrasound, 29–30
    PET/CT for demonstrating tumour
        recurrence, 33
    PET/CT imaging, 31
    ultrasound (US) imaging of ovarian
        cancer, 29–30
ovarian cancer, palliative care for
    bowel obstruction as complication in, 108
    decision making in, 109
    measures used to reduce vomiting, 108
    medications for symptom relief, 109
ovarian cancer, pathology of
    borderline ovarian tumours (BOT) vs.
        low-grade ovarian carcinomas, 109
    borderline ovarian tumours, clinical
        presentation and diagnosis of, 109
    borderline ovarian tumours, pathological
        features of, 109
    clear cell tumours, 100
    endometrioid tumours, 100
    high-grade serous ovarian carcinoma
        (HGSOC) and fallopian tube
        hypothesis, 100–101
    metastases, 100
    mucinous borderline tumours, 109
    mucinous tumours, 100
    serous borderline tumours, 109
    serous ovarian carcinomas (SOC), 100
ovarian cancer, prevention and
        screening for
    BRCA carriers, limited benefits of
        screening of, 99
    BRCA mutations, screening for, 99
    in general population, 100
    and mortality rates, 70
    prevention of, 6–7
    risk-reducing early salpingectomy with
        delayed oophorectomy (RRESDO), for
        epithelial ovarian cancer, 75
    risk-reducing salpingo-oophorectomy
        (RRSO) for women at risk, 74
    risks for, 3
ovarian cancer, staging of
    ascites as predicator for stage IIIB/C, 32
    computerised tomography (CT), as
        primary staging method, 31
    diagrammatic representation of staging
        for ovarian cancer, 104f
    FIGO staging for carcinoma of the ovary,
        200–203
    FIGO system, use of, 31, 104
    malignant ovarian germ cell tumours, as
        stage I cancer in women below 20 years
        of age, 187
    pleural effusion for detection of stage
        IVA, IVB, 32
    radiological and histological staging
        using CT imaging, 104–105
    stage I, 31
    stage II, 31
    stage III, 31

stage IIIA, B, C, 31–32
staging and surgery for advanced ovarian
    cancer, 105
staging surgery for suspected stage,
    elements of, 105
widespread military deposits in case of
    advanced ovarian cancer, 105f
ovarian cancer, treatment of
    bevacizumab, as anti-angiogenic agent
        for advanced-stage epithelial ovarian,
        fallopian tube and primary peritoneal
        cancers, 61
    chemotherapy for advanced-stage
        disease, 107
    chemotherapy for early-stage
        disease, 107
    chemotherapy for recurrent disease,
        107–108
    chemotherapy, description of, 38
    consolidation and maintenance therapy
        for recurrent disease, 108
    cytoreductive surgery (CRS), 38
    cytoreductive surgery (CRS) for
        advanced disease, procedure and terms
        for, 105–106
    cytoreductive surgical approach
        combined with chemotherapy,
        approaches to, 106–107
    fertility-sparing procedures, option for
        patients with borderline tumours, non-
        epithelial ovarian cancers, and early-
        stage 1A epithelial ovarian cancers, 108
    fertility-sparing surgery, elements of, 108
    histological confirmation in, 38
    hyperthermic intraperitoneal
        chemotherapy (HIPEC), 107
    midline incision in non-early stages, use
        of, 38
    palliative chemotherapy in, 38
    palliative radiotherapy in, 38
    primary surgery in, 38
    radical surgery for stage IV, 38
    recurrence rates after chemotherapy,
        107–108
    risk-reducing surgery for BRCA carriers,
        99–100
    secondary cytoreductive surgery for
        recurrent disease after primary
        treatment, 38
    surgery and systemic therapy in, 60
    surgery for recurrent disease, 108
ovarian sex cord stromal tumours
    and genetic mutations, 155
    histopathology diagnosis of, 155
ovarian sex cord stromal tumours, diagnosis
        and investigation of
    association of granulosa cell tumours
        and complex atypical hyperplasia or
        carcinoma of the endometrium, 156
    symptoms of, 155
    tumour markers, 156
ovarian sex cord stromal tumours,
        treatment of
    adjuvant treatment, 156
    of recurrent disease, 156
    surgical management in, 156

palliative care. See also palliative care for
        individual cancers
    anxiety and depression, approach to, 175
    breathlessness, management of, 175
    complex fungating and malodorous
        wounds, management of, 174
    constipation, management and
        prevention of, 172–173
    definition of, 165
    end of life phase in, 177–178
    hypercalcaemia, careful considerations
        for, 173–174
    hypercalcaemia, diagnosis and symptoms
        of, 173
    hypercalcaemia, treatment of, 173
    and nausea/vomiting, 171
    nausea/vomiting, other causes of, 171
    outline of generalist and specialist
        care aspects of problems typical
        of those occurring in women with
        gynaecological malignancies: the
        generalist palliative care, 167t
    pain management in, 168–170
    pain, types of, 170
    partial bowel obstruction, as cause of
        nausea/vomiting, 171
    partial bowel obstruction, management
        of, 171
    practical issues in, 175
palliative care, drugs used in
    anti-emetics, 171–172
    anti-emetics acting on serotonin
        receptors, 172
    anti-emetics acting principally in
        chemoreceptor trigger zone
        (CTZ), 172
    anti-emetics acting principally in the
        vomiting centre in central nervous
        system, 172
    antispasmodic and antisecretory anti-
        emetics, 172
    broad spectrum anti-emetics, 172
    dexamethasone, 172
    pro-kinetic anti-emetics, 172
    symptom control, principles of, 165
    typical prescription for an opioid-naive
        patient with partial bowel obstruction,
        171–172
palliative care, psychosocial issues in
    alienation of patient, 176
    anger of patient and caregiver, 176
    breakdown of relationships, 176–177
    carer distress and exhaustion, 176
pathologists
    and management of malignancies of
        female genital tract, 11–13
    pathologist report for
        gynaecological cancers, required
        information for, 79
pathology of gynaecological cancers.
        See also pathologies of individual cancers
    genetic mutations, role of, 11
    HPV, role of, 11
    neoplasm, role of, 11
patient-centred care
    decision making in, 58

performance status (PS), definition of, 58–59
and quality of life, 59–60
peritoneum tumours, 21
pre-invasive cervical disease
    cervical glandular intraepithelial neoplasia (CGIN), features of, 14, 15t
    cervical glandular intraepithelial neoplasia (CGIN), treatment of, 66
    colposcopy for diagnosis of, 65–66
    cytology results of, 65
    excision biopsy, as treatment of, 66
    hysterectomy, as treatment of, 66
    management of, 65–66
    management of in special circumstances, 67t
    NHSCCP programme standards for management of, 65
    screening protocol algorithm and colposcopy management recommendations for CIN/GIN, 65f
    treatment of with large loop excision of the transformation zone (LLETZ), 66
pre-invasive disease. See also individual pre-invasive diseases
    cervical intraepithelial neoplasia (CIN), definition of, 62
    cervical intraepithelial neoplasia (CIN), grading system of, 62–63
    cervical intraepithelial neoplasia (CIN), risk factors for, 62
    classification of by CIN I-III, Lower Anogenital Squamous Terminology (LAST) project, Bethesda classification, 62
    HPV and pre-invasive cervical disease, 62
pre-invasive endometrial disease. See endometrial hyperplasia
pre-invasive vaginal disease. See vaginal intraepithelial neoplasia (VaIN)
pre-invasive vulvar disease. See vulvar intraepithelial neoplasia (VIN)
preinvasive and neoplastic disease of the female genital tract
    pathology of, 13–17
prevalence, definition of, 3
    complete prevalence, 4
public health, definition of, 1

quality of life
    elements of, 36t
    and living with gynaecological cancer, 184
    measurement of in clinical trials, 185
    in patient-centered care, 59–60
    and radiotherapy, 46
quality-adjusted life-year (lost), calculation of, 4

radiation therapy. See radiotherapy
radiotherapy. See also radiotherapy for individual cancers
    accelerated repopulation as strategy for exploitation of radio-resistant cells, 42
    biological basis of, 42
    for hypoxic areas of tumour, 42

modern high dose rate (HDR) brachytherapy for early-stage endometrial cancer, 43
    pelvic field with suggested field borders for anterior beam arrangement, 45f
    and quality of life, 46
    radiosensitivity of cells, factors of, 42
    radiotherapy, definition and types of, 41
    and redistribution of cells around cell cycle, 42
    for repair of sub-lethal damage, 42
    small lead multi-leaf collimators, use in shaping radiotherapy beam to fit target volume, 42f
    toxicities from, 46
    typical linear accelerator with added cone beam CT for image-guided radiotherapy, 41f
    units of radiation and dose-limiting effects, 42–43
radiotherapy machines, 43

serous tubal intraepitheilial carcinoma (STIC)
    diagnostic criteria of, 70
    imaging of, 70
    lesions of, description, 70
    progression and prognosis of, 70
    sectioning and extensively examining the (SEE-FIM) protocol for fallopian tube histological assessment, 70
sex cord tumours, 20
    fibroma (benign) tumours, 20
specimen pathway
    and fixation of specimen, 21
    request form for, 78
surgery and systemic therapy. See also chemotherapy
    approaches to, 60
    bevacizumab, as anti-angiogenic agent for advanced-stage epithelial ovarian, fallopian tube and primary peritoneal cancers, 61
    CHORUS (chemotherapy or upfront surgery) trial, 60
    clinical trials in, 61
    EORTC 55971 trial, 60
    interval debulking surgery (IDS), 60
    neoadjuvant chemotherapy (NACT), 60
    post-surgery chemotherapy, 60
    primary debulking surgery (PDS), 60
    in treatment of epithelial ovarian, fallopian tube and primary peritoneal cancers, 60
surgery in gynaecological oncology. See also laparoscopic surgery
    abdominal incisions in gynaecological oncology surgery, 83f
    basics of surgical principles, 77–78t
    bladder Injury, as inoperative complication, 79
    bowel injury, as inoperative issue, 79
    bowel preparation for, 79
    and dehydration prevention, 79
    and discussion of patient's needs and expectations, 77

for endometrial cancer in obese women, surgery approaches to, 96
    enhanced recovery programme, 82b
    faecal peritonitis, as inoperative complication, 79
    and haemorrhage, 80
    and importance of knowledge of anatomical structures and individual variations, 80
    incision types, 81
    inoperative issue and complications, 79–81
    mobilization, role in surgical recovery, 80
    open abdominal incisions, risk factors of, 82
    optimization of patient requirements for pre-operative preparation, 78
    and post-operative infection, 80–81
    post-operative pain relief and control methods, 81
    pre-operative investigations to identify risk and clinical condition, 77–79
    pre-operative issues, and impact on fertility, 77
    principles to follow when making choice of approach and site of incision, 82b
    risk factors for post-operative complications, 81t
    thromboprophylaxis and thromboembolic deterrent (TED) stocking, for recovery, 81
    ureter injury, as inoperative complication, 79
    ureteric leak, as inoperative complication, 80
    venous thromboembolism (VTE), as post-operative complication, 81
survival
    definition of, 4
    5-year survival following diagnosis of endometrial cancer, 125t
    5-year survival rate post-exenterative surgery for vaginal cancer, 136
    5-year survival rates of cervical cancer by stage, 44
    5-year survival rates post-treatment of vaginal cancer, 136
    ovarian cancer, survival rates of in UK vs. Canada, Australia, Norway, Sweden, 4
    pan-aortic radiotherapy for cervical cancer, survival rates of, 44
    and recurrence of vaginal cancer, 146
    relative survival, calculation of, 4
    vaginal cancer treated with radiotherapy, survival rates of, 49
    vulval cancer, survival rates of, 50
systemic therapy. See also surgery and systemic therapy
    assessment of response to, 58
    histology report, use of, 57
    radiological assessment of, 58
    single agent as basis of palliative chemotherapy, 58
    single agent vs. combination chemotherapy, 57–58

systemic therapy (*cont.*)
  standardising the assessment of tumour
    response, 58
  summary of the WHO and RECIST 1.1
    Response Criterias, 59*t*

teamwork. *See also* multi-disciplinary team
    (MDT)
  benefits of teamwork in monitoring and
    treatment of cancer, 34–35
  disagreement among multidisciplinary
    teams (MDTs), 35
  working in teams as recommendations of
    the Improving Outcomes Guidance by
    Department of Health, 34
treatment. *See also treatment of individual
    cancers*
  adjuvant treatment, as line of treatment,
    118–119
  approaches to, 34–40
  extent of treatment, local *vs.* systemic,
    36–37
  palliative, as line of treatment, 36
  patient factors, as treatment
    consideration, 37
  radical/curative, as line of treatment, 36
  teamwork, benefits of in monitoring and
    treatment of cancer, 34–35
  therapeutic ratio of intended treatment
    for radical, adjuvant and palliative, 37
  treatment intent, importance of, 36
  tumour factors, as treatment
    consideration, 37
tumour classification
  with Tumour Node Metastatis
    Classification of Malignant Tumours
    (TNM-8), 2
tumour types and abnormalities in disease
    of cervix. *See also* cervical cancer
  cervical adenosquamous carcinoma, 16
  cervical glandular intraepithelial
    neoplasia (CGIN), 14
  cervical intraepithelial neoplasia (CIN), 14
  cervical neuroendocrine carcinoma, 16
  distinguishing CGIN from invasive
    carcinoma, 14
  endocervical epithelium showing
    crowding of nuclei with mitosis and
    apoptotic bodies in high-grade
    CGIN, 15*f*
  features of, 14
  stratified Mucinous Intraepithelial Lesion
    (SMILE), 14–15
tumour types and abnormalities in disease
    of endometrium. *See also* endometrial
    cancer
  endometrial carcinoma, 16
  endometrial carcinoma type 1 and type 2,
    characteristics of, 17*t*
  endometrial hyperplasia, 16
  endometrial hyperplasia distinguished
    from endometrioid carcinoma, 16
  endometrial hyperplasia types and their
    microscopic features, 16*t*
  serous endometrial intraepithelial
    carcinoma (sEIC), 16–17

tumour types and abnormalities in disease
    of vulva. *See also* vulvar cancer
  Bartholins duct and gland neoplasms, 14
  vulval extramammary Paget's disease, 14
  vulval melanoma, 14
  vulval squamous cell carcinoma
    (SCC), 13
tumour types and abnormalities of the
    ovaries and fallopian tubes. *See also*
    ovarian cancer
  borderline ovarian tumours, types of, 19
  carcinomas, 18
  germ cell tumours, types of, 19–20
tumour types and abnormalities of the
    uterine wall
  endometrial stromal sarcoma showing
    typical myometrial vascular
    permeation, 18*f*
  endometrial stromal tumours, 17–18
  smooth muscle tumours of the uterus,
    17, 18*t*
tumours, miscellaneous, 20

uterine sarcomas
  epidemiology of, 147–148
  FIGO staging for uterine sarcomas, 203*b*
  histological assessment of, 147
  origin of, 147
  risk factors for, 147–148
  terminology for, 147
uterine sarcomas, diagnosis and
    investigation of
  assessment of, 148
  MRI of leiomyosarcoma/MRA of benign
    fibroids, 150*f*
  Multidisciplinary team (MDT)
    review, 149
  pre-operative assessment of, 149
  symptoms of, 148–149
uterine sarcomas, treatment of
  adjuvant treatment for uterine
    sarcomas, 151
  chemotherapy, 151
  hormonal treatment, 151
  pelvic radiotherapy, 151
  prognosis following treatment, 151
  surgery for disease confined to uterus,
    149–150
  surgery for disease extending beyond
    uterus, 150
  for women diagnosed after hysterectomy,
    150–151
uterine sarcomas, tumour types in
  endometrial stromal tumours, 147
  smooth muscle tumours of uncertain
    malignant potential (STUMP), 148
  uterine sarcomas *vs.* fibroids, 148
  uterine smooth muscle tumours/
    leiomyosarcomas, 148

vaginal cancer
  and HPV, 49, 126–127, 134
  pathology of, 134
  rate of diagnosis in UK, 133
  statistics of occurrence, 49
  survival rates of with radiotherapy, 49

vaginal cancer, diagnosis and
    investigation of
  examination with colposcopy,
    vaginoscopy, vulvoscopy, 134
  investigation with cystoscopy, 134
  symptoms of, 134
vaginal cancer, diagnostic imaging in
  CT of chest/abdomen to assess spread,
    evaluate lymph node involvement, 134
vaginal cancer, prevention and screening for
  risk factors for, 134
  smoking as risk factor for, 134
vaginal cancer, staging of
  diagrammatic representation of staging
    for vaginal cancer, 135*f*
  FIGO staging for carcinoma of the
    vagina, 205*b*
  lymphatic involvement by stage, 136
vaginal cancer, treatment of
  brachytherapy in treatment of stage I
    tumors, 49
  chemoradiotherapy as most effective,
    morbidity-preventing treatment, 136
  complications of treatment, 136
  diethylstilbestrol (DES) for miscarriage
    avoidance, 134
  5-year survival rate post-exenterative
    surgery, 136
  5-year survival rates post-treatment, 136
  follow-up post-treatment, 137
  palliative treatment for stage IV, 136–137
  pelvic exenteration surgery for patients
    who relapse post-chemoradiotherapy,
    136
  radiotherapy and chemotherapy for,
    135–136
  radiotherapy for stage II–IV tumours, 49
  radiotherapy for treatment of stage I
    tumors, 49
  radiotherapy, side effects of, 49–50
  recurrence rate, 136
  surgical management of, 135
  survival following recurrence, 146
  vault cytology to detect recurrences,
    inappropriateness of, 137
vaginal intraepithelial neoplasia (VaIN)
  biopsy to prevent invasion, 68
  treatment of, 68
vulval cancer. *See also* vulvar intraepithelial
    neoplasia (VIN)
  incidence in younger population, 138
  prevalence among older population in
    UK, 138
  survival rates of, 50
vulval cancer, diagnosis and investigation of
  anatomical considerations for, 138
  clinical examination criteria, 141–142
  diagnosis by needle biopsy, 39, 142
  examination under anaesthesia, 142
  importance of knowledge of anatomy of
    vulva in understanding spread, 138
  Keyes biopsy forceps, 142*f*
  lymphatic drainage of vulva, 139*f*
  and nerve supply, 138
  pictorial representations of vulva,
    helpfulness of, 142

vulval cancer, diagnostic imaging in
  imaging and biopsy of lymph nodes by
    ultrasound of MRI imaging, 142
  imaging for distal disease, 142
vulval cancer, pathology of
  Bartholin's gland cancer, 141
  basal cell carcinoma, 140
  Breslow classification of tumour stage
    in melanoma based on depth of
    invasions, 140, 141t
  chronic lymphoedema of both lower
    limbs, 145f
  comparison of clinicopathological
    features between two vulval
    intraepithelial neoplasias, 140t
  differentiated or keratinizing
    lesions, 140
  HPV-related disease, 139–140
  malignant melanoma, 140
  Paget's disease of the vulva, 141
  sarcoma, 141
  squamous cell carcinoma, 139–141
  squamous cell carcinoma of right
    labia, 142f
  verrucous carcinoma, 140
  in vulval intra-epithelial neoplasia
    (VIN), 140
  vulvar cancer spread, types of, 143
vulval cancer, prevention and
    screening for
  and prevalence of HPV infection, 146
  risk factors for, 138
  strategies for screening, 138
vulval cancer, staging of
  diagrammatic representation of staging
    for vulval cancer, 139f
  FIGO staging for carcinoma of the
    vulva, 205b
  staging and level of depth of
    invasion, 141t
  staging and spread based on
    International Federation of
    Gynecology and Obstetrics
    classification, 142–143

vulval cancer, surgical treatment by stage
  eligible criteria for sentinel lymph node
    (SLN) biopsy, 143
  excision of abnormal skin for minimizing
    risk of further tumours, 143
  locally advanced disease, 144
  primary surgical treatment of the vulval
    lesion, 143
  reconstructive surgical options, 144
  sentinel lymph node (SLN) biopsy for
    early-stage cases, 143
  for stages I and II, 143–144
vulval cancer, treatment of
  adjuvant radiotherapy for node-negative
    disease, 50
  adjuvant radiotherapy for node-positive
    disease, 50
  adjuvant radiotherapy for women with
    close surgical margins, 145
  chemotherapy, recommendations of
    European Society of Gynaecological
    Oncology (ESGO), 145
  complications, chronic problems from
    surgery, 144
  inguino-femoral lymph node dissection
    (LND), 50
  local excision in surgical
    treatment, 50
  management of clinically suspicious
    groin modes, 144
  management of recurrence, 145–146
  and minimization of morbidity, 144
  neoadjuvant chemoradiotherapy for
    locally advanced disease, 50
  palliative radiotherapy, doses of, 51
  palliative resection in, 40
  palliative surgery in, 40
  post-operative radiotherapy for
    metastatic disease, 40
  pre-operative radiotherapy and
    chemotherapy for advanced vulval
    cancer, 40
  primary radiotherapy, 145
  radical wide local excision in (WLE), 39

  radiotherapy for recurrence, 40
  radiotherapy in, 40, 50–51
  radiotherapy technique in, 50–51
  radiotherapy, advances in, 51
  radiotherapy, prescribed doses of, 51
  radiotherapy, side effects of, 51
  sentinel node dissection to reduce risk of
    relapse, 40
  surgical resection for recurrence, 40
  treatment of groin nodes, 143
  tumour removal in, 39
  vulvectomy in, 50
  wide local excision and ipsilateral sentinel
    node dissection or lymphadenectomy
    for stage I, II, 40
  wide local excision for malignant
    melanoma, 40
vulvar cancer. See also vulvar intraepithelial
    neoplasia (VIN)
  aetiology of, 10
  incidence and mortality trends of in UK,
    world, 9–10
  prevention of with HPV vaccine, 10
vulvar cancer, treatment of
  right lymphocoele following
    lymphadenectomy on the same
    side, 145f
vulvar intraepithelial neoplasia (VIN)
  alternative treatments of, 68
  classification of, 66–67
  epidemiology of, 67–68
  histological features of, 13t
  and HPV, 13
  imiquimod cream 5% in treatment
    of, 68
  local excision in treatment of, 68
  National Guidelines on the Management
    of Vulval Conditions, in UK, 68
  vulvectomy in treatment of, 68

World Health Organization (WHO) criteria
  of response, 197–198
World Health Organization (WHO)
  performance status classification, 197